Healing for Body, Soul and Spirit

Healing *for* Body, Soul *and* Spirit

An Introduction to Anthroposophic Medicine

Dr Michael Evans
& Iain Rodger

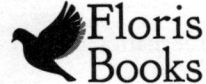

Floris
Books

First Published in Great Britain in 1992
as *Anthroposophical Medicine*
by Thorsons, an Imprint of HarperCollins

Third edition published in 2017 by Floris Books
© Iain Rodger and Michael Evans 1992

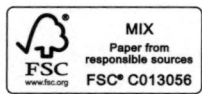

MIX
Paper from
responsible sources
FSC
www.fsc.org   FSC® C013056

British Library CIP Data available
ISBN 978-178250-410-8
Printed in Great Britain by TJ International

Contents

Acknowledgments

The authors would like to thank the following for their invaluable help: Dr James Dyson (without whose encouragement and constructive criticism the book would not have been written), Hazel Adams, Dr Jean Brown, Shirley Chalis, Marah Evans, Dr Michaela Glöckler, Tom Huggon, Adrian Large, Dr Broder von Laue, Dr David McGavin, Thomas McKeen, Joan Marcus, Steven Moore, Dr Frank Mulder, Ruth and Bernard Nesfield-Cookson, Bobbie Pounder, Don Ratcliffe, Jennie Rodger, Joan Smith, Shaena Stoehr, Vera Taberner, Ian Wiggle, the Anthroposophical Medical Council and the Anthroposophical Medical Trust. A debt is also acknowledged to the works of Professor Bernard Lievegoed, Dr Rudolf Treichler and Dr Arie Bos.

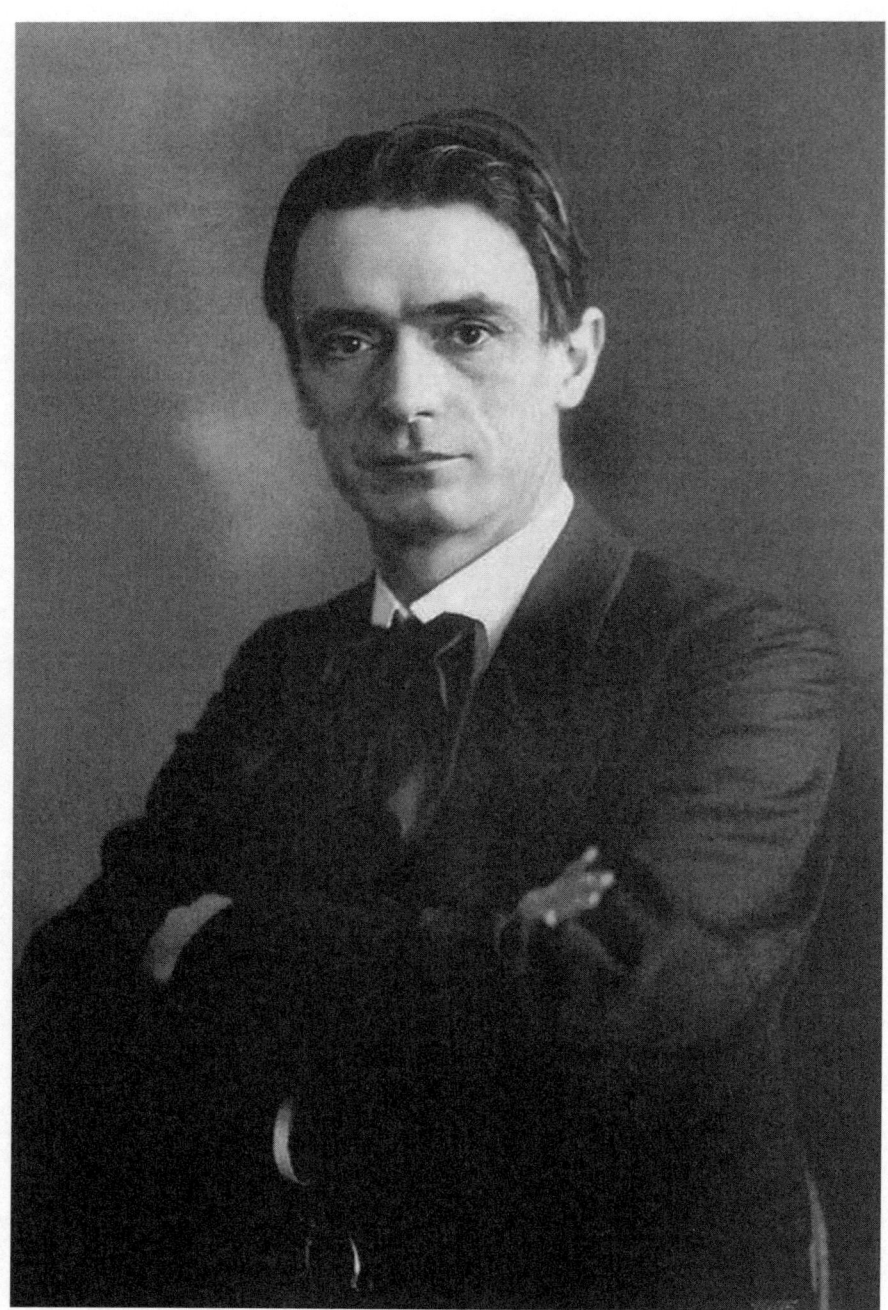

Rudolf Steiner.

Introduction

Recognition of the enormous achievements of conventional medicine has, in recent years, been accompanied by a growing awareness of its limitations and the undesirable side effects of many of its methods of treatment. Patients are less prepared than they were to accept the doctor's prescription without an explanation, and they prefer to have the opportunity to discuss any options which might be available. This more critical appraisal of conventional medicine is reflected in the rapid growth in popularity of alternative approaches, such as homeopathy, herbalism and acupuncture. Most of these are based on philosophies which considerably predate conventional medicine, but they nevertheless benefit many patients.

The conventional approach has advanced medicine in some respects but is based on a limited, materialistic view of the human being which has failed to produce a comprehensive understanding of illness. Some forms of alternative medicine have distinct spiritual philosophies which predate natural science, the study of material phenomena.* Turning to these in search of what is lacking in conventional medicine is like trying to turn the clock back, ignoring what has been gained from natural science. What is needed is not a return to the past, but an extension of conventional medicine to take into account both the spiritual and physical sides of the human.

Precisely this is offered by anthroposophic medicine, one of a number of practical applications of the work of the Austrian scientist and philosopher, Rudolf Steiner (1861–1925), the founder of anthroposophy. The name is derived from the Greek *anthropos* (human) and *sophia* (wisdom), which gives something of an indication that anthroposophy involves the development of spiritual wisdom through human

---

* Natural science (or modern science), which nowadays is generally referred to as just 'science,' is here given its original name to avoid confusion with spiritual science.

self-knowledge. In practice, it is a science of the spirit, extending our knowledge and understanding beyond the foundations laid down by natural science.

Steiner recognised the achievements of natural science in building a picture of the physical world, but sought to go beyond the limits of materialism by rigorously researching the spiritual side of existence. His anthroposophy, or spiritual science, sees humans as beings of body, soul and spirit, and anthroposophic medicine came about as a result of a group of doctors recognising that this extended physiology had remarkable implications for medical treatment.

During the later years of Steiner's life, people from various professions approached him for guidance on how they might apply the principles of anthroposophy to their particular fields. As well as medicine, this gave birth to new forms of education, art, architecture, caring for children with handicaps, agriculture and economics, all of which are now practised worldwide. In the case of medicine, Steiner was invited to address a group of about thirty doctors and medical students who were familiar with anthroposophy. In 1920, he gave a course of lectures which contained insights into human pathology and approaches to therapy, though this could not be considered a systematic introduction to an anthroposophic medicine.[1]

It was through Steiner's collaboration with a Dutch doctor, Ita Wegman (1876–1943), that the foundation for a new medicine was laid. Together, they wrote a book for the medical profession, *Extending Practical Medicine,* and Dr Wegman opened one of the first anthroposophic clinics at Arlesheim, Switzerland, near the worldwide centre for anthroposophy at Dornach.[2] She later became the first leader of the Medical Section of the School of Spiritual Science at Dornach.

As Steiner was not a medical doctor, he worked with qualified practitioners in the development of anthroposophic medicine. He insisted that it should extend conventional practice rather than become an alternative. To that end, all anthroposophic doctors must qualify first in conventional medicine, then do further study to gain an understanding of the human being in health and illness from a spiritual scientific point of view. This widens the scope of their work beyond conventional practice, and means that anthroposophic doctors can be consulted about any medical problem.

The main aim of anthroposophic medicine is to stimulate the natural healing forces in the patient. These are the life forces which maintain the physical body and oppose decay. They comprise a body of non-physical formative forces, called the etheric body by Steiner, and are particularly active in growth and nutrition. Humans are also conscious beings, aware of their environment and emotionally responsive. This awareness comes from having a third *body*, called the astral body, which is particularly active in the nervous system. Finally, people also know themselves to be independent conscious beings, and have the power to change themselves inwardly. This points to the fourth element of the human: the spiritual core, or 'I', which particularly expresses itself in muscular activity and the blood. (All these concepts are explained in detail in the following chapters.)

These four elements interrelate to form a whole, which must be treated as a whole if the patient is to be helped. Anthroposophic doctors seek to understand illnesses in terms of the way the four aspects interrelate. For example, there is a perpetual tendency towards ill-health because the activity of consciousness has a catabolic, or breaking-down, effect on the physical body. The anabolic, or building-up, forces of the etheric body must constantly combat these effects for good health to be maintained. However, if the etheric forces are themselves too powerful, the imbalance again results in illness. Good health is dependent on these opposing tendencies being kept in equilibrium.

The highly complex picture of the human which emerged through Steiner's work can be difficult to grasp. After all, anthroposophic medicine starts with conventional teaching about the physical body and extends this picture with three further elements. But it can easily be understood that everyday experiences of thoughts, feelings and will-power call for an extension of the natural scientific model, simply because natural science excludes anything not physically measurable. This is where spiritual science can build on the understanding of the physical realm gained through natural science, and extend the frontiers of our knowledge.

Physical perception is limited by the bodily senses, but thinking has no such limits. For example, the concepts of mathematics are not sense-perceptible. The spiritual realm might not be perceived directly with the bodily senses but, with careful observation and disciplined thinking, anyone can gain an understanding of spiritual science. However, it is possible to go further. Steiner describes how higher forms of perception can be developed which enable people to perceive the spiritual realm directly. It was through his own development of these faculties that he was able to do the researches on which his descriptions of the spiritual realm were based.

Steiner had the ability to perceive spiritual phenomena in addition to the faculty of perception of the physical environment with which most people are born. He maintained that everyone had latent organs for spiritual perception which they could develop through their own efforts.[3] At present, most people are cut off from direct experience of the spiritual realm in much the same way that visual images of the physical world are denied to the blind. However, just as the blind can have other experiences of the physical world, and can compare these with concepts reported by sighted people, so can those without developed powers of spiritual perception compare their experiences with anthroposophic knowledge.

For example, the ideas that anthroposophic medicine adds to conventional practice might seem strange to someone whose education was based on natural science. But this should encourage neither blind faith nor blind disbelief. If the ideas are thought through with an open mind, they can be assessed on their own merits. The achievements of anthroposophic medicine in practice can also be assessed.

At present, anthroposophic medical work is most widely developed in Germany, the Netherlands and Switzerland, where there are several hospitals and many general practitioners. All are fully recognised and funded by state and private medical insurance schemes. In the English-speaking world, it has taken longer for Steiner's work to become widely known, although interest in this approach is growing steadily. In the UK, anthroposophic medicine is practised both within the National Health Service and privately.

This book has been written to establish a wider understanding of anthroposophic medicine and to meet the demands of growing interest worldwide. It is intended primarily for a general readership but, it is hoped, will also be of use to health care professionals who wish to broaden their approach to therapy. Some concepts have had to be simplified because of limited space but, for the benefit of readers who wish to pursue deeper explanations, comprehensive references to further reading have been given.

It must be understood that this book is not a manual for treatment by unqualified persons. It does not replace proper consultation with a doctor, nor does it serve as a training manual. Comprehensive lists will be found at the back which show how to obtain further information, including where to obtain anthroposophic treatment or apply for training in anthroposophic medical methods.

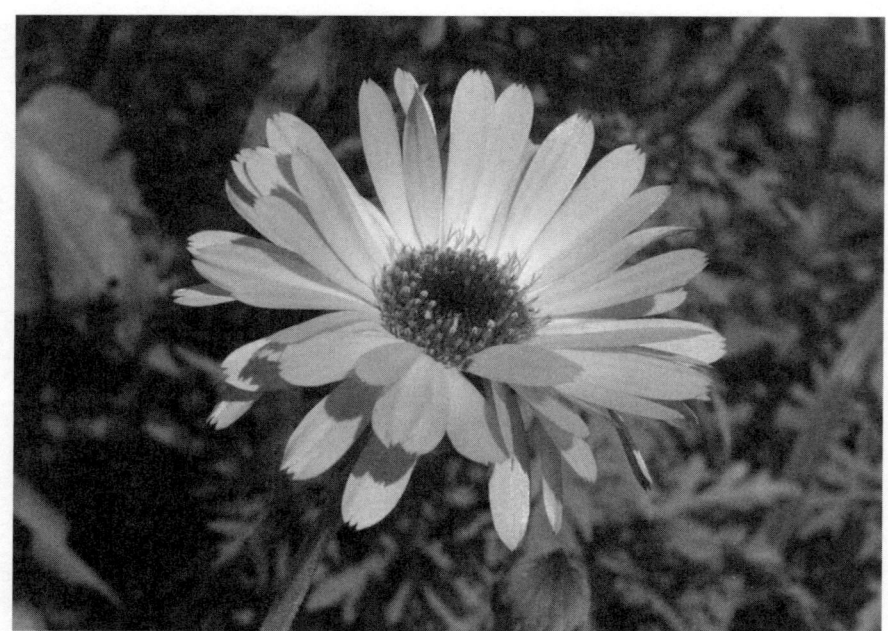

Calendula (marigold) flower.

1. Extending the Art and Science of Medicine

Anthroposophic medicine has a growing reputation for its methods of treatment and offers a new approach to meeting the demands of a rapidly changing world. It should not be confused with alternative therapies, as it is firmly based on the knowledge and experience of conventional medicine. The difference is that anthroposophic practice treats the non-physical (or spiritual) elements of the patient as well as the physical.

Working with such elements to extend the range of conventional practice does not make anthroposophic medicine vague or imprecise. All anthroposophic doctors must first qualify in the conventional training, then complete postgraduate studies which add another three elements to the conventional concept of the physical body. These offer a more complete picture of the human being and are called, in anthroposophic terminology, the etheric body, astral body and 'I'.*

They are non-material, spiritual elements, common to everyone though they cannot be perceived with the physical senses. It should be understood that describing them as spiritual does not imply that anthroposophic medicine is based on beliefs, religious or otherwise. It is based on the methods of spiritual science, which has the same rigour and discipline as natural science, but extends the boundary of what is observed beyond the physical world.

Anatomy, physiology and biochemistry

Conventional medicine as we know it is derived from natural science, the study of material phenomena – whatever can be weighed, measured or

---

* The etheric body, astral body and I are also referred to as the life element, soul element and spirit respectively.

counted. In the last five hundred years, natural science has hugely expanded our understanding of the world around us. Although many of the early scientists were persecuted for their discoveries, they were inspired by this new method of enquiry as they no longer had to rely on traditional religious and philosophical teachings. For us today, this spirit of independent enquiry is as important a legacy as the brilliant achievements of natural science in technology and medicine.

The modern scientific view of the world gradually evolved through one set of discoveries building upon another. The pioneers made their greatest contributions in the fields of astronomy and physics, producing formulae to describe the apparent movements of the planets with respect to the sun. In the seventeenth century, Sir Isaac Newton proposed concepts of force and gravity, through which the movements of the planets were explained by the same formulae that described the way inert objects fell to earth. The basic laws of chemistry began to be formulated when it was discovered that, by weighing inorganic materials before and after chemical reactions had taken place, it was possible to make mathematical descriptions of those reactions.

In Renaissance Italy, an interest in human anatomy prompted artists (notably Leonardo da Vinci) to dissect corpses in order to make the first detailed drawings of the inside of the body. The modern discipline of anatomy grew out of these studies of dead bodies. Similarly, observation and measurement of the functions of human and animal bodies and their organs led to the gradual development of physiology – essentially the methods of physics applied to living organisms. Biochemistry also emerged – essentially the methods of chemistry applied to living things.

These three sciences – anatomy, physiology and biochemistry are taught as basics to all medical students. The principles of each were derived from study of the non-living, but their methods have been applied to the living – to plants, animals and people. Because of this, modern science (including medicine) presents an incomplete picture of the world. As will be seen, the laws that relate to inert matter should only be applied to the physical aspects of living things. They do not take into account their life, soul and spiritual dimensions and, therefore, a further science is called for to complete the picture. This is the role of spiritual science, or anthroposophy.

Life processes

The whole of life is characterised by processes, such as the circulation of the blood, the flow of substances in and out of the liver, and digestive activity. Natural scientific examinations of these processes reduce them to mechanical systems and chemical reactions, typically breaking up the organism to be studied and analysing the parts outside their normal environments. This freezes the physical expression of the process into a form which can be dealt with in the laboratory, but fails to explain fully its role within the living being. It might be said that natural science tends to analyse a snapshot of a process rather than the process itself.

Anthroposophy differs from this approach by regarding the processes as expressions of spiritual principles. It is these higher principles underlying the physical realm that have to be grasped before the life element (or etheric body) can be understood. If the activity involved in a life process is studied, rather than an isolated snapshot, a step is taken towards understanding that element which organises inert matter into a complex living body.

Wherever life prevails, the normal behaviour of matter is modified, or even reversed. For example, lifeless matter tends always towards a state of disorganisation. A stone wall breaks down into dust through erosion; a hot kettle returns to the same temperature as its surroundings when removed from the heat source. However, in plants, animals and humans, matter is organised into complex physical bodies. As long as the life element is present, the high state of organisation is preserved. But when it departs, at death, the matter breaks down again into a disorganised state – it returns to *dust*.

By way of another example of how life modifies the laws of the physical realm, it can be observed that inert matter falls predictably under the influence of gravity. Plants, however, grow up from the ground towards the sun, in opposition to gravity. It is, of course, recognised that they are still subject to gravity, and that ripe apples fall to the ground. The point is that the plant draws mineral substances from the earth, organises them in accordance with a predetermined structure, and endows the whole with an ability to oppose gravity.

At medical school, students learn about the anatomy of the whole body, the physiology of the various organs, the tissues that make up the organs (histology), the cells that form the tissues and the biochemical processes that take place between the molecules that make up the cells. Although not necessarily recognised, there is an acceptance in contemporary medicine that, when an illness can be described on a cellular or molecular level, the explanation in terms of the most minute elements is the most fundamental.

Reductionism

This approach has evolved in tandem with the scientists' ability to analyse ever-smaller constituent parts, and stems particularly from the last century, when refinements in microscope technology made possible the discovery of cells. A German pathologist, Rudolf Virchow, said that all living things, including humans, were made up of cells. When people became ill, he said, it was because their cells had become ill. If we could understand how the cells became ill, we would understand how people became ill.[1] His simplistic ideas formed the basis of modern pathology, the science of bodily diseases.

The tendency to look for an isolated cause of a disease is carried over into diagnosis. What a patient experiences and what the doctor can observe directly form only the starting-point for describing an illness. The more the description is put in terms of minute elements, such as cellular changes, the more fundamental it is judged to be. This determination to seek explanations in terms of the smallest parts falls into a school of thought known as reductionism, and is one of the most characteristic features of conventional medicine.

Let us suppose a patient is losing weight, trembling, has a rapid pulse, is eating more than usual and is possibly rather hyperactive. The illness may be diagnosed as hyperthyroidism (overactivity of the thyroid, a gland in the neck which regulates the rate of metabolism through the production of a hormone, thyroxine). Attention shifts from the patient as a whole to one organ. Blood tests are done to see if thyroxine is present in increased concentrations, and only when this has been demonstrated does the doctor feel they have grasped the diagnosis.

This approach has led to many of the successes of conventional medicine. Natural science has given doctors the ability to intervene on a microscopic level. For example, they can administer chemical substances which inhibit

Realm	Quality	Kingdom of nature	Human element
Spirit	Consciousness of self	Human	I (or self)
Soul	Consciousness	Animal	Astral body
Life	Life	Plant	Etheric body
Material	Weighable and measurable	Mineral	Physical body

Figure 1.

the thyroid's production of thyroxine or, conversely, synthesise thyroxine to give to patients who have insufficient concentrations in their blood. The discovery of an association between bacteria and infections led to research into drugs that would destroy the chemical make-up of the bacteria while interfering very little, or not at all, with the chemistry of the human body. The consequent discovery of antibiotics gave doctors the power to fight infections, and antibiotics are now used whenever bacteria are thought to be involved in disease.

Such advances have been made possible by the discoveries of natural science and may be seen as fruits of the reductionist approach. Perhaps because of its successes, it is an approach which has tended to dominate all others, and has even prevailed in the way medicines are understood and manufactured. Before the twentieth century, medicines were mainly derived from plants but also from some minerals and metals. A herbal remedy would have been prepared as a tincture by standing a finely chopped plant in a mixture of alcohol and water for a set time, before filtering off an extract. By contrast, modern pharmacy isolates individual chemical substances from the original plant and purifies them, with the intention of making more powerful and predictable medicines. The chemical is then often copied or modified, and made artificially. In this way, pharmacy, too, has moved away from the whole organism, the plant, to a single chemical component.

The life body

If one looks at the whole range of applications of conventional medicine, it is clear that it has made possible all manner of life-saving interventions. It has also brought about an enormous number of improvements to people's lives, for example, through the replacement of damaged joints. Anthroposophic doctors do not claim otherwise, and recognise the methods of conventional medicine as sometimes being appropriate. But the fact that anthroposophic medicine offers methods which go beyond treatment of only the physical body is particularly important because the sources of many illnesses lie in the non-physical human elements. This book shows how anthroposophic medicine extends the healing possibilities of conventional therapy, and also how it overcomes the one-sided approach of reductionism.

It is a mistake to assume that the results of observation of inorganic matter can adequately grasp the full nature of living things. The laws applying to the life element are quite different from those of the physical world. Therefore, it is not surprising that life itself is one of the non-physical dimensions conventional medicine fails to grasp. It is understood by modern science that organisms, such as people, use material substances to build their physical bodies, but the living element of a person can never be comprehended by examination of those material components.

It is necessary to look at how the body grows and matures to get a sense of the activity of the life element, or etheric body. On death, the physical body decays back into the earth – it becomes once again the raw materials which had been used to build it up. During life, there were etheric processes holding the materials together, organising them into a highly complex body. This life element can never be understood by the methods of natural science because it is not a material thing. In fact, our understanding of the physical body itself is advanced through a knowledge of the spiritual elements. It then becomes clear that the physical element functions in close relationship with the spiritual elements, subserving the identity of the whole.

The soul

In addition to the concept of the life element, the second area introduced by anthroposophic medicine concerns our feelings, instinctual drives and inner sense of the world around us. Our own inner experiences, such as our feelings, are obvious to ourselves but we cannot observe another's feelings in the way we can see external nature. Therefore, they are not accessible to the techniques of natural science, which limits itself to the observable and measurable. This problem has led to the development of a number of approaches to understanding the inner life, or soul life. For example, the biophysical model looks exclusively for a physical and chemical basis for consciousness, by examining the physiology and biochemistry of the nervous system. Another approach, behaviourism, tries to identify external stimuli which could be responsible for the way humans and animals behave. Psychoanalysis concentrates on unconscious, instinctive urges which express themselves in feelings and thoughts. The existentialist, or phenomenological, approach highlights that aspect of the soul which strives to develop an understanding of the world and itself. And social psychiatry examines the role of the social environment in shaping the soul life.

Anthroposophic medicine acknowledges that these approaches attempt to come to grips with particular aspects of the soul life, but considers that each one fails to describe it in its totality. For example, it is not possible to gain an understanding of the soul while regarding it as merely an expression of physiological processes. The soul world is a realm in its own right and the soul inhabits this realm, just as the physical body exists in the physical world. But this does not mean people's souls are completely separate from their physical bodies. There is a constant connection during life and the soul is deeply affected by the sensations received via the physical body.

The inorganic, physical element is common to humans, animals, plants and minerals. The life element is common to humans, animals and plants. The soul element – characterised by feelings, passions, instincts and consciousness – is common to humans and animals. In addition to these, there is a fourth element that makes us human and separates us from the other three kingdoms. It is a spiritual core which enables us not only to be conscious, but to *know* that we are conscious. In other words, to be self-conscious, or self-aware, beings. That we are self-aware is demonstrated every time we use the word *I* to refer to ourselves. This is only possible if we are aware of our existence as individuals.

The I or self

The third area anthroposophic medicine adds to contemporary medical practice concerns this innermost sense of identity – the *I*, or self. While our thoughts and feelings change from one day to the next, we retain a constant sense of identity throughout. Our physical bodies also change dramatically over a lifetime. The material constituents are constantly being replaced such that, after a number of years, it is unlikely there are many atoms left that were in the body at the beginning of the period. Still, there is a centre we call *I*, which we experience as constant throughout. This inner identity distinguishes us from the outer world and drives us to seek for true knowledge of ourselves and our surroundings, beyond simply fulfilling the physical body's needs. Like animals, humans respond to external events, but only humans are able to conceive and carry out creative acts which go beyond instinct. This centre, this *I*, is the human spirit, and makes each of us unique.★

Treating the whole

A medicine to treat the whole person must be based on knowledge of all four aspects of the human being – the physical, life and soul elements, and the spirit. Each aspect interacts with the others but the whole person cannot be reduced to any one of them. Anthroposophic medicine describes the nature of these aspects and also explains how disturbances in their interrelationships can bring about illness. Conventional doctors know that a patient's emotional state can be the cause of certain physical illnesses, but they understand very little of how this comes about. It is particularly here, in describing how disturbances in the soul life can be expressed as physical symptoms, that anthroposophic medicine is able to offer valuable

★ All three non-physical aspects of the human – the life element, soul element and spirit – may be described as spiritual, but the spirit itself is the central core; the unique inner identity.

new forms of treatment. It aims to treat the causes of such illnesses, rather than simply suppressing their symptoms.

Any treatment which affects one element of the patient may also affect the others. For example, a conventional drug treatment aimed at relieving certain bodily symptoms may have its first effect on the physical body, but then go on to affect the spiritual elements. This secondary effect may not be beneficial. On the other hand, homeopathic medicines – which do not have such a direct chemical effect on the body but tend to stimulate the healing process – can be understood to have their primary action within the life element itself. For this reason, homeopathic medicines and their effects cannot be understood in terms of the measurable laws of natural science. They work on the whole patient via the non-physical life element and can only be understood in terms of the laws applying there.

In addition to remedies which work via the life element, anthroposophic medicine uses a range of artistic therapies which work primarily through the soul element of the patient. Also, through counselling, patients may gain new insights about their lives which lead them to resolve to make beneficial changes to their lifestyles. In this way, the doctor works directly with the patient's spirit, or conscious self.

Of course, anthroposophic medicine does not reject the use of surgery or conventional drugs when appropriate, such as in emergencies. But the spiritual as well as the physical consequences of their use have to be appreciated. Anthroposophic medicine adds to these methods a new range of medicines and therapies which extend the scope of treatment in accordance with its comprehensive picture of the human being. They are not just older, traditional forms of homeopathic or herbal medicine transplanted into the present on the basis that they may work. They are extensions of contemporary medical practice, developed on the basis of a new spiritual scientific understanding which adds enormously to what has been learned through natural science.

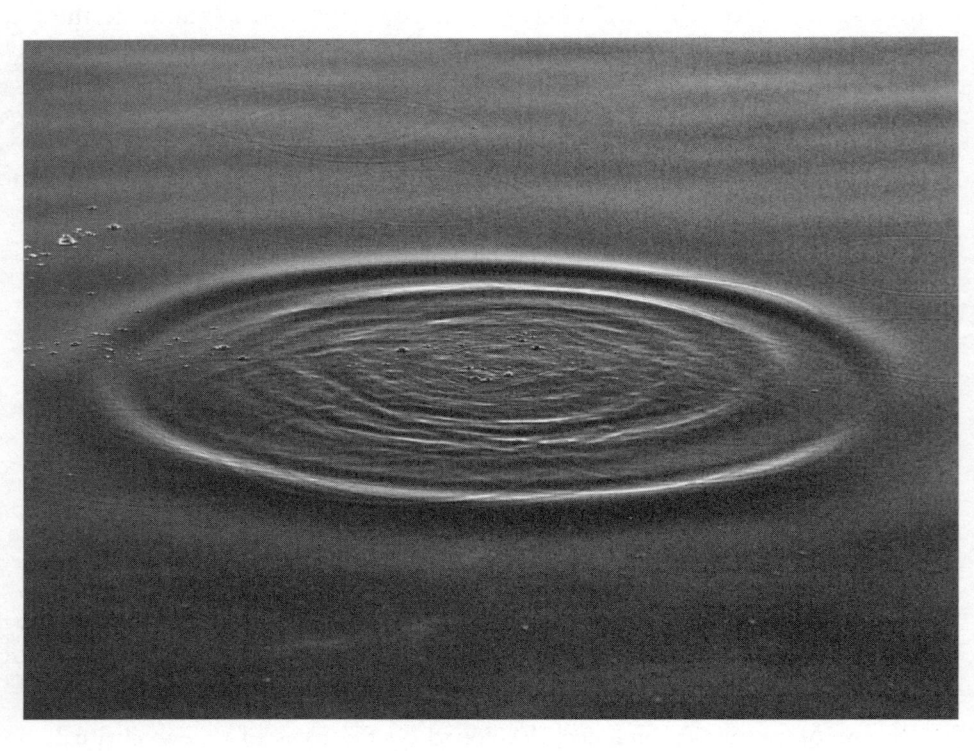

2. A New Study of Life

The life element, or etheric body, consists of formative forces which govern the organisation of the physical body. Left to themselves, the materials that make up the physical body would disintegrate, as happens after death, when the physical body is left under the influence of the laws of the physical world alone. From a purely physical and chemical point of view, there is little difference between the body a moment before and a moment after death. But as soon as the etheric body departs, the physical body starts to decay from a highly organised structure into dust.

Every part of the physical body has a corresponding etheric part underlying it. The etheric body is not only responsible for building the physical parts into a complex whole: it also maintains them, constantly repairing and restructuring them. It strives to keep us in good health and is the source of our natural tendency to recover from less serious ailments in time, whether we see a doctor or not. This self-healing does not happen by chance. It is the result of the etheric body's constant opposition to death and decay in the physical body.

The etheric body is non-physical, so it obviously cannot be understood by examination of the physical body. Looking at the material parts reveals the physical body's form, which is an expression of the etheric body, but not the life element itself. Without an understanding of the etheric body, it is impossible to fully comprehend any organism and its diseases. This can be clearly illustrated using the example of cancer.

Cancer is traditionally understood to be a disease of cells. In a healthy organism, growth comes about through cell reproduction, and development through groups of cells taking on different forms, often of increasing complexity, whereby the different organs and tissues are formed. A fully developed organism contains many types of cells which differ from each other, and from the cells from which they originated. Cancerous tumours, which tend to spread and recur after removal, are made up of cells which multiply far more rapidly than most normal cells. As they grow, they tend to break through the boundaries of the diseased tissues, and even travel around the body via the bloodstream. The cancerous cells often become less differentiated than the normal cells in the affected tissues, as if the cancer had reversed the natural process of differentiation. In general, the less differentiated the cancerous cells are, the more malignant their behaviour.

Conventional treatment, based on this picture, attempts to remove the cancerous cells by surgery, or otherwise to kill them using radiation or cell poisons which, it is hoped, will do only minimal damage to the normal cells. Unfortunately, the chemistry of cancerous cells differs little from that of normal cells – unlike bacteria, which are easily targeted using antibiotics because of significant differences from human cells. A primary characteristic of the cancerous cells is that they tend to reproduce more rapidly than normal cells, so poisons are used which attack the most rapidly dividing cells. But healthy cells that normally reproduce rapidly, such as those in bone marrow (which reproduce to form white blood cells, the component of blood that fights infections) are also poisoned by these medicines.

Understanding the etheric

From the anthroposophic point of view, a kind of template works through the etheric body which guides the cells as they reproduce and differentiate into the groups that make up the different parts of the body. Only through an understanding of how this formative principle is involved in bodily development, from the fertilised egg onwards, can cancer itself be comprehended. It then becomes clear that the cancer arises from a local breakdown in the etheric body, through which the human form is imprinted on the cells. This breakdown allows the cells to reproduce in an uncontrolled way and ultimately to damage the rest of the organism. Therefore, a more appropriate therapy for cancer would be one which helped to restore the formative forces in the area where the cancer had arisen. The forces to be strengthened would obviously have to be those concerned with maintaining the form of the tissues, rather than the forces of cellular vitality. This implies quite different treatment from attempts to kill off the cancerous cells.[1]

It is worth noting that some conventional doctors do not wholly embrace the conventional picture of cancer and have come remarkably close to the anthroposophic view through their own observations and reasoning. Half a century ago Professor David Smithers questioned the conventional view when he was Professor of Radiotherapy at London University in the 1960s. He said that if cells were studied in isolation by, for example, observing single-celled organisms like amoebas, it was apparent that they reproduced as rapidly as their food supplies allowed. They did not limit their own division or movement and, as they divided, the progeny closely resembled their parent cells – they did not differentiate into new types of cells. One could say they remained primitive. Professor Smithers pointed out that this was very similar to the behaviour of cancerous cells – they also reproduced rapidly, moved freely and did not differentiate. So it could be said that, from a cellular point of view, the cancerous cells were the ones that behaved normally.

Pursuing this idea, Smithers wondered why the cells of the body behaved in an apparently unnatural way during embryonic development. Succeeding generations became quite different from their parents and allowed their reproduction to be limited, as if they were subserving some greater function than their inherent tendencies. He thought there had to be forces which guided the cells to develop in such a way that the form of a particular organism arose, and concluded that the given form was the result of 'immaterial controlling forces without which no living organism can exist'.[2]

More recently, this kind of thought was taken further by Soto and Sonnenschein in their 'The tissue of organisation field theory of cancer'.[3]

The nature of the etheric

While natural science attempts to understand living things by studying ever smaller parts – from organs down to molecules and beyond – one fact to have emerged from these studies is that the smaller parts are in a constant state of change. Even the constituents of the skeleton, which appears to be the most permanent part of the body, are continuously changing. The mineral components of the bones are crystals of calcium carbonate and calcium phosphate, and even these hard substances are constantly dissolved and reformed by cells called osteoclasts and osteoblasts. This repeated cycle of change is true of the whole body, with the possible exception of the hardest substance of all, the enamel of the teeth. If we could tag all the molecules in a person's body, we would find that practically every one had been replaced a few years later – even, in some cases, a few hours later. Clearly, the essential nature of an organism is not its material constituents.

The nearest we can get to a realistic physical image of an organism is not a machine but, rather, a moving liquid form such as a river. Looking at the overall form of the river, we can see that it is to some extent stable, at least over a period of weeks. Yet, if we focus on the water itself, and analyse it into drops or molecules, it is immediately clear that these are flowing down the river and are constantly replaced. The contents of the river change all the time, while the overall form remains fairly constant. To take the analogy further, we also know that what determines the form of the river is not the water itself but the influence of the terrain over which it flows.

To search for an understanding of the human form in the body's constantly changing material constituents is as fruitless as it would be to try to understand the river's form by analysing the water molecules. In the case of the river, we could look at the terrain for an explanation, but natural science is of no help in discovering the source of the human form because we cannot perceive the etheric body using our physical senses. However, we could perhaps try to picture it by looking at cases in the physical world where an invisible force imposes forms on material substances.

For example, in the presence of a magnetic field, iron filings are arranged into striking patterns. The patterns cannot be understood simply by looking at the filings themselves. It is only by analysing the nature of the magnetic field that the behaviour of the filings becomes clear. There would appear to be some similarities here with the relationship between the etheric and physical bodies. But the etheric forces still differ markedly from magnetism in that they are not measurable or demonstrable using the techniques of natural science. They are spiritual, not physical, forces. Another approach is needed – one which can lead to direct conscious experience of the etheric realm, in the same way that we are normally directly conscious of the physical world.

Goethe's archetype

In the eighteenth century, the German writer and scientist, Johann Wolfgang von Goethe, said that the life element in plants, animals and humans could not be grasped through what could be directly perceived with the physical senses. He said the real plant was not what could be seen at any given moment in its life cycle – a seed, a seedling, a growing green plant, a flowering plant, a fruit-bearing plant or a withering plant. Its true nature encompassed all of these, but was an invisible archetype which expressed itself in the various physical forms. It was possible to see a momentary manifestation of the plant, but not the archetype itself. Goethe further stated that, while the life element was not visible to the physical senses, it could be grasped in thought, and it was possible for the power of human thinking and reasoning to be transformed into a perceptive faculty. Thinking could be so strengthened that it became another organ of perception, through which the processes of life could be directly perceived.

Rudolf Steiner had this faculty – he was able to be fully conscious in both the physical and spiritual worlds – and was the first to express it with scientific clarity. Though people were normally aware of only the physical world, he said, everyone had the potential to develop consciousness that extended to the spiritual realm.[4] It was not only our physical form that had changed with human evolution, but also our level of consciousness. Such changes had happened throughout history and the time had arrived, he said, when the development of spiritual consciousness was beginning to be possible.

Steiner established spiritual science as a means of coming to know the spiritual realm as well as we know the physical world through natural science.* He described how spiritual perceptions could be at least as vivid as ordinary sense perceptions and, through training, just as reliable. They simply revealed another aspect of existence, as if a veil had been drawn away, rather as an extra dimension would be added to the perception of a blind person by the gift of sight. Consciousness of the etheric realm enables direct perception of the etheric body, just as the physical body is directly perceived with normal consciousness. In the same way that the physical body might be described as a collection of differentiated physical matter residing in the physical world, the etheric body constitutes a specialised organisation of etheric nature inhabiting the etheric world.

* It is clearly difficult to understand the spiritual realm without perceiving it directly, but the same difficulty is encountered by modern science in its investigations of the physical world. In nuclear physics, theoretical particles are studied which are so minute, they can only be 'perceived' at all by their apparent effects on other things. Similarly, phenomena in space have been discovered which have only (so far) been explained by postulating the existence of 'black holes', which again cannot be seen except in their apparent effects on other things. In the same way that the hypotheses of modern science can be used as working models, the results of spiritual science can also be understood and used, even without direct spiritual perception.

Workings of the etheric body

The etheric body is particularly active during the embryonic stage of development, when the human form arises out of a plate of cells called the embryonic disc. It is also particularly active in the processes of nutrition, in which food is used for both growth and continual renewal of the physical body. This constant upbuilding quality of the etheric body is most dramatically expressed in plants which, in conjunction with sunlight, transform water and carbon dioxide into the sugars without which none of the other substances of living organisms could be created. The physical bodies of plants are thus the primary source of nutrition for human and animal life.

The laws of the etheric world are in many ways the inverse of those applying in the physical. For example, physics describes gravitational fields in terms of forces which emanate from points and radiate in all directions towards an infinite periphery. But, while they radiate out from a point, their effect is to pull objects in towards the centre. The etheric world is characterised by forces which emanate from the periphery and radiate in towards a point, while their effect is from the point back to the periphery.[5] This opposite direction of action of etheric forces can be seen in the physical world when, for example, plants oppose gravity by growing up out of the soil towards the sunlight.

The nature of the etheric world is such that it can only be described in physical terminology as infinite space. The etheric body originates in this boundless realm but, when it connects with the physical body at conception, it takes on a bounded quality which relates to the finite nature of the physical world. Goethe described this finite quality as a limited store of creative potential. If organisms had a 'limited budget' of 'creative capital,' as he put it, what was used up in the development of a particular specialisation was no longer available for other creative possibilities. He cited as an example his observation that some animals had horns or antlers, while others had large canine teeth. He thought they could develop one or the other but not both. This is not strictly true – as Figure 2 shows, a number of species do have both. But, on closer examination, it can be seen that the larger the antlers, the smaller the canine teeth and vice versa, in an approximately inverse relationship.

This suggests that Goethe was correct to assume that a relationship existed between canine teeth and antlers, but that it is more subtle than he thought. This principle, known as biological compensation, also shows itself in some of the problems associated with breeding animals. Usually,

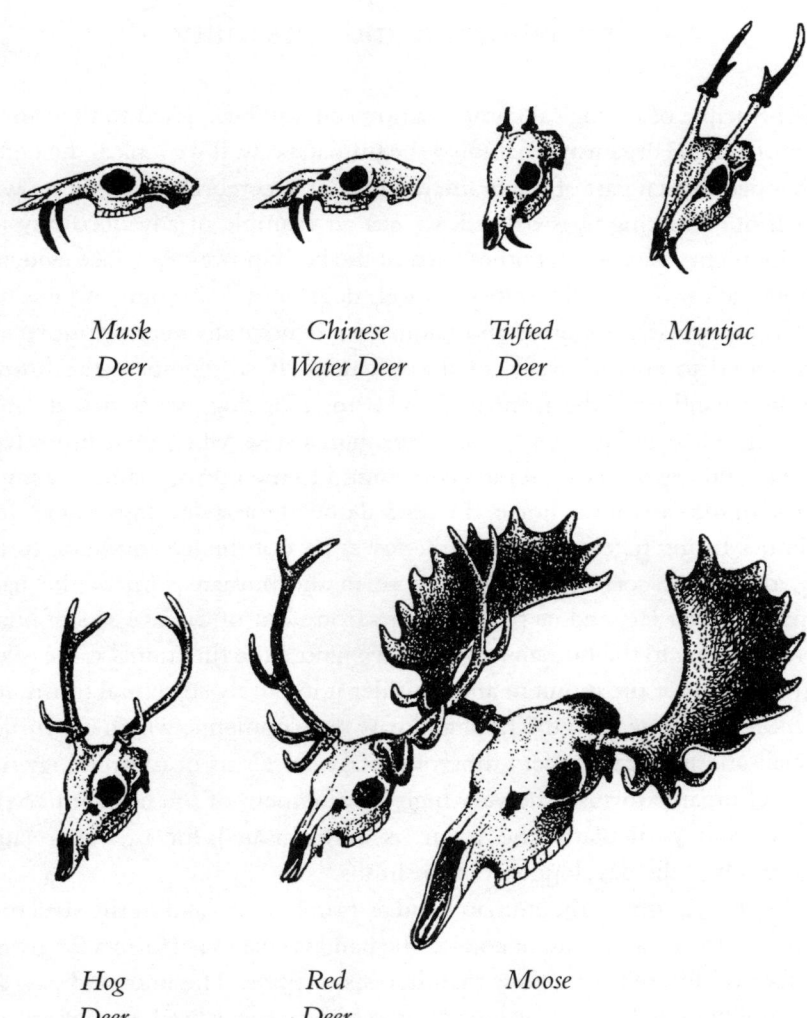

Musk
Deer

Chinese
Water Deer

Tufted
Deer

Muntjac

Hog
Deer

Red
Deer

Moose

Figure 2. Relative sizes of the canines and antlers of the male deer. Illustration from Man and Mammal *by Wolfgang Schad.*

whenever a particular quality is achieved through breeding, other desirable qualities are lost. For example, cows bred to produce very high milk yields have been found to be far more vulnerable to disease and to require more frequent courses of antibiotics.

31

Specialisation and versatility

The principle of biological compensation can also be applied to the various parts of a single organism, including the human body. If we look at the highly developed frontal part of the brain, the two large cerebral hemispheres with which our thinking is associated, we see an example of advanced physical development. If we look at other parts of the body, however, we see evidence of retardation. From the embryological, developmental point of view, the limbs (particularly the arms and hands) are structurally very primitive and correspond to an early stage of development. If we compare the human arm and hand with the front limb of a horse or dog, we find that, quite early on, horse and dog embryos go through a stage when their limbs have five radiating appendages, which correspond to the human hand and finger bones. In the case of the horse, the central one of these develops extensively, its bones fusing together to form the lower part of the leg and hoof. In the dog, the bones corresponding to those in the human palm of the hand form the lower leg, and its paw develops from four of the five sets of bones corresponding to the human fingers. If we ignore the functional value of the human hand for the moment and consider it in purely structural terms, it is far more primitive than the hoof and paw developments, which are further specialisations of the earlier embryonic stage. In terms of morphology (the study of organic forms), the very high development of the human nervous system, and particularly the brain, is compensated for by the relative retardation in the development of the limbs.

The description of the human hand as primitive is valid in the structural terms outlined above, but, of course, the hand is able to perform a far greater number of different functions than hooves or paws. The hoof and paw are structurally more highly developed but also more specialised, so they are less able to fulfil a diversity of requirements. Similarly, the forearm of a mole is superbly developed to function as a spade but this specialisation makes the animal less able to do other things, such as run at great speed.

If we compare different parts of the same organism, it becomes apparent that, in general, there is not only a loss of versatility associated with specialised structural development but also a loss of regenerative ability. A comparison of cells from the nervous system with cells from a metabolic organ such as the liver, shows that the nerve cell is vastly more structurally developed, with up to a million dendrites (branches of the cell which connect to other nerve cells) and an axon (or nerve fibre), which can be more than a metre long. The polyhedral outer form of a relatively unstructured liver cell comes simply from the pressure of other liver cells, and the liver is itself shaped by the organs around it. Functionally, the nerve cell is highly specialised in transmitting and receiving the impulses which are the physical basis of sentience in humans and animals. But this corresponds to the nerve cell's inability to reproduce and a certain lack of adaptability – it is vulnerable to changes in concentration of either glucose or oxygen and is easily damaged or killed. By contrast, the liver cell is able to make a vast number of biochemical transformations, is capable of extensive reproduction and is very resistant to toxic substances, low glucose concentrations and low oxygen concentrations. Its reproductive capacity is so prolific that liver tissue can replace a large part of itself if removed, as opposed to the brain and nervous system which have extremely limited powers of regeneration.

The etheric body

The etheric body can be seen as a body of formative forces which builds up the physical body and supplies a rich but not limitless supply of creative potential. In less differentiated tissues, such as the metabolic and nutritive organs, the creative potential remains available for growth and regeneration. But in highly differentiated tissues such as the nervous system, once a certain degree of maturity has been reached, the capacity for growth and regeneration is limited and, in accordance with the principle of biological compensation, etheric forces are released to be used in some other way. They become forces of thought and mental energy serving the higher function of consciousness, and are then associated with the soul element rather than the life element.

The qualities of the etheric realm are in many ways the opposite of those of the physical world, where order degenerates into disorder. Wherever the etheric principle enters the physical world, it brings about order and form out of disorder and chaos. In the dead physical realm, it makes sense to gain an understanding of an object in terms of its constituent parts. Where physical matter is brought to life by the etheric body of a plant, animal or human, the parts of the organism are better understood in terms of their relationships within the whole.

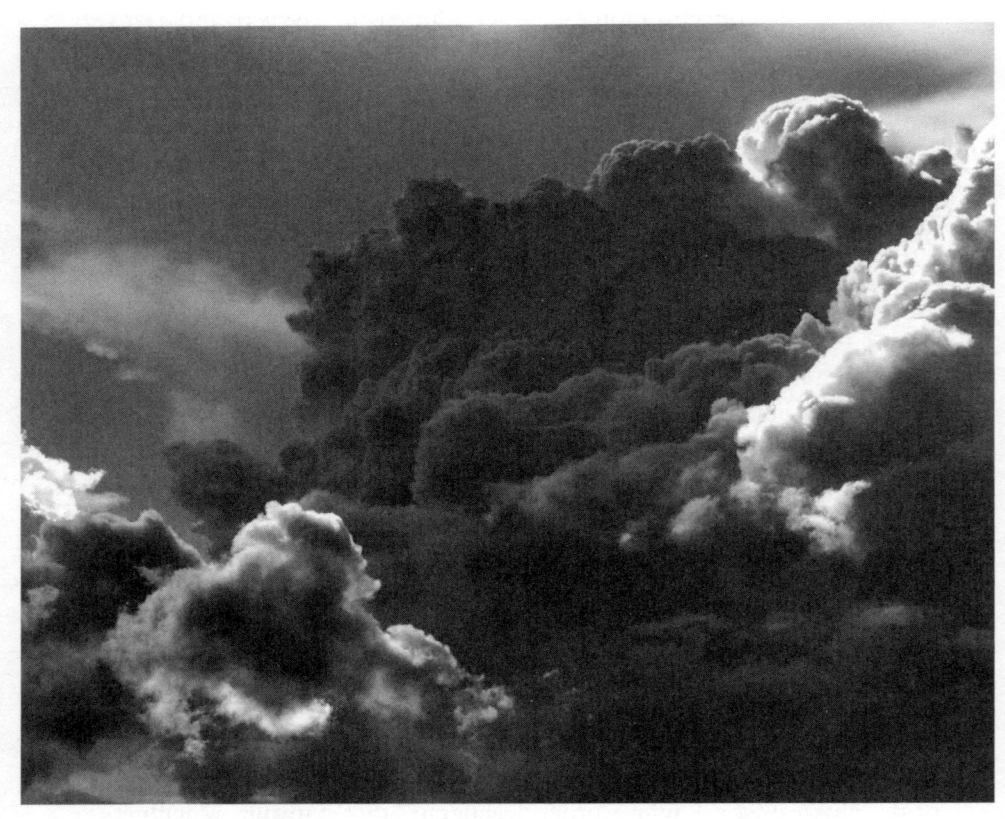

3. The Soul

In addition to having physical and etheric bodies, humans and animals are conscious of the physical world and have inner experiences of instinctive drives. These characteristics are derived from the soul element, or astral body which, working through the etheric body, exerts a formative influence on physical development. This gives rise to internal organs, enclosed cavities within the body and other physical characteristics which distinguish humans and animals from plants. These physical differences may be clearly observed, but the most striking characteristic of the soul element, consciousness, can be more difficult to grasp. Through our consciousness of the physical world, we can be aware of pain when the physical body is damaged, but we are also aware of an inner pain when our feelings are hurt. Unlike the physical pain, these hurt feelings cannot be related to a particular area of the physical body, but they can be every bit as real and, in some circumstances, even harder to endure.

Conventional approaches

Anthroposophic doctors take the soul element, and the way it affects the physical and etheric bodies, as seriously as physical symptoms in understanding an illness and deciding on treatment. By contrast, conventional medicine has largely ignored it, concentrating instead on the physical body, even though the work of psychologists and psychiatrists has shown that emotional problems can play a substantial role in bringing about many physical illnesses. Consequently, modern doctors are ill-equipped to understand the soul element or to take it into account in treatment. Anthroposophic medicine offers a detailed picture of the relationship between the astral and physical bodies, and this is vital for an understanding of how the soul element can be involved in the causation and possible healing of physical illness.

Studying the soul element is made difficult by the fact that people experience their own thoughts and feelings first-hand, but others cannot perceive them directly. Apart from the anthroposophic view, several approaches to overcoming this problem have emerged within the fields of psychiatry and psychology. Perhaps the closest to conventional physical medicine is the biophysical approach to psychiatry, which aims to find the causes of emotional problems in changes in the physical body's biochemistry, in particular in the brain and nervous system. This approach has led to treatments such as electroconvulsive therapy and the use of antidepressant and sedative drugs.

Another approach – behaviourism – tries to identify external stimuli which could be responsible for how animals and humans behave. Through extensive animal experiments, theories of learning were developed which were used to interpret and modify human behaviour. Behavioural therapy can help patients with obsessional problems or certain mild forms of depression. By contrast, the Freudian approach is based on instincts and unconscious processes, which are thought to have a biological foundation but are nevertheless treated as psychological phenomena in their own right. This approach has led to treatment through psychoanalysis, in which the therapist interprets what patients express in a way that aims to help them understand what lies behind their behaviour.

A fourth approach, social psychiatry, emphasises the effects of the social environment on the soul and looks at how social problems can lead to psychiatric illness. Finally, the existential, or phenomenological, approach analyses patients' experiences, their personality and how they make sense of the world. Patients are seen to be continually developing and maturing, and the term *self-actualisation* is used to describe how they determine their own personalities, rather than being mere products of their physical and social environments or unconscious drives. Efforts have been made to integrate these different approaches to understanding the psyche, and most psychiatrists are prepared to use whichever method they think will be most useful for a particular patient.

Consciousness

Anthroposophic medicine recognises that each approach contains an element of truth, but draws attention to the dangers of using any one method exclusively, as each one paints only a small part of the full picture. As one of the non-physical parts of a person, the soul element cannot be reduced to chemical or biological processes in the physical body. It is strongly coloured by the instincts, which have their roots in the unconscious physical and etheric bodies, and is also influenced by the higher element, the spirit, from which is derived a striving for a true understanding of the world and a need to find and fulfil aims in life that go beyond mere bodily needs. Anthroposophic medicine sees life as a process of soul and spiritual development, and crises in the soul, such as emotional problems, can therefore be seen as critical phases in a person's inner development.

The soul element is where consciousness arises, where feelings and thoughts reside. It is also where the impressions of the senses – for example, sight, hearing, smell, touch, taste, balance and temperature are experienced. The physical sense organs make it possible for us to perceive the physical world, but they are just the windows through which physical reality is revealed to the soul. For example, the eye is an instrument which is understood to receive visual images in a similar way to a camera. But it could no more make sense of the light patterns playing on the retina than a camera could understand the photographs it produces.

Contemporary natural science looks to the brain for this centre of consciousness and, certainly, all the electrochemical signals associated with the sense organs are transmitted to it. But there is nothing about the physical brain to make it any more capable of conscious experience of sight than the eyes. It, like them, is an organ consisting of a highly organised arrangement of cells, but neither the organ nor the cells are themselves conscious. The brain and sense organs are instruments of the soul, without which life in the physical world would be impossible.

The interplay of soul and physical body

There is a very fine balance in the relationship between the physical, etheric and astral bodies, and illness results from any breakdown in this balance. Finding where the root of the problem lies is a major part of the anthroposophic doctor's diagnosis. It cannot be assumed that the problem is to be found where the symptoms manifest: physical symptoms often result from disorders of the soul and the way the astral body influences the etheric and physical bodies.

This interplay between physical and psychological causes of illness has been explored by conventional medicine. In the 1940s and 1950s, a group of disorders began to be thought of as being caused by psychological factors, though nearly all of them involved changes in the structure of the physical body. They became known as *psychosomatic* disorders, and included gastric and duodenal ulcers, ulcerative colitis, asthma, rheumatoid arthritis, thyrotoxicosis (overactive thyroid gland), high blood pressure and eczema. Since then, there has been an increasing awareness that the majority of illnesses do not have a single cause, but result from a number of factors. As well as psychological effects, these may include hereditary predispositions, nutrition, reduced immunity and contact with particular viruses or bacteria. It is now accepted by conventional medicine that psychological factors play an important role in bringing about both illnesses which involve structural changes (such as heart attacks, infections, diabetes and cancer) and functional disorders (migraine, indigestion, irritable bowel syndrome, sciatica, stiff neck and lower back pain).

As a result of further study of the role of the psyche in illness, two broad psychological types were described. The Type A personality was thought to predispose to heart disease and was identified in people with very high competitive drives who constantly felt under pressure and found it difficult to relax. Men with this type of personality were found to have twice the risk of a fatal heart attack than had men who were equally outwardly successful, but who were more relaxed and easy-going. The more relaxed nature was called the Type B personality. Even so, the personality type was still recognised to be only one of a number of factors which can predispose to a heart attack. Others include smoking, being overweight, heredity and high blood pressure. Other studies suggested that an inability to express anger increased the likelihood of breast cancer in women under fifty and lung cancer in men. Also, of patients who already had cancer, those who reacted with hopelessness and desperation were found to have a poorer prognosis than those with a fighting spirit.

Another link with psychological factors was found in the case of diabetes. It was only relatively recently discovered that psychological stress can increase the body's need for insulin, though it had long been known that diabetics receiving insulin had difficulty controlling their illness during emotional crises. Previously, it had been thought that they did not pay sufficient attention to their diet and treatment when under emotional strain. Also, it is thought that the onset of diabetes can be triggered by emotional traumas, particularly bereavement, loss and loneliness, though it is again recognised that there are also other factors.

As conventional medicine has come to recognise that habitual psychological attitudes and emotional crises play important parts in bringing about many, if not most, illnesses, attempts have been made to understand the causal relationship. Different people with the same problems react in different ways, so it has to be asked how the psychological factor might contribute to the development of a disorder before attempts can be made at treating these causes. Conventional medicine has discovered that processes in the nervous system influence the regulation of hormones via the pituitary gland, which is directly connected to the lower part of the brain. Also, it is known that branches of the nervous system extend into the thymus and spleen, where certain groups of white blood cells, the lymphocytes, develop. Furthermore, it is known that the nervous system is connected to the adrenal gland and that nervous stimulation thereby leads to increased secretion of adrenaline and corticosteroids, both of which are produced in greatly increased concentrations during severe emotional stress.

It is thought in conventional medicine that the answer to the question of how the psyche can bring about changes in the body's immune system might be found by furthering this knowledge of links between the central nervous system and the rest of the body. But, while these findings are interesting in themselves, this idea assumes that thoughts and feelings are contained within the brain or nervous system, rather than experienced by a non-physical soul which is served by the brain and nerves. Predictably, this line of research has had little success in the development of new treatments. Anthroposophic medicine, on the other hand, offers a description of how the soul works into, and affects, the physical and etheric bodies, both in health and as a cause of disease. It can offer therapies which have direct effects on the astral body and treat the true cause of an illness, rather than focusing on relieving the physical symptoms.

The interplay of astral and etheric bodies

It has already been said that the etheric body is primarily involved with building up the physical body and constantly working to keep it healthy. The astral body, has, in a sense, an opposite effect. It has a breaking-down, or

39

catabolic, effect on the physical body, and thereby imbues a constant tendency towards illness. This contrasting effect comes about because, whereas the etheric body is the basis of life, the astral body is the seat of consciousness, and consciousness in the physical world is bought at the cost of breaking down, or *burning,* physical matter.

One aspect of the destructive effect of the astral body is that consciousness is always accompanied by the breaking down of glucose in the nervous system. This can only happen with the aid of oxygen and is rather like the burning of a flame. Although this burning process takes place in all the cells of the body, the brain and nervous system are the most sensitive, requiring a constant supply of glucose and oxygen from the blood. It is well-known that brain-death occurs within a few minutes if the supply is cut off, whereas the tissues of the limbs, which burn glucose during muscular activity, can survive for as long as an hour. This destructive process, brought about by the astral body, has a proper place within the healthy physical body, as long as it is balanced by the healing effect of the blood, brought about by the etheric body. Any significant imbalance between these two opposing influences will result in illness.

As well as its destructive effect, the astral body can also work in harmony with the etheric body in a forming capacity. It does so particularly during embryonic development, by imposing a human form on the pattern of growth as the etheric body builds up the physical body. However, even this involves a polarity of action. For example, an etheric process produces a limb with a hand 'bud' of solid tissue, then digestive enzymes are made which, in an astral process, break down or 'digest' tissue to introduce the spaces between the fingers. The hand takes shape through an interplay of creative and destructive forces, through the growth and digestion of tissue.

Similarly, in the digestion and assimilation of food, the astral and etheric bodies work together but in opposing directions. Digestive enzymes and acid are secreted in the stomach, and break down the food into manageable components. Only when the food has been sufficiently broken down is the etheric body able to use the components in its constant regeneration of the physical body. The acid and digestive enzymes would break down the lining of the stomach itself if there were not means of protection. A thick mucus is secreted from the lining, and the cells in the stomach wall are especially strongly linked together, preventing any of the juices penetrating through it. The cells are constantly replaced, ensuring that the destructive capability of the acid and enzymes is held in check.

If this equilibrium is lost, either through excessive juices or insufficient protection, the stomach lining is itself digested, producing a hole, or ulcer. The smell of cooking, or the thought of a meal, increases the secretions in the stomach, as do feelings of fear or anger, and these physical responses to psychological changes are well-known to conventional medicine. Doctors are aware that many patients who develop gastric ulcers have been under stress for long periods, often with chronic frustration, but have lacked the means of expressing their feelings. This results in chronic overproduction of acid and enzymes. An anthroposophic doctor would see this as a case of the destructive digestive effect, which is an expression of the astral body, having persistently overpowered the restorative processes of the etheric body. A gastric ulcer is all the more likely to occur if the patient also drinks alcohol excessively, damaging the stomach lining, or smokes, which may impair the healing process by interfering with the blood supply to the stomach wall.

This polarity between the upbuilding life processes and the destructive processes of consciousness goes hand-in-hand with the trade-off between specialisation and vitality described in Chapter 2. Consciousness is associated with the brain, nervous system and sense organs, which centre on the head and upper body. The complexity and specialisation of these organs is characterised by a relative dearth of vitality – the cells are unable to reproduce and are relatively less able to endure adverse conditions. In the lower part of the body are found the organs of reproduction, nutrition and regeneration. The relative simplicity of the cells in the liver or the lining of the stomach is complemented by their tremendous versatility and vitality.

Sleep and being awake

To maintain the balance between the destructive and regenerative processes, there must be alternating times of consciousness and unconsciousness, in other words, wakefulness and sleep. It is common knowledge that sleep is essential for reinvigoration and to assist healing during illnesses and that, as the day progresses, tiredness increases. When we fall asleep, our astral bodies withdraw from our physical and etheric bodies to enable the regenerative processes to work unhindered. At different times of life, the balance between these processes varies. For example, in babyhood, the period of most rapid growth is accompanied by the most sleeping. The etheric processes predominate and there is a great capacity for healing. In old age, growth has long since ceased, the healing capacity is reduced, and periods of sleeping are generally much shorter.

If the daily rhythm of consciousness and reinvigoration is disturbed, the imbalances which result will manifest as disorders. If the disturbance becomes constant, these tend to develop into chronic ailments. Anxiety and fear cause increased bowel action, so diarrhoea can result from attacks of anxiety, as is well-known to many who have taken exams or given public performances. The pulse, breathing rate and blood pressure are also raised by anxiety or fear, muscular tension is increased and more acid is produced in the stomach. If prolonged periods of stress cause chronic anxiety in patients, symptoms more permanent than a short bout of diarrhoea might become apparent. One patient might complain of palpitations on becoming aware of an unusually rapid heartbeat, another of tingles in the limbs as a result of constant excessive breathing. This overbreathing reduces the amount of carbon dioxide in the blood, low levels of which are connected with the feeling of 'pins and needles'.

If the anxiety persists, diarrhoea may become permanent, or alternate with constipation, with abdominal cramps and a bloated feeling, as if the bowel was swinging between overactivity and underactivity (irritable bowel syndrome). When increased muscular tension becomes permanent, it can lead to painful spasms, for example in the neck, and may contribute to an attack of lumbago or sciatica if combined with lifting something awkwardly.

In all these instances, the processes normally brought about for a short time by a strong soul impression begin to manifest more permanently in one or another organ. The astral body's activity is too strong: in a sense, it penetrates more deeply than is appropriate into the particular organ. In these examples, there is not yet a structural change in the physical body – the dyspepsia has not yet become an ulcer, the diarrhoea is not yet colitis – but in many illnesses, structural changes result from an intensification of the same process. Angina – a temporary chemical damage of the heart muscle caused by a lack of oxygen – might be followed by a heart attack, when permanent damage occurs. Frequent diarrhoea might be followed by ulcerative colitis, a chronic inflammation of the bowel lining which results in pain or discomfort and the passing of blood and mucus.

Effects of the astral body on the physical

In the physical world, order tends to degenerate into disorder, and it is only the intervention of the etheric body which reverses this process, bringing order out of chaos. The astral body takes the physical development created by the life element to a higher level, introducing greater differentiation and specialisation into the physical body. Some illnesses can be understood to arise when there is a breakdown in a particular region of this higher ordering, allowing the partial reestablishment of the physical tendency towards degeneration. Such illnesses include those involving the crystallisation of substances which would normally be kept in constant movement and solution, as in the development of gallstones and kidney stones. A crystallisation process might be healthily expressed in the bones as calcification but, following the laying down of fatty substances in the arteries (atheroma), it would bring about a hardening of the arteries (arteriosclerosis) which tends to increase with age. This leads to poor circulation, painful muscular cramps on exertion and, after some time, could result in a stroke, senility, angina or a heart attack.

In oedema – when water collects in the ankles and calves, causing swelling – we have another example of a physical principle dominating the life processes. In the physical world, water collects at the lowest point it can run to under the influence of gravity. Inside the body, it should be in constant circulation, with the etheric forces counteracting the effect of gravity. If this life process breaks down, the water behaves as it would in the outer world, causing oedema. It follows that, if excessive activity of the astral body leads to a breakdown of the etheric processes, an appropriate form of treatment would involve strengthening those etheric forces while at the same time bringing back into balance the excessive astral forces.

The contrast between the anabolic, or upbuilding, influence of the etheric body and the catabolic, or breaking-down, influence of the astral body can be seen in a comparison of animal and plant life. Plants have physical bodies and, as living things, also have etheric bodies. Animals have physical and etheric bodies and, as conscious creatures, also have astral bodies. A comparison therefore offers clear examples of the functional differences introduced by the addition of an astral body.

The special vitality of plants, which have the life element without the opposing processes of consciousness, is demonstrated by their ability to transform inorganic matter into living substance. Animals cannot do this, and are only able to live by eating plants or other animals which themselves eat plants. Generally speaking, plants take in carbon dioxide and build carbohydrates, a fundamental food for animal life. By contrast, animals burn up carbohydrates, using oxygen to do so, and give off carbon dioxide.[1]

It has been described how the interplay of growth and digestion of tissue forms the hand during embryonic development. If this process is compared with the way a plant develops a hand-shaped, or palmate, leaf, the absence of the astral body is again clear. In the plant, the finger shapes arise because of different rates of growth in the developing tissue. The areas of more rapid cell division form the extensions, with the spaces in between brought about by slower growth. In animal (and human) embryos, successive stages of development involve the breaking down of earlier structures so that new ones can be built. Plants lack this possibility of developing by subtracting tissue and can only add – developing by what might be called *positive* growth. They can still change their form – for example their early leaves (cotyledons) may have a quite different structure from the leaves that later unfold – but the cotyledons are not dissolved away and can be seen below, and next to, later leaves. If humans developed in the same way, baby arms would be retained below the adult arms!

Another example of the plant's inability to dissolve its growth is given by the tendency towards woodiness of higher plants which live for more than one or two years. Wood is dead conductive tissue, which the plant lays down each year and grows around, giving rise to the thickening tree trunk and the annual rings which can be seen if the trunk is sawn through. Bark is formed in a similar way but, in this case, the dead material is deposited on the outside of the living tissue.

In the animal kingdom, there is a great range of development of the soul. Without the higher faculty of perception relating to the soul realm, it is not possible to perceive an animal's inner life directly, but it is quite easy to see how much more aware a cat or a dog is than, say, a worm. This observation is supported by the greater complexity of the nervous system in vertebrates and mammals. However, it is not only the nervous systems that become more complex with higher development, but also the systems concerned with breathing and the circulation of blood or equivalent fluids. One of the main tasks of these systems is to transport oxygen to all the tissues of the body and remove carbon dioxide. The increasing complexity allows for higher rates of burning of sugars in the cells (cellular respiration) and, as a generalisation, the higher the development of soul, the greater the rate of burning (metabolic rate). The highest metabolic rates are found in mammals and birds, which are able to maintain a constant inner temperature, irrespective of their environment (warm-bloodedness). This enables mammals and birds to make rapid and powerful muscular actions irrespective of the outside temperature, whereas the activity of cold-blooded animals depends on how warm a day it happens to be.

As well as a higher metabolic rate, the more developed soul brings with it an increased food requirement and a more complex digestion to cope with the food. The complexity of animals' gastro-intestinal tracts ranges from a simple beaker shape in sea anemones, which have one opening as both entrance and exit, to a tube open at both ends in worms, to the much more sophisticated digestions of mammals. Wherever the catabolic, or breaking-down, processes are found in the animal kingdom, they indicate the involvement of a soul. Generally, the more efficient the animals' physical bodies are at utilising nutrients, the greater are their levels of sentience and responsiveness.

Consciousness and vitality

Much as there is an inverse relationship between specialisation and vitality in single organs (see the principle of biological compensation in Chapter 2), there is a trade-off between increased awareness and lowered vitality in animals which may be seen in their powers of healing and regeneration. A damaged limb will heal in mammals, but a limb or tail which is removed cannot be regrown. The cold-blooded lizards, with their lower metabolic rates, are able to regrow their tails and, lower down the hierarchy, a worm can even regrow half of its body. Even simpler flatworms, or planarians, can be split down the middle and regrow into two complete organisms, which is more reminiscent of the regenerative powers of plants than animals. Indeed, the less developed the animal's soul, the more plant-like the qualities of growth and repair become.

The awakening effect of the soul can also be traced chemically in the nervous system. Much information has come to light within the last decades concerning, particularly, the neurotransmitter substances, which are released by one nerve cell and affect another. They are mainly amines, which are derived from, and closely related to, amino acids, the constituents of proteins. One of the main amines is noradrenaline. Its effect is very similar to that of the hormone adrenaline, which is understood to be released into the blood following nervous stimulation of the adrenal gland. Both adrenaline and noradrenaline heighten alertness and awareness. The pulse and metabolic rate are raised, glycogen (the form in which the sugar, glucose, is stored) is broken down, and the concentration of sugar in the blood rises, allowing the cells to burn more glucose to provide more energy.

As well as bringing about heightened awareness, this process increases the body's catabolic rate, the rate at which it breaks down material. In recognition of this, amines which stimulate the catabolism are called catecholamines, and most antidepressant drugs work by indirectly increasing the level of catecholamines in the nervous system. A drug which is chemically very similar to catecholamines is amphetamine, also known as speed. It has a very powerful awakening effect, causing excessive astral activity and 'speeding' thinking. It also causes a feeling of elation, but its effects carry the danger of inducing mania and addiction. Through increasing the speed of metabolism, it also leads to weight loss and, in children, to retardation of growth.

The three main groups of biological substances, which are at the same time the three main groups of foods, are carbohydrates (sugars and starches), oils and fats, and proteins. All three are found in both plants and animals. However, animal substance (meat) is particularly rich in protein, while plant substance (fruit and vegetables) is generally richer in carbohydrates. Bearing in mind the relatively high levels of awareness in animals and protein in meat, it is worth noting that the constituents of protein (amino acids) are chemically very closely related to the catecholamines which stimulate wakefulness.

Another kind of amine which is very closely related to the amino acids is histamine. It is involved in the release of acid and digestive enzymes into the stomach on the one hand, but also in inflammatory reactions on the other. In the former case, it plays a role in the breaking down of food so that it may be safely absorbed into the body. In the latter, it mobilises inflammation, which has a vital role in fighting invasions of bacteria and other foreign bodies. The immune system is stimulated by the process of inflammation to activate phagocytic cells – white blood cells that 'eat' foreign organisms, destroying them by secreting their own digestive enzymes around them.

Acting through the etheric body, the astral body brings about the characteristic physical forms of humans and animals. During embryonic development, it introduces folding processes which give rise to internalised organs and enclosed cavities within the body, and which depart from the predominantly planar development typical of plant organs. These folding processes introduce the nervous and digestive systems into the previously flat embryonic disc.

The development of nervous and digestive systems illustrates the astral body's fundamental qualities. On the one hand, it makes possible conscious experience of both the outer world and an inner realm of feelings and drives. On the other, it enhances the catabolic processes in the body, as typified by the wide-ranging role of digestive enzymes.

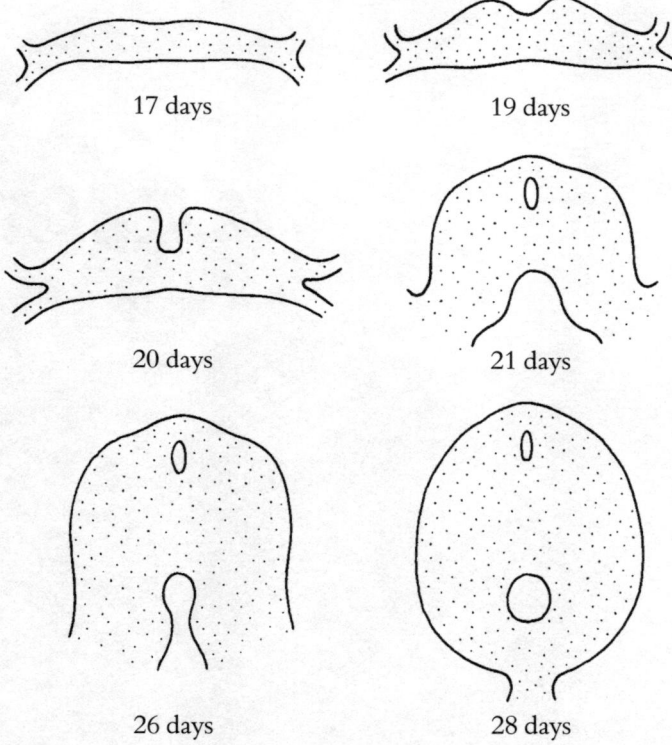

Figure 3. Sections through an embryo showing the early development (in days after conception) of the central nervous system and later the digestive tract.

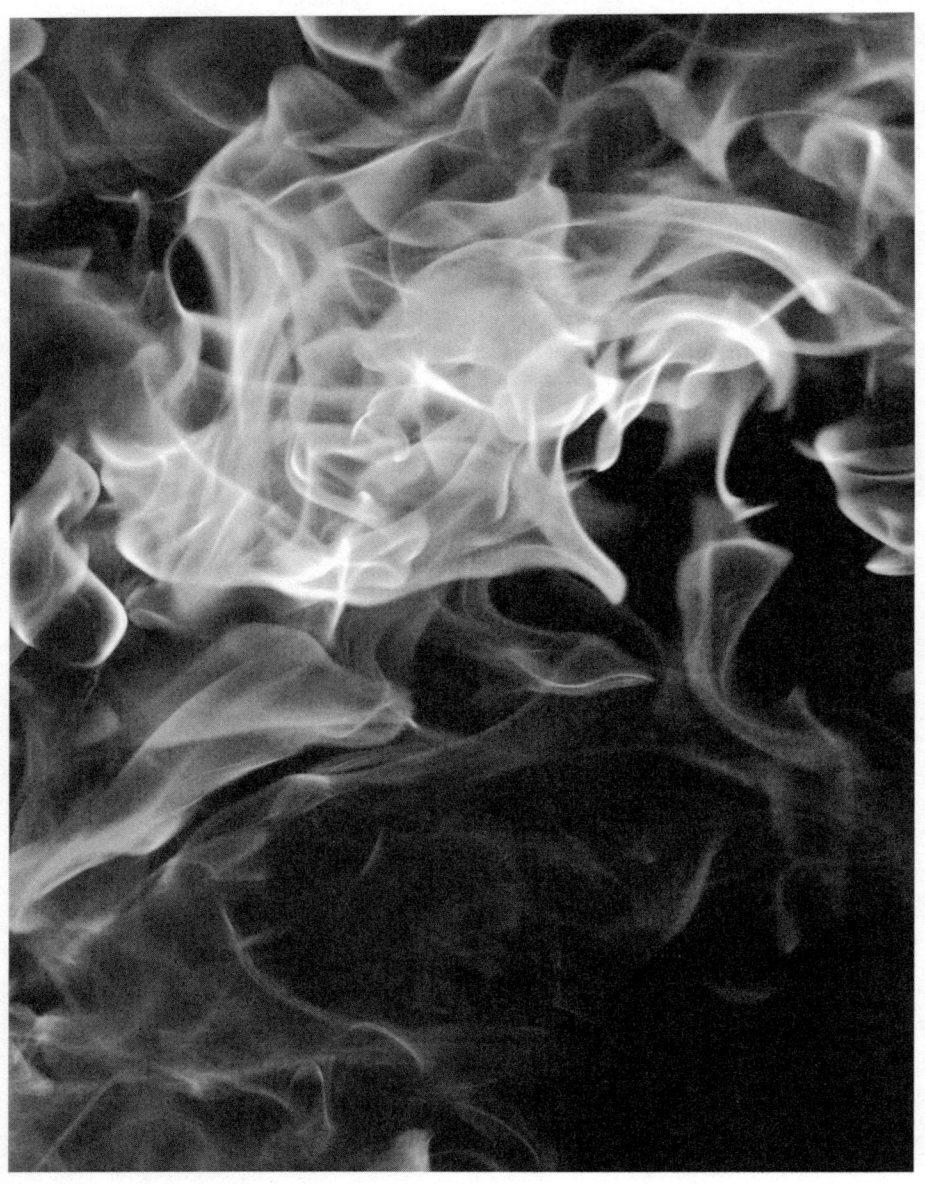

4. The Spirit

Humans and animals are aware of the physical world and are able to experience pleasure and pain because they have astral bodies. However, there is an additional level of consciousness in humans that animals lack – self-awareness. Humans are aware that they are independent conscious beings and, through this self-awareness, are able to distinguish themselves from, and reflect on, the rest of the world. Thinking about the world brings with it the possibility of going beyond the animal's instinctive reactions to events. Humans are able to refrain from instinctive behaviour if their thoughts lead them to consider that it might be better to act in some other way. While animals act out of instinct modified by external conditioning, humans are able to form mental pictures of the consequences of their actions and other considerations, and allow these to influence their decisions.

Anthroposophic medicine describes this extra dimension of consciousness as the activity of the fourth element of the human, the spirit or I. It is a person's inner core, the identity of the self around which thoughts and feelings come and go. The I has a dual effect on the physical body. It works with the astral body in the breaking-down processes and also with the etheric body in the building-up, nutritive processes. It is particularly involved in thinking and, in that capacity, has a destructive effect within the physical body, particularly in the nervous system. It is also associated with the will, and the way volition is expressed through the physical body in movement – for example, the ability to stand upright and walk on two legs is a specifically human attribute.

The I also bestows a sense of continuity and permanence from one hour, day or year to the next, which is made possible by the faculty of memory. Only humans have a true memory. When people wake up, they remember what happened the day before and what they intended to do on the new day. They remember who they are and where they live, and these retained concepts maintain a sense of identity. In animals, however, experiences come and go without being inwardly retained. Their external circumstances can trigger a kind of recollection of similar previous situations, but they have no power within themselves to recall events which are not mirrored in their immediate surroundings. Humans are able to recall past events at will, irrespective of their external circumstances.

Freedom and responsibility

People's ability to think for themselves – to the extent to which they use it – can free them from instinctive behaviour. In so far as freedom is achieved, it is the I which makes it possible. Only humans have the choice between instinctive behaviour – essentially the pursuit of pleasure and avoidance of pain – and higher motives, such as concern for the well-being of others. The ability to choose cannot be separated from responsibility for the consequences of the chosen action. However, not only does the I give people the ability to think for themselves, it also makes it possible for them to transform their own natures.

Some psychological schools acknowledge that freedom is a human characteristic. They generally see the childhood environment as a powerful influence, but assume that people are able to modify their behaviour through their awareness of what they learned when young. Thus, psychologies which include a theme of conscious self-development imply the existence of human freedom. Some go even further and introduce a concept of the spirit. For example, the existentialist, Victor Frankel, described the spirit as the part of a person that searched for, and could perceive, truth and meaning. The soul, he said, might be ill with a neurosis, such as severe depression, and yet the spirit may still be capable of perceiving a situation and grasping the truth. He described patients who endured considerable physical handicaps because of their illnesses, and knew they would die within a short time, who nevertheless used the last days of their lives to help other patients, some directly and others through the example of the way they bore their suffering.

Frankel said the doctor's role went beyond the care of body and soul, and included helping patients to find out what was meaningful for them in what they were going through. He quoted an aphorism from Goethe which he recommended as a maxim for psychotherapy: 'If we take people as they are, we make them worse. If we treat them as if they were what they ought to be, we help them to become what they are capable of becoming'.

By contrast, schools of thought which try to show how animal-like human behaviour is tend to deny the existence of human freedom. For example, in *The Naked Ape,* Desmond Morris makes the case that human behaviour which appears to be for the benefit of others is actually nothing more than a subtle refinement of instinctive drives, such as survival and sexuality. This reduces the human to the level of the animal and, if all actions are deemed to be derived from these urges, freedom and the spirit are denied.

Anthroposophic medicine sees true freedom as a goal which is being worked towards rather than a fully developed, bestowed privilege. The I, or spirit, acts as the agent of transformation in the process of personal development. It exists before birth and after death, and stimulates a departure from the straitjacket of learned, habitual and instinctive forms of behaviour, replacing them with free, conscious acts. This process of personal development is not limited to one lifetime. As has been seen, the physical body is constantly prone to decay, and remains alive only as long as it is maintained by the etheric body. When it dies, the spirit retains the developmental progress made in that lifetime and remains active in the spiritual world while preparing for the next incarnation.*

The consequences of our actions

Through their thoughts and actions, people are constantly shaping the future of the world. The effects of their actions on those around them may be quite obvious, but it can take a long time for some consequences to be recognised. For example, only relatively recently has it become clear, particularly through an increased awareness of pollution, that our chosen way of life has had far more widespread effects on the world than we would have believed possible. Our individual responsibility for everything we have ever done is borne by the spirit, and survives death. Its effect on future lives follows a law which is described by a word borrowed from ancient Eastern teachings – karma.

* This concept of reincarnation should not be confused with the teachings of certain ancient religions which suggest that humans can reincarnate as animals or insects. The human spirit is involved in the development of the human form as a vehicle through which it can act in the physical realm. Animals and insects do not have an individual I, and their bodily organisations are not developed to support them. The only bodily organisation capable of supporting the human I is the one the I is itself active in forming.

In future lives, our karma brings about opportunities for us to develop capacities that had been lacking and to redeem any malevolent influences we had brought into the world. However, we are not normally aware of our karma (unless we have undergone the inner strengthening process required for the development of higher faculties of perception) because if we were, we would cease to be free. The burden of responsibility would be so great, it would impose a course of action which would have to be followed as a predetermined destiny.

This idea of karma is not a concept of retribution, or of being rewarded and punished by a higher authority for good and bad deeds. Its description has been much simplified for the purposes of this book, but the principle that responsibility goes hand-in-hand with self-determination can be understood from examples in everyday life, without having to seek confirmation in the spiritual world. In general, children tend to have a limited awareness of the consequences of their actions and often behave selfishly and irresponsibly as a result. As they mature, they learn through experience how others are affected by their actions and tend to become more altruistic.

When we are preparing to incarnate, our karma influences when and where we are born, to whom, and the circumstances in which we will live. It shapes our constitutions and personalities, and provides the hard lessons in life, which hurt but also stimulate development. Awareness of this karmic element in our development opens up the possibility of finding a meaning underlying major events in our lives, such as illnesses. It becomes possible to see illnesses as more than unfortunate accidents – to see them instead as challenges which are both opportunities for and catalysts of personal development. This is, of course, very different from the contemporary view of the human as an advanced animal, who comes into being at conception and ceases to exist at death, and gives rise to a very different form of therapy.

From the anthroposophic doctor's point of view, the first step is to be aware of the possibility that an illness may have some significant meaning for the patient. By discussing the problem with the patient, the doctor might be able to help discover its meaning. What emerges may be quite mundane or very profound. A relatively mundane example might result from the experience of a short bout of flu or a flu-like illness. Although not very severe in patients in their twenties or thirties, it may be enough to bring it home to them that they have been exhausting themselves, perhaps through working too hard and by not maintaining a healthy balance of activity. They may decide that it is time to restore that balance and adjust their lives accordingly. There follow some more profound examples, taken from work at Park Attwood Clinic, a former anthroposophic medical centre in England.

Examples of life changes

A severe case concerned a man who placed very great value on his physical fitness and sporting achievements, and who developed a disabling arthritis. This forced him to re-examine his values and priorities. In time, he was able to find a new basis for his life but such a process, when forced upon a patient in this way, can be terribly traumatic; the patient requires a great deal of support while an adjustment to a new way of life is taking place.

A woman in her mid-thirties, who had put most of her energy into being a successful wife and mother, felt she could never live up to the standards she expected of herself, which were based on what she thought others expected of her. She became severely depressed and anxious, and was then incapable of running a home at all. This confirmed her feeling that she could not cope, and the depression and anxiety deepened in a vicious cycle. During this crisis, she needed a lot of support. For a while, she was given anthroposophic medicines and conventional sedatives, and was further supported by nursing and artistic therapy. The corner was turned when she began to let go of the expectations she had of herself. Gradually, she began to feel that she should accept herself for what she was, rather than measure herself against some arbitrarily imposed scale. This led to a feeling that she should act out of her own volition rather than her idea of what others expected and, by this time, the recovery was well in hand. After some months, she was able to resume her life with her family, and soon reported that she felt far more fulfilled as she had become more true to herself. Later, she said it had been worth suffering the pain of the illness for the transformation it had brought to her life.

A fifty-two-year-old man suffered a sudden onset of severe eczema, which strong steroid treatment from his family doctor did little to alleviate. Outwardly, he was a rather tough character, who had tended to use his fists to sort out disputes. He was an expert teacher of karate and greatly enjoyed the martial arts. Out-patient treatment with anthroposophic medicines brought no obvious improvement, so he was admitted to Park Attwood. Initially, he continued to be aggressive and showed no empathy for patients suffering from depression, saying he could not imagine what depression was. He made it clear that he regarded talk of feelings as unmanly and not for him. The atmosphere of the centre he said he found strangely serene, and therefore unreal, and he was very derisory about the custom of saying grace before meals. He was started on painting therapy and therapeutic eurythmy (see Chapter 7), despite his protestations that it was a waste of time, and was given anthroposophic medicines and ointment to apply to the eczema.

The centre offered a very supportive social atmosphere, and there was plenty of time for him to talk to the staff, or co-workers, as they were called. After a while in this environment, he appeared to be softening slightly and, one day, in conversation with a nurse, he suddenly burst into tears when describing his experiences in the Korean War. He had never described these to anyone before and, by crying in front of the nurse, openly transgressed his taboo over feelings. It emerged that he had witnessed great cruelty and suffering in the war, and had been badly burned by napalm. He had never suffered from eczema before, and the areas now affected coincided exactly with where he had been burned thirty-four years earlier. It further emerged that he had been emotionally deprived as a child and had developed an aggressive show of strength by way of compensation. This adolescent way of behaving seemed to have been fixed in him by his experiences in the war, which he had been unable to deal with, and had remained ever since.

He attended a lecture at the centre about Leonardo's mural painting, *The Last Supper,* after which the depicted gestures of Christ and His disciples were discussed. The following night, he had a very moving dream in which he opened his arms to the position of Christ's in the mural, and felt as if energy was streaming from one arm to the other via the heart region. He woke up feeling certain that he would start to get better and, from then on, his eczema did improve steadily. He was by this time behaving quite differently, showing considerable sympathy and understanding for other patients, especially those with emotional problems. He also expressed a genuine respect for the work at the centre. His condition improved sufficiently for him to be discharged and, quite soon afterwards, he was able to return to work. It was clear that he had not only recovered from the eczema but had also undergone a considerable inner transformation. It seemed it was only through the acute and very uncomfortable illness that he was able to confront, and ultimately overcome, his facade of aggression and begin to express himself. The eczema had been a symptom of a deep emotional problem and had also played a part in a major step in his personal development.

In cases of illness in old age, when the patient is nearer to death, or perhaps suffering from a terminal disease, the significance may be more difficult to deduce because it may not be experienced fully until after death. It would be difficult to see how a terminal illness could have a positive meaning at all within the ideology of conventional medicine. However, anthroposophic doctors consider that there is still a meaning within the context of karma and personal development, but accept that its assessment has to be more tentative.

A woman in her mid-fifties developed symptoms of a very advanced cancer of the ovary. Her abdomen was markedly distended with fluid as a result of the spreading of the tumour, and she died within three months of the discovery of the illness. Her life had been characterised by considerable disappointments. She had been brought up by her grandparents, because her own parents had had more children than they could cope with, and had always seen this as rejection by her parents. She was a gifted person, and was a qualified nurse and movement therapist. Though attractive, she had never married or had any children of her own, and this was also deeply disappointing to her. She never stayed very long in one place, though generally well-liked, and consequently had few close friends. In her forties, she had cared for her aged mother until her death and, during this time, had felt a degree of appreciation from her that she had not felt before. She inherited her mother's house and lived there alone, estranged from her brothers and sisters, who were all married with children.

During her cancer, which she knew was terminal, she was able to express some of her deep disappointments. Early on, there had been great fear and panic associated with the illness, made worse by the fact that the pressure from her swollen abdomen made breathing difficult. But she developed close ties with nurses and other co-workers at the centre and, after considerable outpourings of anger at the difficulties she had endured in her life, including the cancer itself, she came to a remarkable degree of acceptance and inner tranquillity. She died soon afterwards, but those caring for her felt that her chronic 'inner sores' had been healed before she had died, and that they would not be taken unresolved into the spiritual life after death. She had not only come to terms with her approaching death, but also with her life.

In these examples, the illnesses enabled the patients to take significant steps in their personal development. Anthroposophic medicine aims to heal illness in a way which supports, rather than suppresses, such development. Through counselling, a deeper meaning to the experience of an illness may become apparent to both doctor and patient.

Four states and four elements

Now that the characteristics of the four human elements have been outlined, it is possible to see a more comprehensive picture of nature emerging. It can be seen that spiritual science is compatible with natural science, but adds another dimension to its concept of the world. In particular, the qualitative approach of spiritual science extends the quantitative parameters of natural science. For example, spiritual science identifies a qualitative relationship between the four human elements and the four natural elements – earth, water, air and fire. More specifically, it relates the human elements to the four fundamental states of matter or energy – solid, liquid, gas and warmth. By applying heat, the densest form of matter, a solid, can be made into a liquid. The heating makes the molecules of the solid more energetic until a threshold is passed when it 'melts' into liquid form. Similarly, a liquid can be made into a gas by applying heat. Warmth itself might be thought of as a *condition* of a solid, liquid or gas, which it is, but it can also exist in its own right, as radiant heat from the sun for example. In this sense, it is pure energy, rather than matter with more energetic molecules.

The physical body relates to the solid state, the etheric to the liquid, the astral to the gaseous and the I to warmth. The relevance of this for anthroposophic medicine is that the I expresses itself in the physical world through warmth, the astral through gases and the etheric through liquids. When student doctors study anatomy, they dissect corpses that have been pickled for a year. This gives the impression that the body is a quite solid structure because the pickling turns soft, virtually fluid organs, like the liver,

Human element	State	Natural element
I	Warmth	Fire
Astral body	Gas	Air
Etheric body	Liquid	Water
Physical body	Solid	Earth

Figure 4.

into fairly firm structures. The living body consists very largely of water and is, in fact, far more fluid than solid, the firmest parts being the bones. Gases are dissolved in the fluids and tissues of the body, as well as being present in the intestines and lungs, and the whole body is warm, with the deep tissues maintained at a mean temperature of about 37 °C (98.5 °F). In fact, closer examination reveals that some parts are warmer than others, and the temperatures of one organ and another, or different areas of skin can vary considerably. Using modern techniques of thermography, it is possible to produce a colourful image of the pattern of warmth of the skin. The *warmth body* can be imagined by picturing this kind of representation of the distribution of warmth throughout the body.

Looking at the apparently solid physical body gives the impression of a clear boundary between the person and the outside world. Everything inside the skin is seen as part of the person, everything outside it as part of the outer world. But this boundary is less clear when considering the *fluid body*. A certain amount of moisture is constantly excreted from the entire skin surface, which evaporates into the air. The boundary is still less clear in the case of the *gaseous body,* as there is a constant exchange of internal and external substances in the process of breathing. On breathing in, what had been outside is taken into the body via the lungs. Similarly, on breathing out, gases which had been dissolved in the blood become part of the outer air. The boundary is most diffuse in the case of bodily warmth, as there is a constant exchange of warmth with the environment.

Starting with relatively simple life forms, such as sea anemones and sponges living in salt water, it can be seen that the concentration of salts in them is close to that in the surrounding sea, and that they are very dependent on this level for their survival. They absorb oxygen dissolved in the water and give off dissolved carbon dioxide, and their temperatures are the same as the surrounding water. Slightly higher life forms, like worms, possess a rudimentary circulation which regulates the level of salts (solids) in the organism, allowing them to maintain a mineral content which is independent of their environment. However, their skin has to be kept moist so that they can absorb oxygen from the air. They remain dependent on external water, without which they would eventually die from dehydration.

Amphibians, like frogs and toads, also need moist skins to absorb oxygen, but they have lungs as well, making them somewhat less dependent on water (liquid) in their immediate environment. Reptiles, too, have lungs, indicating an internalisation of the airy (gaseous) element. But amphibians and reptiles are cold-blooded: they are still dependent on the ambient temperature to determine their body temperatures. Apart from humans, only birds and mammals regulate their own temperatures, indicating an internalisation of the warmth element. (The fact that birds and mammals are warm-blooded does not imply that they have an independent I.)

The independent warmth element acts as the physical medium through which the I works into the body, creating self-awareness. The gaseous element (particularly oxygen) is the physical medium for astral activity in the body, which brings about consciousness. The etheric body depends on the liquid element (particularly water) in its work to maintain life. Without water, there is no life – only the inorganic mineral element, as in a desert. When a person dies, the bodily warmth is quickly lost, breathing ceases and the lungs collapse. Eventually, after the bodily organisation has broken down and decomposition has taken place, all that is left is the mineral element, the skeleton.

While the element of warmth is the vehicle for the physical activity of the I, there are also many other characteristics of the presence of an I. Self-awareness, free-will, independent thinking, the ability to remember events at will and an upright posture have already been mentioned. The power of speech and the absence of fur or feathers (nakedness) might be added to the list. These are differences between human and animal forms as viewed at a given time, but there are also differences which become revealed when the life cycle is taken into account.

One distinguishing characteristic of humans is a very prolonged childhood. Most mammals also have periods of caring for their young, but they are always much shorter in relation to their lifespans. Another reflection of the presence of an I can be seen in growth and development. The peak of an animal's physical growth coincides with reproductive maturity. However, in humans, growth continues after this point is reached in the early teens, and is not completed until the early twenties. Reproductive maturity can be seen as the coming of age of the astral body, or animal principle, but the coming of age of the I, or human principle, comes later, at about twenty-one.

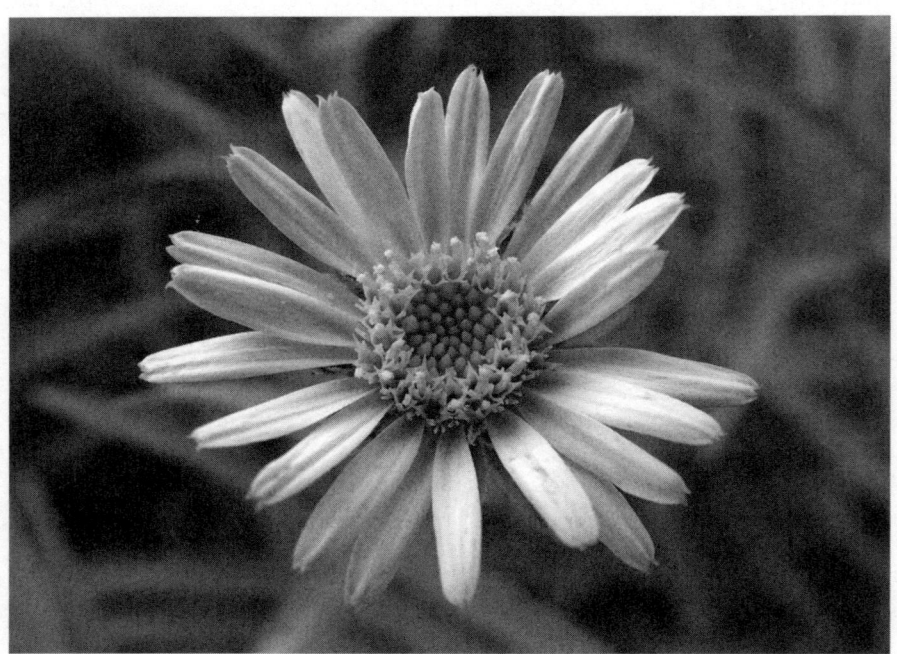

Arnica flower.

5. The Two Main Types of Illness

It has been seen how spiritual science, or anthroposophy, extends the view of the human being from a purely physical organism to a broader picture including life, soul and spiritual elements. In the anthroposophic picture, there is a delicate balance between the processes producing consciousness, which have a destructive effect on the physical body, and the upbuilding, regenerative processes of the life element. It is unhealthy for either the destructive or the upbuilding processes to predominate, and illness can result. Typical symptoms can be identified which characterise overactivity of the catabolic or anabolic processes but, before elaborating on this, it is necessary to delve a little deeper into anthroposophic physiology.

In conventional medical studies, the human organism is differentiated into a number of systems, such as the nervous system, the circulation and the respiratory system. Anthroposophic medicine describes three main systems, which are characterised by the way the three non-material elements of the human work into the physical body. The nerve-sense system includes the activity of all the nerves, the brain, the spinal cord and the sense organs. The metabolic-limb system includes the assimilation of nourishment, the metabolism and the activity of the limbs. The third, the rhythmic system, includes the breathing and the pulse.

The nerve-sense system

The nerve-sense system is obviously concentrated in the head, where the brain and most of the sense organs are to be found, and radiates throughout the body from there. It has already been seen that the nerve-sense system is associated with consciousness, catabolic processes, lowered vitality and more highly specialised bodily structures. Where these characteristics are observed, the spirit has a destructive effect on the body whereas, in the unconscious, restorative processes, the spirit works harmoniously through the astral, etheric and physical bodies. The most sophisticated structures in the body are to be found in the nerve-sense system – for example, the three tiny bones that link the eardrum to the inner ear which are so delicate they can transmit the minutest movements of the eardrum. A similar microscopic complexity can be found in the structure of the eye. The low capacity for regeneration of these organs goes hand-in-hand with a withdrawal of the etheric processes from them. In accordance with the principle of biological compensation, these etheric forces become available for other activity, and are transferred from their upbuilding activity to the activity of thinking.

The structures of the sense organs come closer than any others in the body to the inorganic, purely physical element, almost as if they were machines. Therefore, it is easy to see how these organs lend themselves to comparison with man-made instruments. The pupil, lens and retina of the eye may be compared directly with the aperture, lens and image sensor or film of a camera; similarly, the hairs of the inner ear may be compared with the strings of a piano. Virtually the whole body is infused with blood, carried in minute capillaries so that it is in almost direct contact with the cells of the body, only separated by the thin capillary wall. But the inside of the eye is an exception. Although most of the eye wall is richly supplied with blood, the interior is filled with a transparent fluid. The cornea (the clear part in front of the pupil and iris) and the lens are completely without a blood supply. The oxygen and nourishment they need must be dissolved through the clear fluids of the eye. As they are cut off from the vitalising effects of the blood, they are particularly vulnerable to damage or ageing as in a cataract, for example, when the lens becomes progressively more opaque. As well as in the sense organs, the fine sculpting effect associated with the nerve-sense system may also be seen in the remarkably complex shape of the skull. Its detailed structure contrasts with the relatively simple form of a limb bone.

The metabolic-limb system

The metabolic-limb system includes the stomach and intestines, in which food is broken down and absorbed into the blood and lymphatic systems. The blood then passes first to the liver, where many of the newly absorbed substances are taken into liver tissue. The liver cells change glucose and other simple sugars into glycogen, and in this form they can be stored until needed. Amino acids are transformed into the protein albumen, a fundamental component of the liquid part of the blood. As organic substances are digested, the specific qualities they held through having been part of a particular animal or vegetable are destroyed in stages until they have a 'neutral' or virtually lifeless quality.

It is the liver that starts the process of rebuilding them into components of the human body, with the stamp of the human organism. From the liver, they are carried to all other parts of the body via the bloodstream. Hence the process of nourishment can be seen as a flow, through the bloodstream, into almost all the cells of the body. This metabolic process is centred on the digestive organs and the liver, from where it radiates throughout the body. The metabolic-limb system also includes the limbs, which bring the body into movement. In the muscles of the limbs, which have rich blood supplies, many of the substances brought by the blood are transformed into the energy expended in movement. All muscular activity also generates warmth, which is distributed to the rest of the body via the blood.

In direct contrast to the nerve-sense system, the metabolic-limb system is characterised by unconsciousness. We are not aware of the upbuilding processes taking place within us unless something goes wrong and starts to cause pain. The exercising of the will through movement is also unconscious. The idea, for instance, to walk across a room occurs in our thinking but the walking itself follows unconsciously. If it were necessary to think out the required movements of all the different muscles involved in walking across the room, we would soon fall over! By observing our own inner experiences, it is possible to make a distinction between thinking of something we intend to do and actually doing it. For example, this may be quite apparent first thing in the morning, when there can be a considerable delay between deciding to get up and actually doing so. On beginning to rise, we can get an impression that the source of the movement is not the mind, which so rapidly conceived the idea, but some deeply unconscious part of the soul. This unconsciousness is a characteristic of both volition and the whole activity of the metabolic system.

Whereas the nerve-sense system connects us to the outer world through awareness, the metabolic-limb system connects us physically. Our legs, in particular, resist gravity and make us mobile. Our arms and hands enable us to work on our surroundings and to be creative in the world. Through the metabolic-limb system, physical substance is taken in as food and we are able to be active in the physical world. Through the nerve-sense system, our physical bodies are linked to the spiritual activity of consciousness, which senses the physical world but does not directly affect it. The metabolic-limb system has an upbuilding and warming effect on the body; the nerve-sense system has a breaking-down effect and its organs are characterised by relative coolness.

The rhythmic system

In the middle, between these two *poles* of the organism, is the rhythmic system, which is expressed in all the rhythms of the body but especially in breathing and the pulse. It is centred on the heart and lungs, and hence the thorax. While the nerve-sense system, or head pole, is associated with thinking and the metabolic pole with the will, the rhythmic system is particularly associated with feelings. The heart is traditionally seen as the seat of the feelings, and a physical expression of this may be observed in the immediate changes of breathing rate and pulse which are commonly experienced when emotions such as anger and fear arise.

Rhythm offers a means of mediating between opposites, for example in breathing in and breathing out, or in the cycle of sleeping and waking. Checking the regularity of a patient's bodily rhythms is an important part of diagnosis. Most obviously, the pulse is checked but light may also be thrown on the cause of an illness by disturbances in the sleep cycle, the menstrual cycle, or the regularity of bowel movements. In terms of consciousness, we are aware of our feelings but less so than our thoughts. There is a dreamy quality to them which falls between the sharp awareness of thoughts and the unconsciousness of volition.

The mediation between the two poles may also be seen anatomically. Whereas the head pole has the bone on the outside with the soft brain tissue within it, the metabolic pole has soft muscle tissue on the outside, arranged around the bone. In the chest, there is an alternation of bone and muscle on the outside (the rib-cage), becoming more open at the lower end, which encases various soft organs arranged around the spine. Thus both structural aspects of the poles are incorporated in the rhythmic system, where the extremes of the poles meet and merge.

Bodily system	Inner activity	Level of awareness	Physical effects
Nerve-sense	Thinking	Conscious	Cooling, catabolic, hardening
Rhythmic	Feeling	Dream-like	Balancing, mediating
Metabolic-limb	Volition	Unconscious	Warming, anabolic, softening

Figure 5.

The two poles meet where the bloodstream and the lungs come together. The bloodstream is associated predominantly with the upbuilding, warm, metabolic processes, and breathing, which has a cooling effect on the blood, more with the sensory processes. Breathing takes place through the head and, although it normally happens unconsciously, is more easy to regulate consciously than the pulse. The relative speed of the pulse (in an adult, typically about seventy-two beats per minute at rest), compared with the breathing rate (about eighteen breaths per minute), also reflects the contrast between the dynamic physical activity of the metabolic pole and the relative physical stillness of the head pole.

Balance and illness

The maintenance of health is very much a matter of keeping the metabolic and nerve-sense processes in equilibrium. As the rhythmic system is particularly involved in maintaining this balance, it has a special role in healing. Throughout life there can be inherent tendencies towards predominant activity of one or the other pole without necessarily causing illness. For example, there is a gradual shift in emphasis between birth and death. The early months after birth are taken up with feeding, sleeping and growing, the baby's body is softer than in later life, and its pulse is more rapid than an adult's all typical characteristics of the metabolic pole. In old age there is a tendency to *drying up* – the skin loses its suppleness and the hands and face become wizened. Old people generally sleep and eat less than when they were younger, and there tends to be a loss of mobility and increased vulnerability to cold. These are all characteristics of the head pole.

There is also an emphasis on either nerve-sense or metabolic-limb activity which is associated with constitution. People with dominant nerve-sense systems tend to be thin, with a more angular body, and to look older than their years. If the metabolic-limb system predominates, the tendency is towards a rounder shape, even plumpness, and to look younger than they are. There may also be a tendency to a relative emotional and intellectual immaturity. These descriptions are of contrasting constitutional types, but there is no implication that illness will develop unless the predominance of one pole over the other becomes too extreme. If this happens, two main forms of illness can arise which are specifically associated with the two poles. An unhealthy excess of the activity of the metabolic-limb system is characterised by an increase in warmth and an excess of fluid (swelling) – the essential features of fever and inflammation. An unhealthy excess of nerve-sense activity is characterised by a loss of fluid, excessive hardening, a loss of mobility and flexibility, and a build-up of mineral deposits in the body. These are the features of degenerative or sclerotic illnesses, such as osteoarthritis or arteriosclerosis.

In anthroposophic medicine, these are the two main types of illness – the feverish and inflammatory on the one hand, the degenerative and sclerotic on the other. However, to see any illness as purely one or the other type is almost always an oversimplification, and usually both tendencies are involved. Rheumatoid arthritis, for example, begins with marked inflammation in the joints and they may become red, swollen, painful and hot. As the disease progresses over the years, degenerative tendencies appear, such as chronically deformed joints. Tuberculosis, which is essentially an infectious inflammatory disease, also tends to last a long time and leaves hardened tissue and scars in the lungs, which are characteristic of sclerosis.

The symptoms of the common cold include excretion of mucus from the sinuses, which are inflamed and red, with inflammation of the throat and a higher temperature than normal, particularly in the first couple of days. Although the symptoms are of the metabolic type, the area most affected is the head, the opposite pole. People tend to be predisposed to catching a cold by being run-down or getting chilled. The chill can be seen as an invasion of the body by a foreign element, the outer coldness. The run-down condition, in an otherwise healthy person, is indicative of a lack of the restorative processes through too much 'head' work or insufficient sleep. Both the coolness and the 'excessive consciousness' are typical of the head pole, but the symptoms of the cold are characteristic of the metabolic pole. This not only serves as another example of the interplay of the two poles m a disease, but also shows how the physical symptoms can be more related to the body's healing processes than to the underlying cause of the illness.

In any given illness, characteristics can be identified of unhealthy overactivity of either of the two opposing systems. These are indicative of the relationships between the spirit, soul, life and physical elements in the patient. Such indications are essential if the doctor is to make as complete a diagnosis as possible and prescribe appropriate treatment.

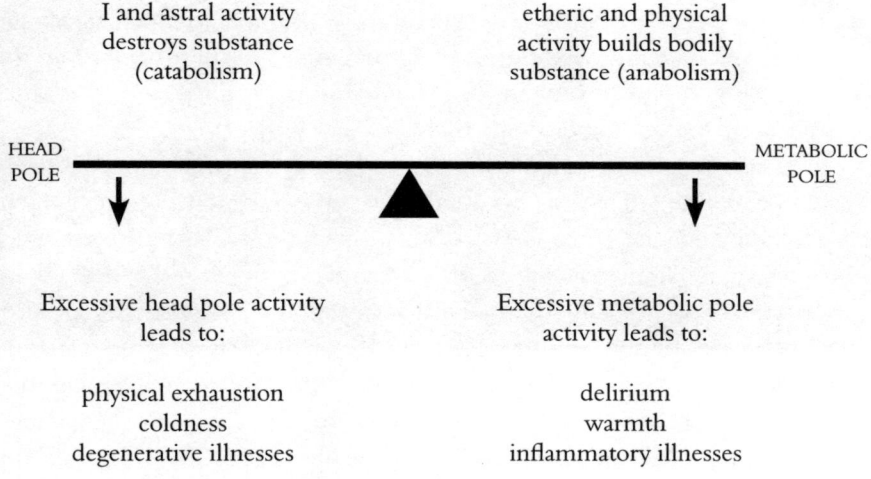

I and astral activity destroys substance (catabolism)

etheric and physical activity builds bodily substance (anabolism)

HEAD POLE

METABOLIC POLE

Excessive head pole activity leads to:

physical exhaustion
coldness
degenerative illnesses

Excessive metabolic pole activity leads to:

delirium
warmth
inflammatory illnesses

Figure 6.

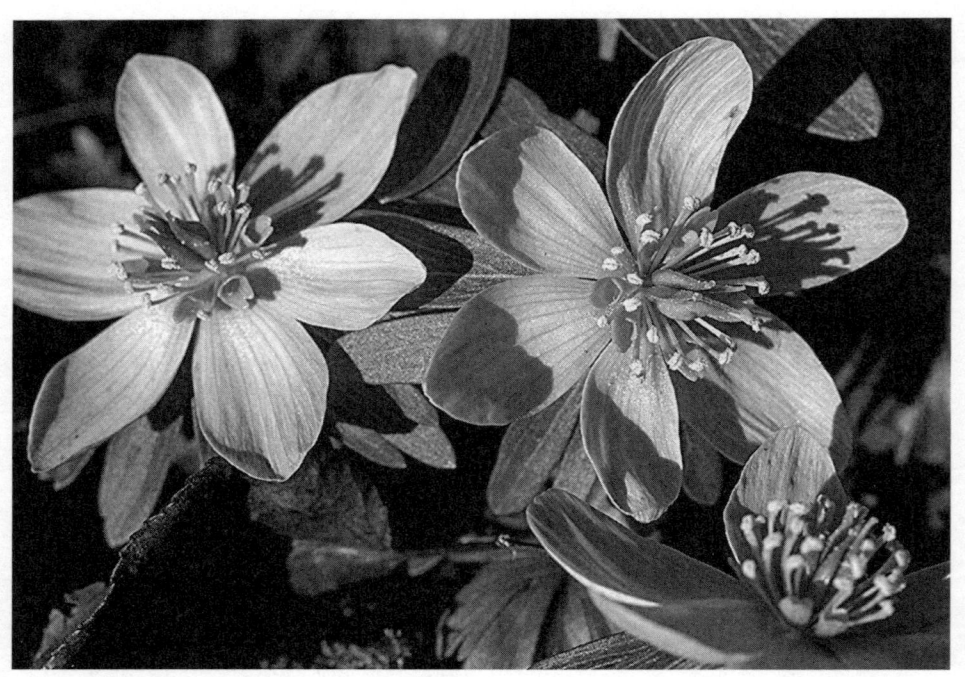

Winter aconite.

6. The Use of Medicines

When an illness arises from an imbalance of the nerve-sense and metabolic-limb systems, a means of restoring balance is required to effect a cure. Anthroposophic medicine looks for examples in nature of similar life processes to those in the human organism, and uses animal, plant and mineral substances to make remedies. By contrast, conventional medicine looks at diseases in terms of molecular changes in the physical body, and isolates chemical drugs from substances occurring in nature.

All life consists of processes, such as growth, nutrition, digestion and respiration, which are physical expressions of the activity of the spiritual elements. Life cannot be regarded as a static state – it is created and constantly maintained by the dynamic activity involved in these processes. Consider, for example, a plant. What can be seen at any given time as the form of the plant is an organisation of physical material which has been built up by the life processes within it. The process of photosynthesis, for example, when inorganic substances are brought to life with the aid of sunlight, is vital to the plant's ability to sustain itself and grow. Wherever life is present, such upbuilding (etheric) processes will be found; wherever consciousness is present, breaking-down (astral) processes will be found, such as the burning of sugars.

Conventional medicine analyses diseases in terms of molecular changes and develops chemical drugs aimed at counteracting the molecular changes to alleviate the physical symptoms. Anthroposophic medicine looks at the interplay of processes which cause the molecular changes associated with the symptoms. It aims to harness related processes in, say, plants within medicines which may then be used to stimulate a return to the proper balance of processes in the patient.

Plant remedies

As plants have physical and etheric bodies, but not astral bodies with their destructive influence, they are particularly related to the regenerative, healing processes of the human etheric body. The plant's most characteristic organ is the leaf, which is where, in green plants, photosynthesis takes place. Leaves have flat, open forms and are typically located in the middle part of the plant, between the 'poles' of the roots and the flowers. Relatively high levels of organisation and more complex forms can be seen in the flowers, whereas the roots tend to be relatively simple structures which have the *metabolic* role of absorbing nourishment for the whole plant.

In the plant, the flower is related to the animal kingdom, and the roots have a similar relationship to the mineral world. The flower demonstrates the greater complexity of form which is a characteristic normally associated with animals. Also, it is through the flower, with its colours and scent, that the plant relates to the animal world, for example when pollinated by bees. The roots, on the other hand, grow in the ground, and absorb minerals and water from the soil. The middle, or leafy, part of the plant is the most completely *plant-like,* demonstrating great vitality but less complex forms than the flowers.

The pinnacle of the plant's growth is the seed, which is one stage on from the flower. The seed itself tends to be a simple structure but it bears within it the potential for a whole new plant. This suggests a similarity to the I, which is like the spiritual kernel, or seed, of the human, and contains the potential for the future development of the person. It can be seen from this very brief illustration that, in its form, the plant displays expressions of the mineral, plant, animal and human kingdoms in its roots, leaves, flowers and seeds respectively.

Although the plant does not have its own astral body, there is a slight penetration of astral forces into the flower, and this brings about its more complex form. In the flower, most plants just touch the astral, or animal, realm. But, in some, the astral element penetrates rather more deeply and this gives rise to poisonous substances within the plant, such as atropine in deadly nightshade. Just as the astral activity in the nervous system goes hand-in-hand with a destructive tendency, an equivalent astral activity in plants gives rise to substances which have a destructive effect if ingested by animals or humans. The poisonous plants have an *abnormal* level of astral activity, and this mirrors the state of illness in humans which is brought about by excessive activity of the nerve-sense pole.

Homeopathic principles

In this way, it is possible to trace relationships between processes which give rise to certain substances in plants, and processes which bring about illnesses in people. Substances may then be identified which can be used as remedies. An important aid to this way of working is to study a plant in the context of its whole family, in order to discover the characteristics of that family. Not only do these characteristics reveal the expression of the family as a whole, but they also show which species are typical of the family and which manifest the more extreme characteristics. The latter can often be of medicinal value.

This technique differs greatly from conventional medicine, or allopathy, which generally aims to employ particular chemical substances to bring about a direct effect on the chemistry and functioning of the physical body. They are usually very direct effects, such as the use of steroids to suppress inflammation, or drugs to stimulate the production of insulin when this is considered to be lacking. The fundamental principle is to use drugs that cause the opposite effect to the symptom – if the illness involves what is considered to be too much inflammation, treatment is given to reduce the inflammation; if there is too little insulin, more is given or drugs are used to stimulate the body to produce more.

The principle of homeopathic medicine is the opposite of allopathy.* Here, the motto is 'like cures like'. Medicines are tested by giving them to healthy people and noting the symptoms produced. When a patient presents a set of symptoms to the doctor, a medicine is chosen which would produce the same symptoms in a healthy person. Homeopaths maintain that the medicine stimulates the body's own powers of self-healing, but it has to be said that homeopathy is based on many years of experience that it works in practice rather than on a detailed picture of exactly how it works.

---

* The words homeopathy and allopathy are both derived from Greek, the prefixes *homeo-* meaning like and *allo-* unlike, while the suffix *-pathy* means suffering.

The homeopathic way of preparing medicines also differs from conventional methods. A solution is generally made from whole plants or minerals and put through a process of dilution in steps, known as potentisation. At each step, the solution is agitated, or succussed, before being again diluted. In a medicine which is specified as 6C (sixth centesimal), for example, the original tincture would have been diluted to one part per hundred, and succussed, six times over. It seems strange that the more the tincture is diluted, the more powerful the medicine becomes, but homeopaths have found this to be the case through many years of observation and experience of treatment.

The homeopathic doctor aims to select for the patient the medicine which has a symptom-picture most closely resembling the symptoms of the illness. To that end, the doctor is interested in aspects of the patient's mental state and general constitution which may be of little interest to a conventional physician. For example, it is useful to know if the symptoms are influenced by being warm or cold, or by any particular action or bodily function. In so far as the homeopath is concerned with a wealth of detail about the patient, and does not reduce the illness to a cellular cause, the approach may be termed holistic – the symptoms are related to the person as a whole, rather than being considered in isolation. However, homeopathy lacks an understanding of the causes of illness, of why a remedy has a particular symptom-picture, and of how the medicines actually work. Strictly speaking, it is not even necessary for the homeopath to know whether the remedy is from a plant or a mineral, let alone the specific nature of the plant or mineral, as long as the symptom-picture is known.

Herbal medicine offers another approach to the prescribing of medicines based on the cumulative knowledge of hundreds of years of use of herbs as remedies. Generally, unpotentised preparations from the whole plant are used rather than specific chemicals, and herbalists often use the remedies to promote excretory functions, such as sweating, urination and the purging of the bowels, in the belief that these indirectly aid healing. The medicines offer many effective and gentler alternatives to conventional synthetic drugs and herbalists prefer to use these in most cases, reserving the more powerful drugs for occasions when they are essential. However, some herbalists have adopted the conventional, allopathic view of disease and seek to integrate the use of herbal medicines into conventional practice.

Anthroposophic medicine accepts that both the homeopathic and allopathic approaches are valid, and uses both potentised homeopathic medicines and unpotentised herbal medicines. It also recognises the homeopath's and the medical herbalist's valuable observations of the effects of particular medicines. However, anthroposophic medicine aims to deepen the understanding of illness and medicinal substances by extending natural science with the understanding gained through spiritual science.

Examples from the buttercup family

One plant that is used in the preparation of anthroposophic, homeopathic and herbal medicines, *Aconitum napellus,* provides a good example of how a qualitative anthroposophic understanding of a plant may be derived through studying it in the context of its family.[1] *Aconitum,* or monkshood, is a genus within the buttercup family *(Ranunculaceae).* This family can be divided into three main groups: *Thalictrinae* containing clematis, actaeas and thalictrums; *Adoninae* containing ranunculi (buttercups), adonis and pulsatillas; and *Helleborinae* containing delphiniums, aquilegias and aconitums.

The *Thalictrinae* are generally woody climbing plants, or large plants with branching stems and many small, whitish flowers. The *Helleborinae* tend to have strong, straight flower stems, with single, or few, large coloured flowers. They have underground tubers or creeping stems and are often poisonous. The *Adoninae* are low to medium-sized plants, with branching stems and coloured flowers. If the formation and development of the leaves of all the plants within the family is examined, two distinct types emerge. In the first, particularly found in clematis, the leaves are divided into leaflets by stem-like structures, but these minor stems and leaflets still represent one leaf. In the second type, typical of aconitum, the leaves differentiate by developing deep incisions from the edge.

From wider anthroposophic studies of plants, it is known that the clematis leaf expresses a preponderance of development of the lower part of the plant, the root and stem. The aconitum leaf is more typical of the upper part of the plant in the sense that it has the appearance of having been eaten away as if by a similar astral activity to that which produces

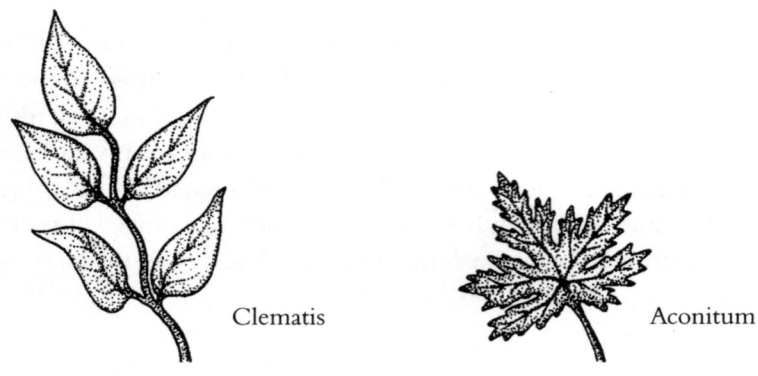

Clematis

Aconitum

Thalictrinae	Adoninae	Helleborinae
Clematis	Ranunculi	Aconitums
Actaea	Adonis	Delphiniums
Thalictrums	Pulsatillas	Aquilegias

Figure 7. Each clematis has three to four leaflets separated by stems. The leaves of aconitum are deeply incised.

the fingers of the human hand (see Chapter 3). The *Adoninae,* the middle group of the family, may have either the clematis or aconitum types of leaves, both characteristics combined, or neither.

Working from the stem upwards, flowers generally consist of a ring of sepals, called the calyx, then a ring of petals, called the corolla. Within the petals there may be a ring of nectaries, which produce nectar, and within this the stamens, the male part of the flower. Within the stamens there is the pistil, the female part of the flower.

In *Thalictrinae,* and particularly clematis, there are generally no petals, just sepals, and a ring of stamens, which take on the display function of the corolla. In this case, the stamens take on the role normally performed by an organ found lower down the flower structure (nearer the stem). In *Helleborinae,* such as aconitum, petals are again lacking but, this time, the calyx takes on the display function of the corolla. Once again, we see in *Helleborinae* the opposite tendency to that expressed in *Thalictrinae,* with an organ from lower down the structure being, as it were, elevated to the

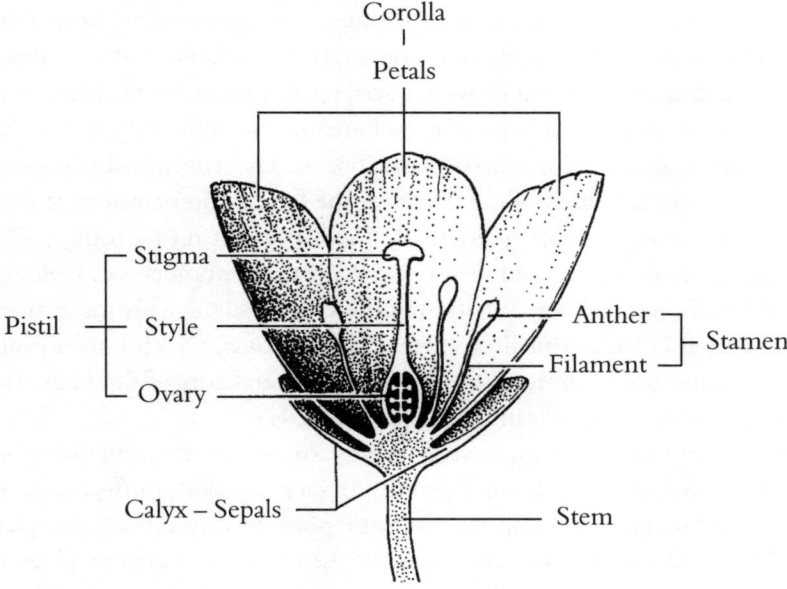

Figure 8. The parts of a flower.

function of a higher part. As might be expected, in the *Adoninae* several variations between the two forms may be found – adonis itself having real petals and sepals.

The upper parts of *Thalictrinae* are dominated by functions associated with the lower parts of the plants, while the reverse is true of *Helleborinae*. Expressed qualitatively, this means that *Helleborinae* tend to have stronger flower development, with the astral element extending beyond its normal province, and *Thalictrinae* tend to have stronger stem development. This picture is supported by the observation that *Helleborinae* have a preponderance of growth leading to flowering, or sexual reproduction (a higher and more animal-like process), while *Thalictrinae* have a preponderance of vegetative growth. Within the middle group *(Adoninae)*, buttercups fall closest to *Helleborinae* and pulsatilla closest to *Thalictrinae*. The most extreme of the *Thalictrinae* is clematis; the most extreme of the *Helleborinae* is aconitum.

From this description, it might be expected that a destructive quality would be found in aconitum and, indeed, it is one of the most poisonous plants. The poison is distributed throughout the plant, but is concentrated and stored in its thick underground tubers. It might also be expected that aconitum would have a special relationship with the nerve-sense system. The empirical findings of both homeopathy and medical herbalism have shown that aconitum is particularly indicated for trigeminal neuralgia, a very painful inflammation of the nerves of the face. In homeopathy, it is also indicated for feverish colds, particularly those brought on by being chilled, perhaps by exposure to cold wind. By contrast, a number of *Thalictrinae* are indicated for conditions of the reproductive system, with the extreme, clematis, used in male genital problems. The *Adoninae,* which hold a central position in the plant family, also relate to the central part of the body, with adonis having its main indication as a heart remedy.

The picture of aconitum reveals a very strong astral influence which descends into the sepals, raising them to a higher function, forms the deeply incised leaves and gives rise to powerful poisons throughout the plant. The flower's shape and the positioning of the stamens (which produce the pollen) are specifically developed such that only bumble-bees can pollinate them, indicating a heightened level of specialisation through the astral activity in the flower.

The qualitative, comparative study of plant forms given above is a greatly simplified version of the much more detailed investigation which is required in practice, but it does give an idea of the way possible links with formative and spiritual processes in humans may be discovered.★ The study is pursued as far as possible before any conclusions are tested in clinical practice, and only if this brings confirmation are the links considered to have been demonstrated.

This emphasis on the study of processes, for example the process which produces a toxic chemical in aconitum, contrasts sharply with conventional medicine, which concentrates exclusively on the chemical itself. Anthroposophic medicine looks at the particular qualities of the processes because, in so doing, it indirectly observes the spiritual activity behind the substances produced. The physical substances themselves are simply end products of the processes, and can be seen as processes brought

★ There is no suggestion here of following some kind of doctrine of signatures – an approach which has been rightly discredited. This doctrine is what remains of what may once have been a deeper art, but which degenerated into the idea that plants which look like a particular human organ are good for treating that organ. The anthroposophic study of plants as remedies looks at the underlying formative processes, rather than particular physical features, in order to make connections with related processes at work in humans.

to rest, or dynamic activity made static. Plant sugars (physical substances) are end products of photosynthesis (a life process), which takes carbon dioxide and water and transforms them into substances which are characteristic of plant life.

Mineral substances

Similarly, bark and wood are dead materials, but their source is the life processes of the plant of which they were once living elements. It is quite well-known that the source of coal, a mineral, is plant life, but it is not so widely appreciated that the thick layers of limestone which make up many mountains were formed from the calcium contained in tiny ancient animals. Their minute calcareous shells were deposited on the seabed when they died and, in time, became hardened into rock. Many minerals, which are rightly considered part of the inorganic realm, had their origins in living creatures. The transformation of carbon into various forms may be traced in its passage from the fluid organic activity of tree sap, to the hardened wood (when it is still part of the organism, though dead), to the fossilised fixed form of coal (when it has become completely mineralised). The study of substances in fixed forms (as in natural science) is the study of the dead end products of creative processes. If the life and soul elements are to be comprehended at all, the study of living things must be the study of the processes themselves.

Grinding a mineral substance into a powder and dissolving it – common steps in the preparation of medicines from mineral sources – can be seen as a kind of reversal of the process by which it came about. When dissolved, the substance is in a state more akin to its origin and can more easily be taken into the body as medicine, as all substances have to be dissolved in the breaking-down processes before being absorbed. If it also potentised, the chemical strength of the substance is reduced, but the spiritual process associated with its origin is enhanced. When a potentised medicine is given to a patient, the therapeutic effect of the spiritual process is taken in through the etheric body, the organisation of life processes (whereas the remedial effects of artistic therapies are taken in through the soul and, in counselling, the I is dealt with directly). The spiritual processes associated with the medicine can then have a harmonising effect, restoring balance to the relative activities of the physical, etheric and astral bodies and I.

In the human body, there are areas where hardening is healthy, such as in the bones, and areas where it is a symptom of disease or decay, as in the walls of the blood vessels. In old age, there is a calcification of the walls of the arteries (arteriosclerosis) and, at the same time, a loss of calcium from where it should be, in the bones (osteoporosis). A plant with formative processes which create a marked separation of the soft, fluid element and the hard, woody element is the silver birch. Its spring leaves display a delicate softness, while its bark is strongly mineralised, giving it a silvery appearance. The waterproof property of the bark, even when thin, made birch highly prized for canoe construction.

The soft young leaves can be used effectively in the treatment of arteriosclerosis when prepared as an infusion. Hence, to prepare the leaves for use against a hardening, mineralising process, they are subjected to the opposite – to warming and dissolving in the preparation as an infusion. By contrast, the mineralised bark and wood can be used to treat inflammatory conditions and bowel problems when the motions are too fluid, as in diarrhoea. The hardening and forming qualities of the wood can be accentuated by turning it into charcoal (further mineralising it) before preparing it as a medicine.

Like the birch leaves, a mixture of herbs called Menodoron, which is used to help regulate the menstrual cycle, is prepared by the warming process of cooking. Medicines prepared in this way are called decoctions, and the warming helps to prepare the medicine to act on the metabolic pole. Conversely, when aconite is prepared for the treatment of conditions of the nerve-sense system, cold processes are used, which help to prepare the medicine to act on the head pole.

The importance of warming is also seen when ethereal, or essential, oils from plants are prepared for medicinal application. Plants such as lavender, rosemary, thyme, sage, marjoram, peppermint and lemon balm all have aromatic, warming qualities. They often benefit people suffering from sclerotic (hardening) diseases through their warming effect. In anthroposophic medicine, they are given in potentised form by mouth or injection, but their most widespread use is applied to the skin as massage oil or finely dispersed in water in an oil bath.

The mode of thinking involved in the anthroposophical way of relating substances to disease processes differs markedly from that associated with modern chemistry and physics and, for this reason, it can prove difficult to grasp. It should be remembered that the links can be seen directly with spiritual perception but, lacking this, it is necessary to develop a discipline of thinking which is able to go beyond the limitations of natural science described earlier. This is not to belittle the considerable achievements of chemistry and physics, but these achievements should not be allowed to give the impression that the nature of substance may not be approached in any other way.

Alchemy

Modern scientists are justified in criticising the inexactitudes of the alchemy of the Middle Ages, but it is fair to say that the alchemists were not so much engaged in early attempts at analytical chemistry as in discovering qualitative connections between the chemical elements and the human soul and spirit.[2] Modern chemistry regards substances as purely objects of the material world. That the alchemists had a quite different attitude is made clear by their religious reverence towards the substances they studied. While it would be inappropriate to return to the ways of the alchemists, it would be quite wrong to think of them as completely misguided because subsequent research has invalidated some of their work. Theirs was a qualitative approach to the study of matter, and a modern qualitative approach is needed to balance the one-sidedness of the quantitative approach of natural science.

It is this qualitative aspect which is at work in the prescription of potentised medicines, as opposed to the techniques of conventional medicine, which tend to be too heavily based on evidence from the laboratory. For example, in conventional medicine, an antacid is given for indigestion. This simply uses an alkali to neutralise acid in the stomach, just as can be done in a test-tube in a laboratory experiment, but takes no account of what may be behind the symptom of the indigestion.

For the alchemists, there were three main chemical principles, represented by sulfur, mercury and salt. Sulfur is associated with the combustible, potentially volatile state; mercury with the fluid, mediating state; and salt with the crystalline, fixed state. The combustible tendency of sulfur is related to the warming activity of the metabolic-limb system; the mediating tendency of mercury is related to the harmonising activity of the rhythmic system; and the crystallising tendency associated with salt is related to the hardening, sclerotic processes of the nerve-sense system.

79

A crystalline substance which particularly represents the salt principle is silica, which composes about ninety-five per cent of the earth's crust. It is present in small concentrations in the body, especially in the skin and hair. As the main constituent of glass, silica displays the quality of transparency, like the lens in the eye. It also fulfils a key role in modern communication and information technology in the form of silicon chips and fibre optics. These relationships can be pursued, but it can already be seen that, both within the body and in the external world, silica is associated with nerve-sense activity. It comes as no surprise then, to find that classical homeopathy regards silica as the prime remedy for treating weak, neurasthenic states, sensitivity to cold and susceptibility to overstimulation of the nervous system. In anthroposophic medicine, it is also used to treat a tendency to recurrent colds and sinusitis. These conditions all represent an excessive activity of the nerve-sense system.

Sulfur is itself a prime example of the sulfur principle. It is a vital component of proteins, the main structural element of human and animal bodies, and is essential for the building up of the body, a major task of the metabolic system. When life ceases, and decomposition of the organic material ensues, sulfur is one of the first elements to separate, which contributes to the characteristic smell of decomposition. In medicinal applications, sulfur stimulates the metabolic processes. For example, in an infection, if the inflammation threatens to become chronic, sulfur can be used to reactivate it and, thereby, bring the infection to a resolution. In conventional medicines sulfur is used as an ointment to soften the skin in treating conditions like acne.

Calcium and magnesium

Two remedies from the mineral kingdom which are very closely related from a conventional chemical point of view are calcium and magnesium. Calcium, which bridges the animal and mineral worlds, is a major constituent of animal shells and of human and animal bones. Magnesium, on the other hand, has a greater role in plant life. It is the central element in the chlorophyll molecule, which lies at the heart of the plant's ability to photosynthesise, and thus transform inorganic material into living tissue. This strong association with plants, and their ability to create organic substance, demonstrates its relationship to the etheric, upbuilding processes in humans. Magnesium can be used to treat both depressed vitality and emotional depression.

Calcium plays a central role in animal and human locomotion, not only as a component of bones but also because it is involved in muscular contraction. Its closer relationship to the astral body is also reflected in its ability to counteract overactive etheric processes in patients. In anthroposophic medicine, it is used to treat excessive inflammatory or allergic responses, and also overactive fluid tendencies, such as excessive growth in children, which is accompanied by overdevelopment of the lymphatic tissue of the neck and throat, and can predispose to chronic tonsillitis.

In anthroposophic practice, the doctor may use a remedy to counterbalance the illness process (the allopathic principle) or a remedy with qualities which match the tendencies of the illness (the homeopathic principle). Or a combination of substances may be prescribed which will work on the illness in different, complementary ways. For example, migraine headaches are thought to be caused by the blood vessels of the brain at first narrowing in spasm, then becoming dilated, with a seeping of fluid into the surrounding tissue. In coming to a qualitative understanding of such an illness, it may be noted that the problem involves a blood process (related to the metabolic system) in the brain (nerve-sense system). The initial symptom is a contraction and tightening (characteristic of the nerve-sense system), followed by an excessive dilation of the blood vessels (metabolic system).

In many cases, attacks follow periods of mental strain, which supports the idea that the cause lies in the nerve-sense system, but the end result is a predominance of the metabolic processes in the head – the centre of the nerve-sense system. This picture may be further complicated by the additional symptom of nausea, which can be regarded as a pathological consciousness in the metabolic region. In good health, the processes of the stomach are deeply unconscious – we are unaware of them until something goes wrong. The therapeutic aim is to reduce the excess of metabolic activity in the head and nerve-sense activity in the stomach. For this, an anthroposophic preparation called Bidor is used. It contains silica to harmonise the nerve-sense system, and sulfur combined with iron, which balances the metabolic and respiratory functions, alleviating the overflow of the metabolic processes into the head.

Medicines in anthroposophic practice

As all anthroposophic doctors are first trained in conventional medicines they are also able to prescribe conventional drugs when appropriate. Many of these drugs are extremely powerful and their use in emergencies can be very valuable, even life-saving. However, their equally powerful and damaging side effects are also becoming increasingly recognised by both the public and conventional doctors. For example, steroids are known to cause osteoporosis (weakening of the bones) and adrenal problems, and some non-steroid anti-rheumatic drugs predispose to irritation and possible haemorrhage in the stomach. Less widely recognised are the more subtle and long-term effects, which may not show up until much later in life. Many conventional drugs suppress the symptoms of specific illnesses. For example, painkillers and anti-inflammatory drugs used to treat osteoarthritis can temporarily alleviate pain and reduce swelling, but it is becoming apparent that they have no positive effect on the long-term outcome of the illness, and may worsen its progression.

Antibiotics can be life-saving in very severe infections, but they are used by most family doctors to treat a myriad of minor infections which would resolve themselves if given a little time. It is acknowledged by conventional medicine that this practice has led to strains of bacteria developing which are resistant to antibiotics, but the likelihood that indiscriminate use of antibiotics reduces the body's own ability to fight infections has been overlooked. The main cause of most infections is the patient's susceptibility to them, rather than the mere presence of the bacteria or virus. While the use of antibiotics shortens the period of infection by killing the offending bacteria, it does nothing for the patient's susceptibility to infection. Anthroposophic medicine offers a wide range of preparations which stimulate and enhance the body's own healing response rather than killing off the foreign elements for it. Antibiotics can then be reserved for more serious infections, when they might be essential.

While anthroposophic doctors certainly do not claim that conventional medicines should not be used under any circumstances, and prescribe them when they feel their use is appropriate, they are aware of the one-sidedness of their effects and the problems which might result from their use. The need for conventional drugs can often be obviated by the use of anthroposophic medicines, sometimes to a remarkable degree. For example, at one anthroposophically orientated National Health Service general practice in England, the quantity of conventional medicines prescribed has been reduced to twenty-five per cent of what the average family doctor uses in a comparably sized practice. This has been achieved despite having the usual cross-section of patients found in any NHS surgery, and despite the fact that only a minority of the patients specifically chose the practice because of its anthroposophic orientation. Clearly, the principles of anthroposophic medicine have a major role to play, even within contemporary general practice.

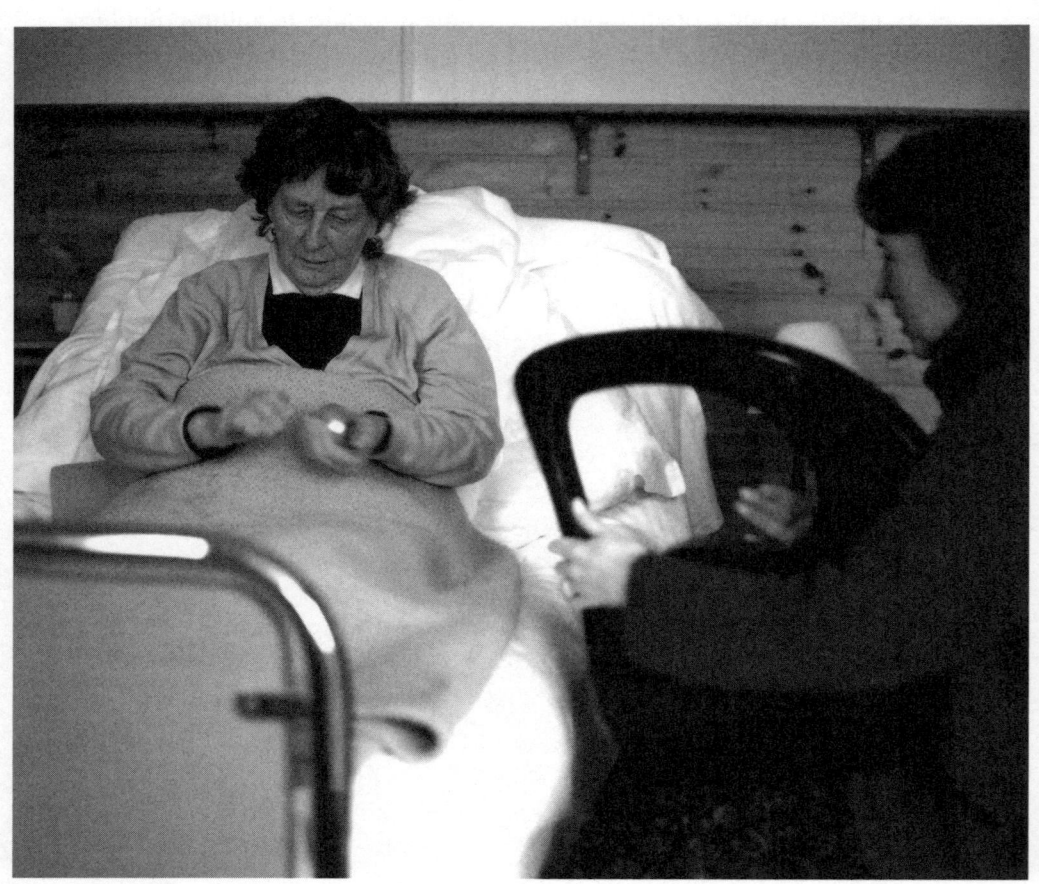

Music eurythmy therapy.

7. Artistic Therapies

In modern society, art is commonly regarded as a luxury or optional extra, with science more highly valued, especially for its technical applications. In past societies, for example in the Middle Ages, religion and art were inseparable, and played much greater roles in people's lives. Painting, music, sculpture and architecture were considered to be sacred activities. The substance of the physical world is transformed in artistic creation in such a way that it takes on a special value for people. In this sense the development of the arts through the different cultural periods of history may be seen as a reflection of humanity's changing consciousness.

Different times have given rise to characteristic forms of expression – the harmonious proportions of Greek architecture and sculpture, the two-dimensional painting of the early Christian era, the first vivid expression of personality in the faces painted by Rembrandt, the formal structures of classical music and the self-expression in the music of the Romantic period. Artistic activity also plays an important part in the further development of consciousness, for both the individual and society as a whole.

With a knowledge of how the four human elements are involved in artistic activity, it is possible to develop exercises which work in a specific way on those aspects of a patient. The emphasis in such exercises is on the effect on the patient rather than the final artistic creation, and this distinguishes artistic therapy from other artistic pursuits. The way particular artistic activities relate to the different human elements can be understood most readily in the cases of music, painting, sculpture and modelling. Lovers of music may well have had the feeling that something of a higher or spiritual nature is expressed in, for example, a symphony. And everyone will be aware of the powerful effect music has on the feelings. It can evoke profound moods of sadness or joy, and span the extremes of passion and pensiveness. This is one indication that, in music, the laws of the spirit express themselves in the realm of the soul – the human identity, the I, is expressed in the realm of the astral body, the seat of feelings and emotions.

Painting is a manifestation of the laws of the astral body expressed in the etheric realm. Colours, like music, can evoke powerful feelings, for example through the beauty of a sunset, a landscape or a flower. Whereas music is expressed in time and sculpture in three-dimensional space, painting uses planar surfaces. Flat surfaces are particularly associated with the life element and the etheric realm. The main organs of the plant world, leaves, are roughly two-dimensional and, on the microscopic level, the primary organs for life processes are two-dimensional cell membranes. In painting, characteristics of the astral realm, colours are expressed in fluids on a two-dimensional surface, the medium of the etheric realm.

The principle of form in sculpture does not have the dramatic effect on our emotions that music or colour do, indicating that the astral body is not involved in the same way. The sculptor works physical material into the desired three-dimensional form just as the etheric body constantly builds up physical substances into a human form. In sculpture and modelling, the laws of the etheric body are expressed in the physical realm.

An art of movement called eurythmy was devised by Rudolf Steiner to express the forms of movement of the etheric body in the physical realm. This, too, has a therapeutic application when exercises are designed to work back into the patient's inner nature. The etheric movement can be seen physically in the way the tissues and fluids of an embryo extend and fold to build up the human body from what is initially a simple ball of cells. The etheric body is a medium for the expression of the I and astral body as well

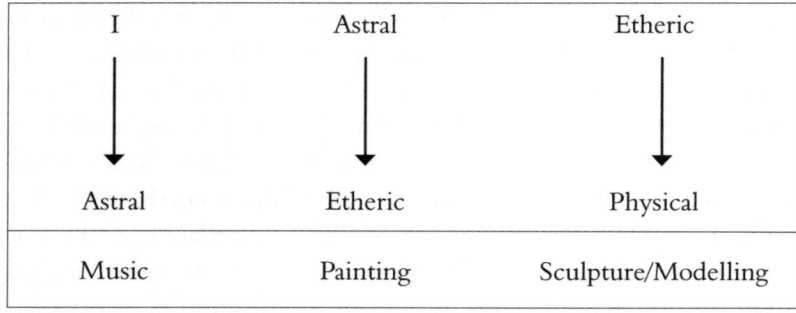

Figure 9.

as its own inherent movements, so the forms and gestures of eurythmy also relate to music and to the ways the sounds of speech are formed by the larynx, tongue, teeth and lips. In this way, the movements of eurythmy are able to be an expression of the whole human being through the medium of the physical body.

Therapies

Anthroposophic medicine seeks to understand a patient's illness in terms of the interrelationships between the I, astral body, etheric body and physical body. The therapeutic aim is to influence the activity of one or more of these elements in order to regain a healthy balance. As described above, the different arts arise through the interplay of two or more of these elements. By developing artistic activity that works back into the elements concerned, a therapeutic influence can be achieved. The value of a course of artistic therapy can be specific or general. It may support a specific bodily process but, in addition, the new experiences introduced by the therapy can strengthen self-confidence generally, and this can be helpful in both physical and psychiatric disorders. Also, it is often found that the process of overcoming artistic problems that arise during treatment produces indications and encouragement for the overcoming of fundamental problems in the patient's life and health.

The therapists, who are trained in both the art form and its therapeutic application, practise in close conjunction with anthroposophic doctors. Treatment is normally one-to-one but can also be in groups when necessary. Initial exercises reveal to the therapist the nature of any one-sided tendencies in the patient. Along with the medical picture described by the doctor, this helps the therapist to create a sequence of artistic exercises to meet the particular needs of the patient.

Sculpture or modelling

Sculpture or modelling therapy relates particularly to the working of the etheric body into the physical body, and is strongly indicated when the illness is expressed as a problem of forming. For example, in ulcerative colitis, the forming activity of the bowel is weakened. In psychiatric disorders, weakness in the form-giving processes may be expressed as an inability to structure thoughts properly or, when the etheric forces lose their normal connection with particular organs, in hallucinations (see Chapter 12). The artistic therapist creates a series of exercises to counter the disorder and bring about the necessary change in the patient's constitution, guided by both the medical understanding of the illness and what is expressed in the patient's artistic work. Other approaches to artistic therapy lay great emphasis on catharsis, self-expression and the psychoanalytical interpretation of the patient's creations. In anthroposophic artistic therapy, the emphasis is on stimulating and encouraging therapeutic effects in the patient's whole constitution.

One patient, whose diagnosis included a predominance of nerve-sense activity, began his modelling therapy by making numerous little cubes and stalactite shapes which were very intellectually thought-out. He was given the exercise of creating a large plane of clay containing wave forms as this encourages a greater affinity with the watery element and a less intellectual frame of mind. Another patient, who was just beginning to recover from acute schizophrenia, was still very anxious and was having difficulty concentrating. He was asked to fashion a sphere with his hands, then to form geometrical shapes such as a large cube. The forming aspect of this treatment helped his concentration and had a calming effect. These exercises should not be thought of as specific prescriptions, but as examples of tasks the therapists can give to patients as part of an individualised course of treatment. The course not only relates to the illness in question, but also to how it affects the patient's particular constitution and how that is expressed artistically.

Painting

In painting therapy, the qualities of light and colour are expressed via a watery medium. As air is the carrier of light, we can see how in watercolour painting the natural elements of air and water come together. Air and water are related to the astral and etheric bodies respectively, and the interplay between these bodies is central to the harmonious function of all four elements of the human being. In the physical body, the meeting of the airy and watery elements is most clearly expressed in the lungs, where inhaled air interacts with the blood. Oxygen is dissolved into the blood from the air, while carbon dioxide is released from the blood and breathed out. This process takes place in the rhythmic system, which has a special relationship with feelings.

Painting therapy may be used to treat a wide range of physical and psychological disorders, and is particularly indicated for disorders of the rhythmic system, such as breathing problems. In asthma, for example, the rhythm of the breathing is impaired because the airways become partially blocked by an inflammatory process that causes swelling and an excessive build-up of fluid. The balance between the airy and watery elements has been lost and, in this case, the artistic therapist would look for ways to balance the predominance of etheric (watery) activity. Painting therapy can also be used to treat conditions characterised by excessive dryness and hardening, such as the sclerotic diseases, osteoarthritis and arteriosclerosis (hardening of the arteries). In psychiatric treatment, it can be used to treat such disorders as obsessional problems and depression (see Chapter 12).

In fact, very diverse possibilities for treatment are offered by painting therapy. The colours themselves have a therapeutic effect, such as the inherent qualities of warmth, activity and expansion in the reds, oranges and yellows, or the coolness, passivity and contraction of the blues and greens. Unconsciously, we are constantly affected by colours, and the therapist tries to work with these effects in the course of treatment. The polarities of light and dark or form and fantasy may also be used to good effect. Painting techniques offer further therapeutic opportunities, for example working on wet paper, which can stimulate spontaneity, or applying fine layers of colour to dry paper, which tends to encourage a quieter, more reflective mood. The activity of painting normally involves short periods of total involvement interspersed with moments of standing back to observe and reflect. In this way, it can be seen to mirror the rhythmic cycle of breathing – *breathing out* the creative activity and *breathing in* the quieter moments of observation.

Eurythmy

Another form of artistic treatment, which stimulates an inner process through external activity, is eurythmy therapy. In modern life, people are often engaged in several activities at once, for example driving while listening to music and thinking about work. The thoughts tend to be unrelated to the feelings created by the music, and the actions involved in driving the car tend to be unrelated to both. When the pressures of modern life cause thoughts, feelings and actions to be fragmented in this way, the soul activity also becomes fragmented. This leads to a poor union between the soul and the physical body which, in advanced cases, may manifest as disturbances in bodily movement as well as illness. Eurythmy treatment is particularly valuable in such illnesses when, for example, the posture may have become distorted, the gait unnaturally heavy or light, or the breathing shallow and unrhythmical. Eurythmy therapy aims to restore a healthy relationship between the soul and the physical body, and to correct any disturbances in movement. It also works towards a reunion of the patient's thoughts, feelings and actions.

The bodily movements or gestures which are used as exercises are related to the vowel and consonant sounds that are made when speaking. The sounds of speech are formed by relative movements of the larynx, lips, teeth and tongue, in conjunction with the flow of breath. The gestures are imbued with the same character as these subtler movements of the speech organs, and patients are encouraged to try to be aware of the inner expression which is associated with a given sound. For example, when making the vowel sound *ah,* the lips and teeth are open. The gesture associated with this sound is also open, and the sense of wonder or understanding, which it may convey in speech, is cultivated in the patient. By contrast, the mouth is more closed in the sound *oo,* and a quite different feeling is associated with it.

The sense of rhythm in speech, particularly as it is expressed in poetry, is also used therapeutically. Some rhythms express an extrovert quality, some a more inward contemplation, others more of a martial character. The proper balance of rhythms in the body is one of the hallmarks of health, and loss of rhythm is often part of the development of a disease. Therefore, the enlivenment of rhythm in the soul can have a very useful therapeutic effect. There are also exercises which can help a patient who is lacking a healthy sense of three-dimensional space. These are particularly useful when dealing with excessively introverted and sedentary people who may have withdrawn from full engagement with their immediate environment. Experiences of the six directions of three-dimensional space (up, down, left, right, forward and back) may be accentuated by these exercises, which strengthen the activity of the I and re-establish a confident connection with the environment in people with agoraphobia and other irrational fears.

Artistic therapists work together with doctors, nurses, therapeutic masseurs and hydrotherapists in anthroposophic practices and hospitals. Methods of working together have been developed, such as case conferences (see Chapter 16), so that the picture of the patient which is used as the basis for a powerful, integrated programme of treatment is as full as possible. The training undertaken by artistic therapists covers the various effects of the many forms of their particular therapy. In practice, they have to be creative themselves in evolving a series of exercises individually tailored to the needs of the patient. The exercise programme must be designed in such a way that it can respond to the patient's progress, or to any difficulties that may arise during treatment.

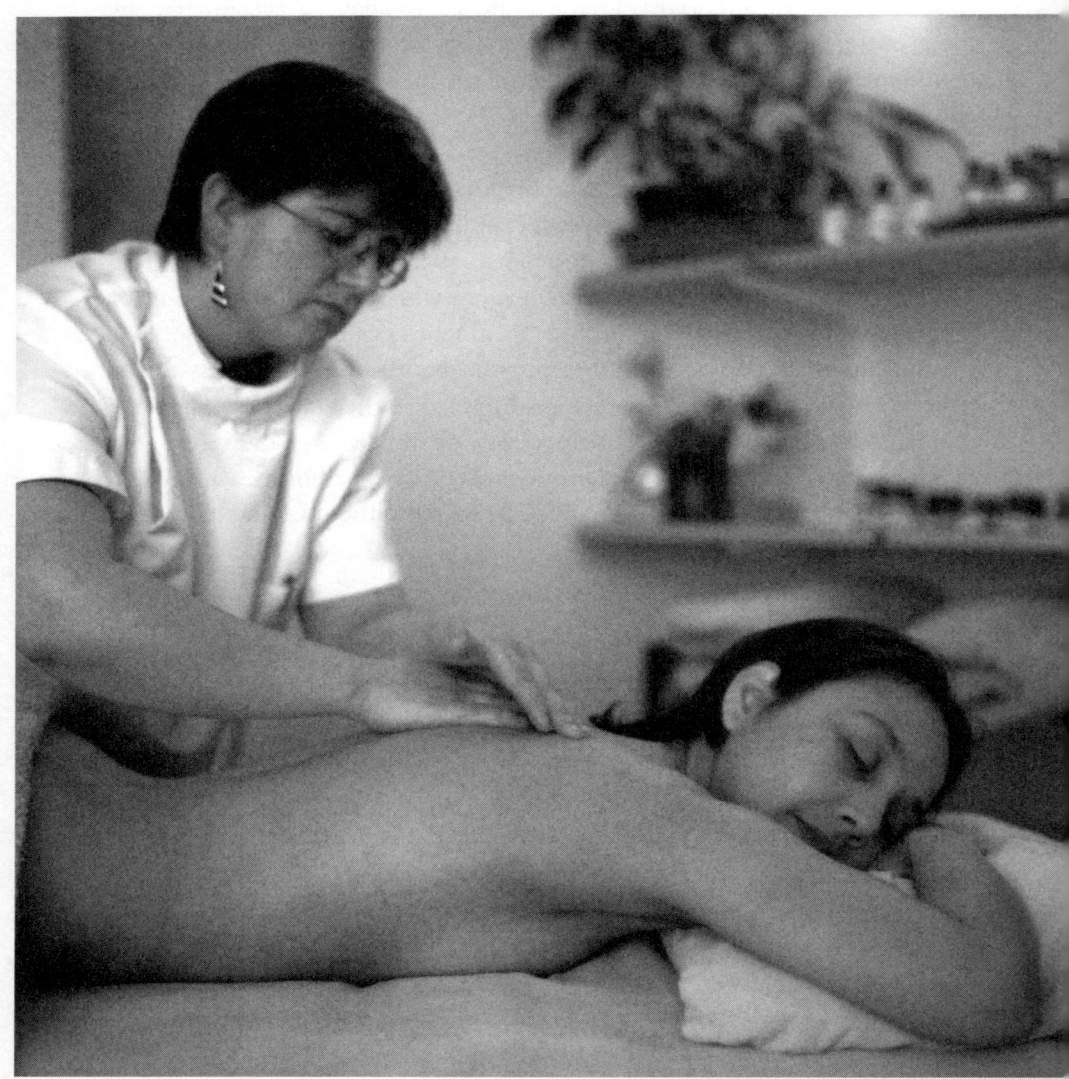

Massage.

8. Therapeutic Massage and Hydrotherapy

All massage affects the skin and also the underlying muscles and soft tissue, which have a semi-fluid quality. The fluid parts of the body are where the etheric upbuilding processes express themselves most directly, but there is also an interplay of nervous stimulation in the muscles, and emotional disturbances can lead to subconscious muscular tension. In this sense, the muscular tension can be seen as an expression of the emotional and nervous condition of the patient. The tension, as is typical of the astral influence, consists of a loss of fluidity and a tendency towards rigidity. In an extreme form, it constitutes an illness.

The rhythmic system brings the head pole and metabolic pole into harmony. The rhythmic quality of natural cycles of activity – such as breathing in and out, and the systole and diastole of the heart's action – harmonise the opposing etheric and astral activities. With that in mind, Dr Ita Wegman and Dr Margarethe Hauschka developed a strongly rhythmical form of therapeutic massage. The rhythm in breathing tends to follow a pattern of in-breath and out-breath, with a pause before the next in-breath. In the massage, the kneading takes a progressively stronger hold of the tissue, then relaxes the hold, then there is a pause before the next stroke. There is an association between breathing in and waking up, and breathing out and relaxing. The kneading of the first part of the massage has a wakening quality, and the softer movement of the second, a quality more akin to going to sleep. This means there is first a predominance of astral activity (waking up), then of etheric activity (relaxing). Through the rhythmical alternation of the two in the tissues, a powerful local harmonising effect can be achieved.

Massage

The natural movement of water is in curves, not straight lines. The curves may be gentle or strong, and they may develop into spirals or vortices. The etheric body, or body of formative life forces, is strongly related to the watery, fluid element and has a natural kinship with curving forms. This expresses itself formatively in the curves and rounded shapes of the body, and it may be noted that people who have a constitutional predominance of metabolic (etheric) activity have more rounded bodies than those with predominant head (astral) activity, who tend to have more angular bodily features. The movements in the massage also take on this curved quality. Around the joints of the body, the curves may be quite tight, and form spiral movements. When massaging the back, they might follow a figure of eight and include the rhythmic alternation.

Sometimes the tips of the fingers are used during a massage, and the concentrated pressure this can produce makes the patient strongly aware of the affected area. This stimulates a breaking-down, dissolving effect in areas of hardening. On other occasions, when the palm of the hand is used, a much softer effect is achieved. As the pressure is released, the palm can be used to lift the tissues, with a kind of sucking effect. This creates a feeling of lightening and gives a strong sense of release.

The etheric forces have a unifying effect on the body. One of the hallmarks of living things, as opposed to purely mechanical systems, is that an activity or change in one area always exerts some influence on every other part of the organism. That the organs and tissues are not isolated in separate compartments has long been recognised and put to use in treatment by ancient eastern forms of medicine, such as acupuncture and reflexology. Acupuncturists use needles to stimulate a healing response in the body, but the needles tend to be inserted some way away from the site of the symptoms. In reflexology, the processes of the whole body are considered to be reflected in various parts of the feet. Reflexologists treat the feet to exert healing influences on problems elsewhere in the body. Conventional medicine cannot comprehend this, as it limits itself to treatment of the local pathological process.

Rhythmical massage often works on one part of the body in order to influence another. An excess of astral activity in one part of the body is likely to be accompanied by a deficit in another. For example, in tension headaches, it may be possible to relieve the headache by vigorously kneading the calves and feet. This is aimed at diverting the excess astral activity causing the spasm into the lower part of the body by stimulating astral activity in that area, and can bring a degree of relief immediately. Massage of the neck and the whole back, following a downward movement from the neck along the spine, may also help to relieve the neck and shoulder tension typical of these headaches.

During treatment, the masseur picks up many indications about the patient's bodily condition, which the physician would be unlikely to perceive in the same way. The distribution of muscular tension throughout the body becomes clear. A common finding is extreme tension and spasm in the neck and shoulders, perhaps extending down to the waist, with a relative lack of tension below the waist. The lack of tension can be just as extreme as the tension in the upper body and, in some cases, just as unhealthy. The masseur develops sensitivity to the condition and tone of the skin and soft tissues. In some patients, these may feel loose and unformed while, in others there is a sense of dried, hardened tautness. Considerable variations in the temperature of the skin are also noted.

A female patient might be referred to a therapeutic masseur with a band of extreme tension in the middle of her back, circling the trunk, muscular flaccidity and a marked coldness below it, and normal warmth in the upper body. The masseur might know from the doctor who referred the patient that she has suffered from a long-standing disorder of the reproductive organs since having had sexual and marital difficulties. When the doctor and masseur confer on their perceptions of the problem, an extended picture arises. It becomes clear that the knot of muscular tension around the trunk, the coldness and lack of tone below the waist, the chronic gynaecological problems, and the sexual and marital anxieties are all different expressions of the same problem. The conventional medical diagnosis could be that she has a chronic pelvic inflammatory disease, for example a longstanding, low-grade infection of the fallopian tubes. Adding to this diagnosis, the anthroposophic understanding of what lies behind the infection would be that the unconscious activity of the patient's I is deficient in the pelvic region, as expressed in the lack of warmth.

Therapeutic help may be given on several levels, including massage, medicines and counselling. The massage might be aimed at bringing warmth and tone to the lower half of the body and releasing the knot of tension in the trunk. Breathing becomes more relaxed when this tension is relieved, and that releases a spontaneous flow of warmth into the lower body. Such an improvement may initially be temporary, and require a series of treatments to become self-sustaining. Once this point has been reached, improvements in the gynaecological symptoms are likely to follow. Medicines and counselling may be required to help achieve these changes.

Quite similar findings might arise for a patient suffering from illnesses of other organs in the lower abdomen, as in ulcerative colitis, which affects the large bowel. The masseur's observations assist the doctor in developing a detailed picture of the patient, and can directly indicate therapeutic possibilities by what they add to the overall picture.

The masseur is very conscious during treatment of the distribution of warmth in the body. In anthroposophic medicine, a disturbance in the warmth organisation can be seen as a cause as well as a symptom, of illness. The warmth organisation is the physical medium for the activity of the I, and it has a potential for healing which can be exploited. To that end, warm, draught-free rooms are used for therapeutic massage, with only as much uncovering of the patient as is required for the treatment. Plant oils are used which lubricate the skin but also induce a warming effect on the body, and this effect can be enhanced by the inclusion of aromatic oils in a mixture. The masseur selects oils most suited to the patient and the type of healing response which is sought.

Oil-dispersion baths

In conventional medicine, the use of preparations applied to the skin has been largely restricted to the use of ointments for local skin conditions. Only relatively recently have medicines been deliberately applied to the skin to be absorbed into the bloodstream as a way of treating internal conditions, such as angina. Anthroposophic medicine applies many substances externally for the purposes of influencing the body as a whole. For example, ethereal plant oils may be used which are related to the mild catabolic, breaking-down processes the astral element introduces into the flower. These oils, such as rosemary or lavender, can stimulate a response from the whole metabolic system if applied to the skin during baths.

Of course, oil and water do not mix but, in treatment, an apparatus is used which draws a thin stream of oil into a vortex of water, creating a fine dispersion. The oil droplets are so fine that they remain dispersed for a considerable time before separating out. When patients are immersed in these oil-dispersion baths, the whole skin is affected. They emerge with a very fine layer of oil all over, which continues to have an effect if they are carefully wrapped in a cotton sheet and blankets rather than dried off. After spending about a quarter of an hour in the bath, and resting, wrapped up, for another three-quarters of an hour, patients usually feel the warming effect of the oils for many more hours. The bath itself is roughly body temperature, so it is the quality of the oil, rather than the heat of the water, which brings about the profound warming. The effect of the treatment is that the I is better able to exert its influence within the physical body and, as a result, the patient feels inwardly quiet and composed. This form of treatment is an anthroposophic development of hydrotherapy.

In addition to the warming quality of an oil-bath, each of the ethereal oils has a specific effect. For example, lavender, with its relaxing, soporific qualities, contrasts with rosemary, which has a stronger toning, awakening effect. Rosemary also strongly stimulates the peripheral circulation, and for this reason can be used as a local treatment in footbaths, when a warming effect in the feet and legs is required.

Irregularities in the warmth organisation can also be helped by hydrotherapy. Cold areas in the lower body, especially in the pelvic region as described above, often accompany gynaecological problems and these are particularly helped by baths containing melissa (lemon balm) oil, which has a refreshing and gentle warming effect. Anxiety is often accompanied by areas of coldness (as in a cold sweat), particularly in the legs and feet. This can be helped by footbaths up to the knees containing rosemary. Warm footbaths with mustard can be used in addition to vigorous massage of the calves and feet in treating migraine attacks. The mustard reddens and mildly irritates the skin, diverting the excessive metabolic activity from the head into the calves and feet. In a similar way, warming footbaths can help to relieve an asthma attack.

Pyrogenic baths

A profound and long-standing problem with warmth is often found in patients with illnesses such as cancer and M.E. (myalgic encephalomyelitis, or post-viral fatigue syndrome). Such patients often have body temperatures nearer to 35 °C (95 °F) than the normal 37 °C (98.5 °F). In healthy people, there is generally a rhythmical variation of their temperatures, most people being slightly warmer in the evening than they are first thing in the morning. Patients whose body temperatures are reduced tend to lack this regular rhythmical quality. Medical treatments for cancer and immune problems are dealt with in Chapter 13, but within the context of hydrotherapy special 'pyrogenic' baths can help by supporting a normalisation of body temperature. The patient is immersed in water up to the chin for an hour, during which time the water is kept at, or just above, body temperature. The warming effect is not from the water but, in this case, from removing the body's ability to cool itself. The main method of cooling is the evaporation of sweat from the skin but, in the bath, the sweat goes into the bath instead of evaporating, and the cooling effect is lost.

A pyrogenic bath can raise the body temperature as high as 39 or 40 °C (102–104 °F) and, if the patient has not had a feverish illness for years and has a subnormal temperature, is quite strenuous for the body. The patient's pulse and blood pressure must be carefully observed during the bath, and for an hour afterwards while resting in bed. It is not suitable for severely debilitated patients or those with serious heart problems, but its profound warming effect can make a valuable contribution to re-establishing a normal body temperature when this is lacking. To the anthroposophic doctor, it is important that the warmth is produced within the body rather than from outside. This is because the body's own warmth organisation is an integral part of the whole person, just as much as the physical structure of the body. Warmth or cold forcibly introduced from outside is foreign to this organisation in much the same way as a splinter is foreign to the physical structure.

Lying in baths, patients experience a degree of weightlessness through the buoyancy of the water, and this is helpful when there is difficulty in standing or walking, as in arthritis or following a stroke. However, hydrotherapy's primary effect is on bodily functions, such as the circulation, muscular tone and the distribution of warmth. Indirectly, it can also affect the soul, as there can be emotional reactions to the profound relaxing and warming effects. Similarly, in massage, the release of muscular tension can bring with it a release of pent-up or buried emotions.

The medium of hydrotherapy, water, is the medium in which we are suspended before birth. As the medium of the etheric forces, it has a special relationship with the healing processes of the body. The therapeutic potential of baths has been recognised since the time of Ancient Greece, when Hippocrates, who is known as the father of modern medicine, established a healing centre on the island of Cos, which included elaborate bathing facilities. Throughout Europe, recognition of the healing effects of bathing in water from certain springs led to the development of many spa towns, which still flourish in central Europe. Traditional medicine is less respected in Britain, where the therapeutic use of spas all but died out in the early twentieth century. The conventional medical view, which rapidly dominated British culture, regarded the main use of hot spas, such as at Bath, to be as primitive sources of hot water, and their therapeutic value was lost to conventional practice.

Cultural factors have also played a part in bringing about a disregard for the importance of warmth in the maintenance of health. In winter, it is common to see men outdoors in shirtsleeves and women with little or no covering on their legs. Many offices and public buildings are kept very warm and, when people go in and out of such buildings, they often pay little attention to extreme temperature changes. Anthroposophic medicine sees the human warmth organisation as the physical carrier of I-activity, with great importance for the maintenance of health. It is possible that the widespread inattention to keeping warm is a factor in the development of the many degenerative and sclerotic diseases, such as arteriosclerosis and osteoarthritis, which are the predominant contemporary health problems of the western world. The range of hydrotherapy treatments can contribute to alleviating this damage. They can also give patients the opportunity to become more aware of their bodily warmth as a step towards becoming more responsible for their own health.

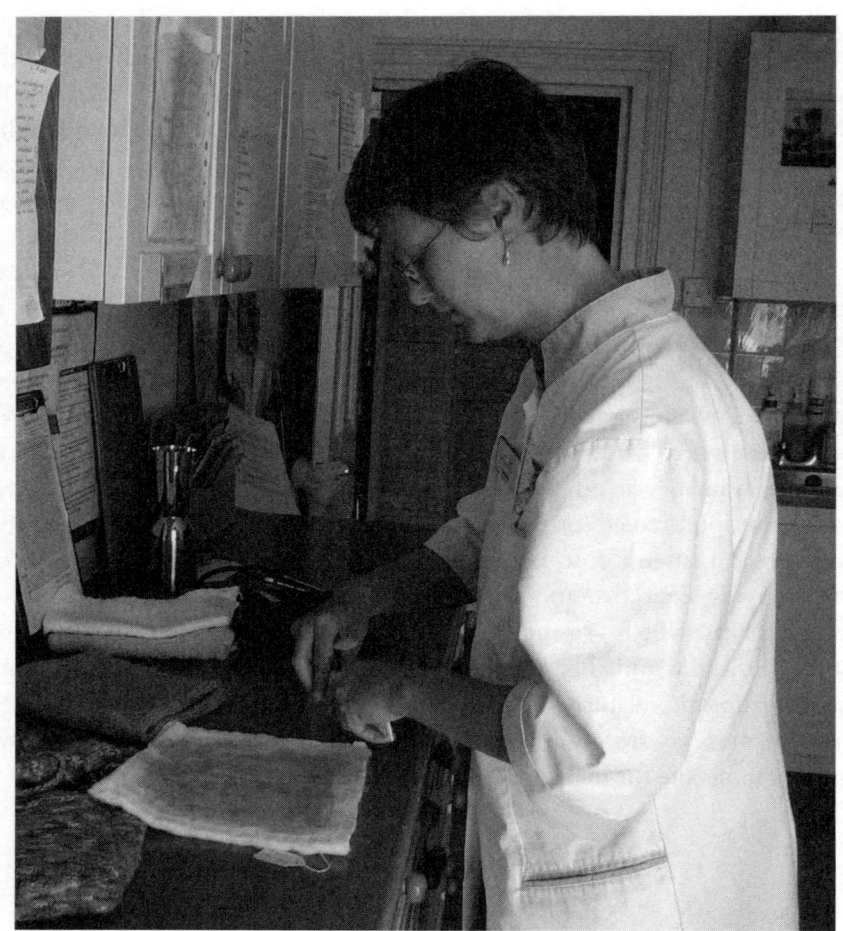

Preparing a compress.

9. The Art of Nursing

Nurses have been deeply affected by the technical advances of conventional medicine. Their work has become increasingly specialised and, thereby, has been divided up. They have become responsible for technical tasks, such as measuring blood pressure and checking heart monitors, leaving many of the more personal aspects of their role to assistants and auxiliaries. There has also been an escalation of time-consuming paperwork in conventional medicine through the need to keep detailed records of the results of technical tests. While much good has come from the technical aspects of modern medicine, these developments have made it increasingly difficult for nurses to find enough time to establish personal contact with each patient and to give the care that good nursing demands.

Anthroposophy is able to integrate an understanding of the physical body and its ailments with an understanding of the spiritual element of the patient, and this has practical implications for nurses. For example, one of the differences between the nurse's role and the doctor's is that the nursing team cares for the patient twenty-four hours a day, seven days a week, whereas the doctor normally has contact with the patient only for short periods. Through this extended contact, nurses have a special responsibility for supporting the rhythmical functions of the patient. The cycles of sleeping and waking, eating and bowel movements, activity and rest, when properly regulated, support the healing process. Neglect can have the opposite effect because, in times of illness, patients may not be able to maintain healthy rhythms themselves.

Nurses who wish to practise anthroposophic med medicine must complete a conventional nursing qualification before supplementing it with anthroposophic training. In many ways, the anthroposophic approach is in accordance with the best of conventional nursing philosophy, but it tends to lay greater emphasis on particular areas. The nurse's task is defined as assisting people in those activities which contribute to health, or to its recovery, or to a peaceful death, which the patients would do for themselves if they had the necessary strength, will or knowledge. Nursing also helps patients to follow prescribed therapy and to become independent of assistance as quickly as possible.

Nursing practice

In practice, nursing generally involves caring for the physical environment of the patient. This may include ensuring that the bed gives adequate support, the surroundings are clean and warm, and there is plenty of fresh air. An anthroposophic nurse will also be aware of what might be described as the patient's soul environment. This includes everything taken in by the senses – the quality of light in the room, the colours, sounds and smells, and also the aesthetic quality of the surroundings, as it is beneficial for the patient to have things of beauty to focus on. It also includes the avoidance, if possible, of anything lacking in aesthetic quality, which can have a far stronger effect on someone lying ill in bed than it would on a healthy person.

The soul environment also includes the mood the nurse brings to the patient and, for this reason, it is important what frame of mind the nurse is in when entering the sick room. It may be necessary to pause in order to adopt the calmness and openness necessary to allow an appropriate response to the patient's needs. A state of hurry or irritation or, for that matter, an exaggerated geniality, would get in the way of being receptive to the patient. On the level of the soul, patients need emotional warmth and support from their nurses just as much as, on the physical level, they need a warm room to assist recovery.

The nurse also needs to help the patient in a social sense. At a given time, there may be a need for peace, privacy and rest but, depending on the patient and the stage of the illness, at another time it may be important to mix with other patients and to be involved in social and cultural activities. Attending stimulating talks or musical evenings, for example, or going for walks in the countryside can rekindle an interest in life, which may be therapeutic in itself.

The patient's warmth organisation can be greatly supported by the application of ethereal plant oils by the nurse. In their training, anthroposophic nurses learn a technique of application of these oils which is similar to therapeutic massage (described in the previous chapter). It tends to concentrate on the soothing, balancing movements which encourage the flow of the etheric, upbuilding processes, rather than the more vigorous kneading actions associated with stimulating consciousness in a particular area. Use of the oils can stimulate warmth in areas where it may well be deficient, such as the neck, shoulders, back, abdomen, feet and lower legs. It can also produce a feeling of well-being and provide great comfort to patients who are dying and feeling lonely or frightened about what they are facing, particularly at the stage when words are inadequate. Such treatment often helps to provide a feeling of security in which deep-seated fears can be released and discussed in a way that would not come about in normal conversation.

Oils, or ointments, are chosen according to the particular needs and condition of each patient. During their application, the nurse gains a sense of the patient's skin and muscle tone areas of relative warmth and cold in the body, and also indications of the patient's emotional state. As with the similar observations of the therapeutic masseur, these indications are very helpful to the doctor, particularly as many of the nursing treatments are given on a daily basis.

Such treatments are usually prescribed by the doctor, but nurses might also apply oils on their own initiative. For example, if a patient has difficulty getting to sleep at night, a nurse might apply a back massage of lavender oil, as this has a very relaxing effect. The personal contact between nurse and patient is also important because it adds an invaluable emotional warmth to the treatment. Not only can the use of lavender oil obviate the need for a sleeping tablet, but it is also an entirely different experience for both patient and nurse. The application of oils has a special role in supporting the treatment of patients with symptoms of anxiety and other emotional problems, and also patients who are physically very weak and may be bed-bound.

The nurse further complements the work of the therapeutic masseur and the hydrotherapist in the administration of baths and footbaths. Stimulating footbaths containing rosemary in the morning and relaxing ones with lavender in the evening form a regular part of nursing treatment. Mustard footbaths may be administered by nurses to alleviate certain kinds of headaches, asthmatic attacks and bronchitis, and at the first signs of a panic attack. They may also be used at the first signs of the onset of a headache or a cold. As it is so important to apply the treatment early in the development of the symptoms, nurses are often called upon to act promptly on their own initiative in such cases.

Nurses must have a good knowledge of the characteristics of the substances they use in treatment, particularly herbs. Each one needs to be used in a specific way to release the healing properties to the maximum effect. For example, flowers need delicate handling if their therapeutic properties are to be enhanced rather than destroyed by insensitive preparation, such as infusing them for too long. Infusions made from roots, stems, seeds and leaves each require a particular simmering time. Mechanical or unthinking preparation reduces, and can even nullify, the therapeutic effect, and the nurse must be familiar with each remedy to get the best from it.

Knowledge of plant remedies

A plant with many therapeutic uses is camomile, which is particularly effective as a soothing agent. An infusion of the flowers can be given as an inhalation to help relieve and clear sinusitis or bronchitis, or as a gargle and mouthwash for mouth infections. In a hip bath it is good for soothing the genital region after childbirth. Camomile may also be used in a compress prepared from an infusion of the flowers. It is applied to the patient's skin as hot as possible without being painful, and covered with another cloth before a third, woollen layer is wrapped around the body and secured with safety pins. This keeps the compress in position and helps to retain the heat. A hot-water bottle placed on top of the woollen layer adds to the warmth, and the patient is tucked up in bed to rest for at least half an hour. Used on the abdomen, such a compress can be very helpful in a variety of metabolic and digestive disturbances. Camomile is strongly indicated when there are spasms or cramps, especially as in indigestion or period pains.

By contrast, a lemon compress is prepared in lukewarm water. Applied to the feet and calves, it can help limit the extent of a high fever when there is a risk of the patient becoming delirious or, in children, when there is a risk of febrile convulsions. Such treatment can help to avoid the automatic use of paracetamol and similar drugs, whose dangers for health in the long-term are described in Chapter 10.

Compresses, oils and ointments are also regularly applied by nurses to have an effect on the major organs. A warm cloth with an ointment containing lavender and rose oil placed over the heart helps to calm palpitations in cases of anxiety or in the heart conditions of the elderly. Copper ointment applied over the kidneys also has a local warming effect and helps to restore harmony to their activity. Compresses are often applied over the liver for patients with problems in that area, and also in some cases of depression, when it is beneficial to stimulate the vitality of the metabolic organs.

Anthroposophic nurses are trained in the techniques of preparing and administering all these treatments, many of which would appear quite foreign to nurses who are only conventionally trained. Through extending their skills with such practical techniques, nurses often find they get much more fulfilment from their work. As well as more personal contact with patients, anthroposophic nursing involves much more direct contact with the materials, such as plants, from which remedies are made.

In anthroposophic hospitals and clinics, the nurses administer the medicines prescribed by doctors, just as they would in conventional practice. Above and beyond the concentration and accuracy required for this, anthroposophic nurses cultivate a reverence and deep feeling for the qualities of the medicinal substances. They do not need the detailed knowledge the doctor must have to prescribe the medicines, but it is important that they understand some of the fundamental principles if they are to administer the medicines effectively. Whether the treatment involves giving a medicine, applying an oil, or any other techniques the nurse concentrates outwardly on performing the task correctly, and inwardly on the qualities of the substances being used and the nature of the treatment.

Communication

Nurses work together as a team providing twenty-four-hour care, and the provision of consistency and continuity in treatment is dependent on their ability to communicate accurately and effectively with one another. Their role as communicators, combined with their observations of patients over long periods, also enables them to assist in the doctor's meetings with patients. Often, patients need to hear what the doctor has to say several times before grasping it fully, and nurses may be able to explain it more personally through the closer relationships they have built up with them. Similarly, patients sometimes find it easier to discuss with nurses certain matters which the doctor ought to know and, in these cases, the nurse can tactfully pass on the information. The vital communicative role also applies in sharing knowledge with other therapists, such as a therapeutic masseur or artistic therapist who, like the doctor, might see the patient for shorter periods. The nurse keeps them informed of the patient's mental and physical state, and ensures that periods of therapy do not adversely affect important aspects of the patient's daily rhythm. The closer contact nurses have with patients also means that they are often able to help in difficult communications with friends and relatives.

Anthroposophic nurses fulfil a central role by bringing all the individual aspects of treatment together and ensuring that they form a harmonious whole rather than, through poor communication, working against each other. The anthroposophic approach aims to humanise every aspect of the nurse's work, restoring the personal contact that has been lost in the technical specialisation of conventional nursing. Each and every activity is accompanied by an awareness of, and reverence for, the task of caring for a patient who is not just another physical body in a bed, but someone who has a soul and a spirit.

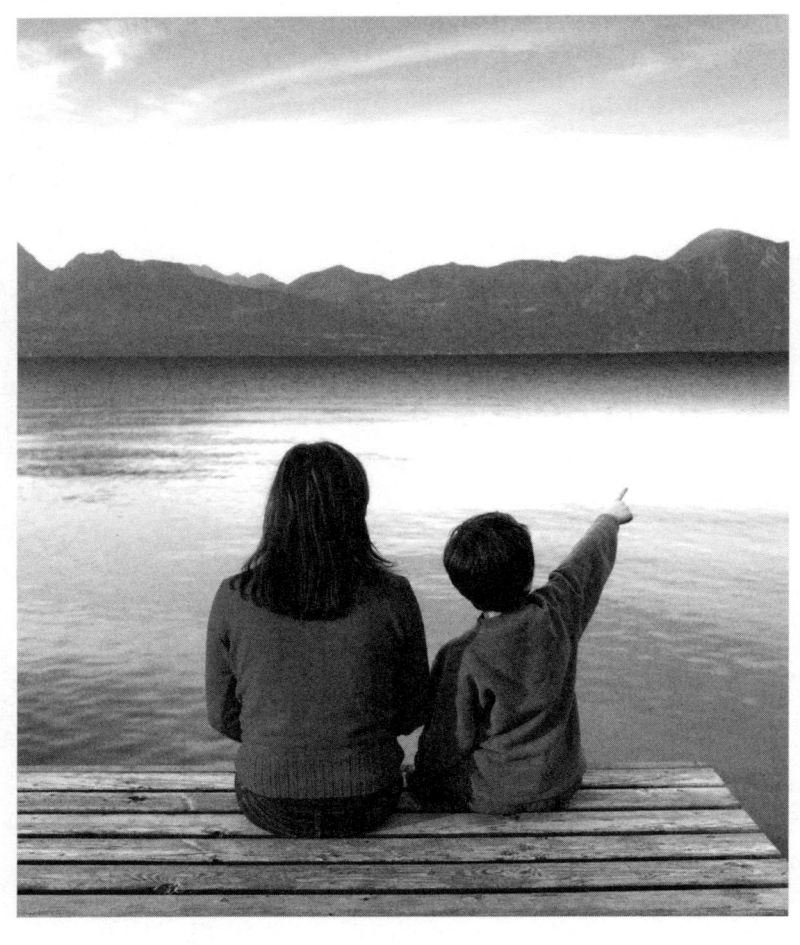

10. Childhood Illnesses

From conception and on into childhood, the human spirit is involved in shaping the physical body which is to be its vehicle for a life on earth. This activity is particularly intense between conception and birth, and in the first few years of life – the time of maximum growth and maturation. While this is happening, eating and sleeping dominate the infant's daily life. Through the newly formed physical body, the child is influenced by heredity and environmental factors. At birth, these influences are very strong and the body is, to some extent, foreign to the spirit incarnating into it. The spirit must increasingly make the body its own, especially in the first seven years, when it remoulds it in a way that might be compared to the breaking in of new shoes.

This first seven-year phase of childhood is concluded by the change of teeth, which is a dramatic expression of the extent of the remoulding process. The enamel of the teeth is the hardest substance in the human body, and in later life cannot be renewed. Only this once does the renewal of the constituents of the body include the teeth. The second phase of childhood leads to puberty, at around twelve to fourteen. The third leads to adulthood, at about eighteen to twenty-two, when the process of physical maturity is complete. These phases of bodily development are accompanied by changes in the development of the person as a whole.

Following the change of teeth, the formative life forces (etheric forces), which were previously so involved in reshaping the body, become partially freed from this role, particularly in the case of the system of nerves and senses. They then become available as forces of mental creativity and can be applied to, for example, the formal learning of reading, writing and arithmetic. This allows more serious teaching to begin, replacing the learning by imitation of the earlier phase. The emancipation of the etheric body represents a step in the process of the child's independence from its parents. The predominance of the physical body in the first phase, when it is being remoulded, is replaced by a predominance of the etheric processes during the second phase As they are also the processes of healing and revitalisation, this phase tends to be a time of particularly good health.

At puberty, there is an awakening of sexual drives and turbulent emotions. From the anthroposophic point of view, this is the time of the awakening, or freeing, of the astral body, which had previously been bound up with the processes of growth and development. During this third phase, there is a powerful demand for personal independence, but without the developed sense of responsibility, which tends to come later (about eighteen to twenty-one) with the awakening of the I. This is generally recognised in so far as adult rights and responsibilities are given at this time, rather than at the time of reproductive maturity in the early teens.

The role of illness in development

As can be seen from the above, only the physical body becomes completely independent at birth and there is a kind of birth of the etheric body around seven, of the astral body around fourteen and the I at about twenty-one. These ages are by no means fixed and individual paths of development can vary widely. Also, this does not mean that a young child does not already have its own etheric body, astral body or I, but that they are partially freed from their unconscious activity in the processes of growth and maturation at around these ages and become more available to the personality. Before puberty, for example, the astral forces are particularly involved in maturing the reproductive organs. Afterwards, they arouse powerful emotions and desires and produce a determination to make decisions for oneself.

Against this background, the role of illness during childhood, particularly in the first seven years, can be seen in a quite different light from the conventional view. The opportunity for remoulding the physical body is provided by the constant dissolving and reforming of its structures. During feverish illnesses, all the metabolic processes speed up and the high temperatures can offer a special opportunity for a more intensive reshaping. Fevers are often accompanied by a loss of weight, reflecting the preponderance of breaking-down processes that take place. Many observant parents and teachers notice that children look a little more mature after such an illness. They may also seem more composed and less prone to irritability than before the illness.[1]

Young children often have very many feverish infections, especially soon after starting at a playgroup or school. This is generally recognised to be the result of meeting many of the bacteria and viruses carried by humans for the first time, and needing to build up immunity to them. For some time after birth, particularly if the baby is breast-fed, the child is protected by the mother's immunity, but the time comes when the child must develop its own immunity. In measles especially, there is a profound activation of the immune system, with many antibodies produced. In the past, when children got measles it was common for doctors to regard it as the coming to maturity of the immune system. They would tell parents of children who were having many minor illnesses that they would be much more resistant once they had recovered from measles. Nowadays, virtually all conventional doctors try to prevent the major childhood infections, such as measles, mumps and whooping cough, through an extensive vaccination programme.

Doctors still recognise that the many coughs and colds that appear when children start school are part of this developing maturity and not a sign of serious ill-health, but they still have the tendency to over-prescribe medicines like paracetamol (acetaminophen) to suppress the fever, and antibiotics to kill the bacteria on the body's behalf. This is in spite of the fact that, in seventy-five to eighty per cent of cases, the body would have been capable of overcoming the infection itself. Only the minority requires medical treatment. There is now a large body of scientific research documenting the positive role of fever in overcoming infection. It needs to be seen as supporting the healing process rather than a dangerous activity needing suppression. In recent years the official guidelines in the UK have been changed to avoid using antipyretics (drugs suppressing fever) in order merely to suppress fever or to avoid febrile convulsions.[2]

It is becoming apparent that this use of medicines discourages the body's own healing processes and even, in the case of the suppression of fever, weakens them. Antibiotics have been widely used to treat infections since the 1940s and 1950s (though there is now widespread awareness that antibiotic resistance has been caused by over-prescribing antibiotics). Since then, the medical profession has become increasingly aware of a wide variety of diseases caused by abnormal immune responses, but few conventional doctors have questioned whether these two facts might be connected. The abnormal responses can take the form of auto-immunity, when the immune system attacks the tissues of the body itself, or there may be an excessive response to foreign substances in the form of an allergy.

For example, hayfever is an excessive reaction by the immune system to pollen in the eyes and nasal membranes. Asthma is also thought to be caused by this kind of mechanism. Not only is asthma becoming more common, but more children and adults are dying from it, despite ever-stronger drugs becoming available to control it. The appearance of what seems to be a completely new illness in which the immune system breaks down – acquired immune deficiency syndrome, or Aids – might also be taken to suggest that the increasing number of people suffering from such disorders may be connected with the widespread and indiscriminate use of antibiotics and paracetamol, which weaken the immune system.

At the centre of the immune system is the body's ability to distinguish between foreign substances and the bodily tissues. This can only be achieved by having a highly developed sense of identity which extends right down to the molecular level, as the immune system must be able to distinguish the bodily tissues from inorganic material, from substances originating in plants and animals, and also from substances originating in other humans. This ability is therefore specific to the individual concerned. During childhood, the immune system is maturing at the same time as the I is working to make the physical body its own, putting its own stamp of identity on the mixture of inherited characteristics. The inflammatory childhood infections offer special opportunities for the individual identity to be stamped more deeply into the substance of the body. The warmth of the fever is analogous to the warmth that melts sealing wax and allows the impression of a signet ring to be stamped into it as a sign of the owner's identity.

It follows from this that a suppression of the natural course of an infection will have detrimental consequences as well as short-term benefits. The same will be the case with the artificial prevention of diseases like measles, mumps and whooping cough, which used to be thought of as the normal illnesses of childhood. If the I is prevented from making the body its own during early childhood, a foreign element remains for the rest of the life. Foreign substances and processes within the body are characteristic of the sclerotic (hardening) and degenerative diseases of later life, and an increase in these is to be expected as a result of such interference with the development of the immune system. The link would appear to be supported by a study published in *The Lancet* which found that children who have measles with a rash (i.e. the illness develops fully) have a lower incidence of cancer and degenerative joint disease in later life than those who do not develop a rash.[3] It is perhaps no coincidence that the sclerotic and degenerative diseases, such as cancer, heart attacks and strokes, are the main causes of death in the Western world, where vaccination against measles routinely takes place.

Anthroposophic medicine offers a range of remedies aimed at stimulating and supporting the body's own healing response to infection. For example, homeopathically prepared belladonna (deadly nightshade) or argentum (silver) can be used to moderate excessive fever without completely suppressing it. This may be particularly important in cases where there is a risk of febrile convulsions or if the fever makes the child delirious. Lemon compresses applied to the calves and feet can also be used to control a fever. In the majority of infections, the child recovers without the use of antibiotics or fever-suppressing drugs. When the infection is more serious, antibiotics may be required. For example, in severe illnesses such as bacterial meningitis, antibiotics are essential to save the child's life.

Some home remedies

Space does not allow for a detailed account of the various childhood illnesses, many of which require medical attention. However, there follow some examples of how home remedies can be used to treat common complaints.[4] The examples of home remedies are not alternatives to proper supervision by a doctor. Chapter 14 has further details of dosages and methods of treatment.

Teething tends to be a cause of considerable discomfort for children. It can usually be relieved by giving babies something hard to bite on, and Camomile D3 pills dissolved in a teaspoon of water every couple of hours. Alternatively, the gums can be massaged with Weleda mouthwash.

Colds can be treated with Ferrum Phos. comp. pills which, again, may be dissolved in a teaspoon of water for babies.[5]

Middle-ear infections are often very painful, and should always be referred to a doctor, but they do not usually require antibiotics. They can be relieved by applying a warm onion compress to the ear and giving medicine such as Apis/Levisticum, as prescribed. To make a compress, finely chop a medium-sized onion, tie or fold it inside a cloth, warm it on a hot-water bottle and secure it against the ear with a woollen scarf or balaclava. If the child is old enough to co-operate, it helps to have the affected side of the head laid against a hot-water bottle to keep the compress and the ear warm.

Sore throats can be treated by gargling with sage tea or Weleda mouthwash, by sucking sage pastilles, or by taking Cinnabar/Pyrites tablets. Again, in most cases, antibiotics are not necessary.

Education

Younger children are obviously very dependent on other people to look after them, particularly their mother. Only by example do they learn to stand, walk and talk. Their dependency on, and sensitivity to, their environment mean they are very easily influenced by the moods and attitudes of others, especially their parents. They are also strongly influenced by sense impressions from the world around them. Because of this, anthroposophic doctors emphasise the importance of natural and aesthetic environments for young children. It is also important that they exercise their imaginations by playing with simple toys made from natural materials. These require the child's active participation to make them represent cars or babies, rather than synthetic toys, which are more exact copies of the real thing and therefore demand less of the imagination.

Consciousness has a destructive effect on the body, but this is greatly reduced during sleep. Daydreaming, creative play and fantasy fall between the fully awake state and the sleeping state of dreaming, and also have a less catabolic effect on the body. Especially in the first seven years of childhood, healthy development requires that the upbuilding, anabolic forces predominate. Only after the ages of six or seven should the etheric forces – which are involved in growth, including the development of the nervous system – begin to be called upon for intellectual work as part of a more formal education. Until then, children should be involved in creative play, practical activities such as baking, and artistic activities such as painting, singing and eurythmy. It is also beneficial for them to be told imaginative stories. This is the approach adopted by Rudolf Steiner schools (also known as Waldorf schools). If children are encouraged to learn reading, writing and arithmetic before they are ready, their etheric forces are called upon to fulfil an intellectual role before they have completed their formative work on the physical body. This weakens the physical constitution, which may result in tiredness, poor concentration, headaches, a proneness to recurrent infections and a tendency to degenerative diseases in later life. The untimely intellectual development brings on a premature ageing process which can have harmful effects throughout life.

When reading, writing, arithmetic and foreign languages begin to be learnt, they should be taught in as imaginative and artistic a fashion as possible to children from six or seven up to about fourteen. This helps to prevent an overburdening of the body with the catabolic effects of abstract thought by balancing it with imaginative and creative activity. It also helps to produce a more balanced person in later life who is still able to be creative, and has a developed aesthetic sense as well as a capacity for clear thought. This approach to education, which began in the 1920s, is followed by Steiner Waldorf schools throughout the world. Although there has been a recognition in state education of the importance of balancing factual learning with the active participation of children finding things out for themselves, there remains a short-sighted conviction that the earlier children learn to read and write, the better.

Anthroposophic doctors regard an education which works in harmony with the natural development of children as one of the most important elements of preventive medicine. The contribution an appropriate education can make to health, in both childhood and adulthood, is enormous. It was described earlier how an imbalance in the soul can cause illness. A teacher in a Steiner Waldorf school aims to spot such tendencies as they begin to appear and to find a way to harmonise them. An excessively slow and dreamy child would need a quite different educational approach from a prematurely intellectual and hyperactive one. Whenever possible, anthroposophic doctors work alongside the teachers, supporting the preventive medical aspect of their work.

The main contribution of anthroposophic medicine to the treatment of childhood illnesses comes from the understanding gained by regarding childhood as a time when the I is remoulding the physical body. Parents, doctors and teachers can help this process so that children's bodies become vehicles which are able to serve the I healthily throughout life. The way children's own healing forces are supported by doctors during illness is seen to have consequences for the rest of their lives. However, love and wise care from parents and teachers can have an even more profound effect on children's health than medical treatment. Doctors, therefore, also have a special role as advisors to the parents and teachers on the medical aspects of children's development.

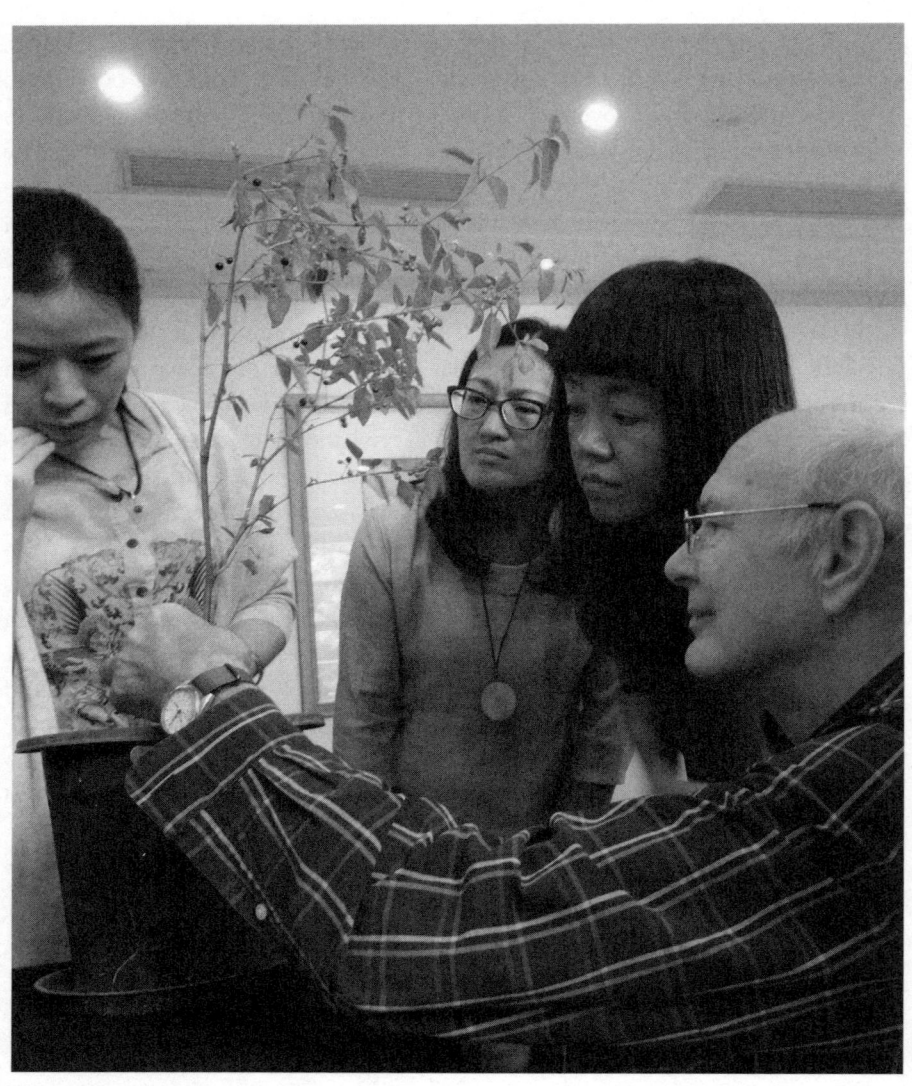

Plant study with Michael Evans.

11. Inner Development

The growth and development that takes place during childhood is obvious, particularly because the physical changes are so dramatic. Although not so outwardly obvious, the rest of life continues this process of development. From the age of thirty, a noticeable physical decline can be observed, but there need not be a similar decline in the development of the soul and spirit. Our inner development, which is observable to an extent in personality, is increasingly in our own hands as we mature. Through anthroposophy, we can become more aware of how to take responsibility for it.

Many opportunities for development arise in life, which often come in the form of crises or problems. These challenges may be unique to the person concerned or, because life is also strongly coloured by natural biological changes that affect us all, they may be common to everyone. There are certain spiritual and psychological stages of development that are typical of particular phases in life, and an understanding of these can help enormously in coming to terms with the problems as they arise

Phases of adult life

The first phase of adult life runs through the twenties, from about twenty-one to twenty-eight, and tends to be very strongly influenced by the powerful feelings and emotions which began to stir during puberty. It is a time of searching for an identity and direction in life, and perhaps also for a life partner. There is usually a great amount of energy – all-night parties are perfectly manageable, and the prospect of back-packing around the world holds no fears. This phase is also generally the time when the career begins and the first home is established. The process of finding the right work, and the right partner, is at the same time a process of finding oneself and a set of values and aims to live by.

In the next phase, from about twenty-eight to thirty-five, a more serious note generally appears, with the direction in life becoming clearer. Priorities which may have been worked out during the twenties now become more important. The vitality of youth begins to be limited, and illnesses often occur at this time if a continuation of the lifestyle of the twenties is attempted. Exhaustion, anxiety or mild depression may force a recognition of the priorities in life and the realisation that they should be upheld more earnestly. Life is no longer a game. There is also a need to organise, to achieve advancement at work perhaps, or to keep on top of running a home. Different needs have to be balanced in an increasingly busy life, especially if, as is often the case, there are small children to look after. The twenty-one to twenty-eight period is characterised by the sensitivity of the emotional aspect of the soul, and is called in anthroposophy the phase of the *sentient soul*. The twenty-eight to thirty-five period is associated with the practical application of the intellect, and is called the phase of the *intellectual soul*.

By the time of the next phase, around thirty-five to forty-two, people have often mastered many of the demands of their work, and may even have attained their career goals. However, this is a time when nagging doubts often arise. There tends to be a questioning of whether it would be fulfilling to continue in the same career for the next twenty or twenty-five years, and long-standing relationships might seem stale. Deeper questions about the meaning of life may also arise, representing a more spiritual appraisal of the life to date. These questions are concerned with a greater objectivity and awareness of the implications of one's actions, and are related to a third aspect of the soul, the will. The thirty-five to forty-two phase is called the period of the *consciousness soul*.

The physical decline becomes more apparent from forty-two to forty-nine, most dramatically for women in the menopause. The challenge of this phase is to identify with wider needs and interests; for example, looking beyond what has already been achieved in the career, or finding a new role as young children mature and leave home. The more there is an identification with the needs and concerns of others, the more spiritual advancement takes place. This personal development can, to an extent, bring an inner freedom from the physical body's decline.

In the next phase, from forty-nine to fifty-six, much depends on whether this development has taken place, because clinging to past achievements inevitably brings painful experiences. For example, at work, people in this phase often feel increasingly threatened by rising younger colleagues. It is much better all round for the older person to act as mentor and benefactor to the younger ones rather than to try to hold them back for fear of competition.

Between fifty-six and sixty-three, the experiences of the previous phase are intensified as the prospect of retirement looms. Thoughts of death bring on a questioning of values and priorities, and of what has been achieved in life. The progress made in earlier periods towards a true wisdom and understanding increasingly influences how older people are able to handle what life brings them.

After sixty-three, and particularly after seventy, what is achieved has more significance for humanity as a whole than for the individual's personal development. The differences between the lives led by old people can be very striking, with some able to be highly creative and inwardly active despite the physical body's degeneration, while others succumb inwardly to the physical decline. Once again, this has much to do with the development achieved in earlier phases.

Self development

From birth to death, we are all undergoing a process of inner development, even though we are generally unaware of its full significance. The situations we face on a daily basis make demands of us that act as a kind of schooling. However, throughout history, there have been methods of training which have focused on particular aspects of inner development, in some cases leading to direct perception of the spiritual realm. In Ancient Egypt, for example, there were schools teaching this knowledge. A master guided a chosen pupil through an arduous series of inner exercises aimed at purification of the soul. The training usually required withdrawal from everyday life into a temple, and took place in great secrecy. The insights gained through spiritual perceptions were generally used to benefit the culture as a whole, rather than the individual. For example, methods of cultivation were discovered and improved in this way.

Various forms of training for inner development have been practised down the centuries, particularly by religious orders. In the Middle Ages, Christians established monasteries and convents where they upheld strict vows and practised rigorous meditative exercises. But a significant change had taken place between the time of the Ancient Egyptian temple schools and the later Christian practices. It is not only the human physical form that has been affected by evolution: consciousness itself has also changed. Before the time of Christ, the human I was not sufficiently developed for people to be able to bring about their own inner development. Hence, the Ancient Egyptian training required the complete submission of the pupil, who was prepared by others in such a way that spiritual perception was eventually attained.

Since the time of Christ, the I has become capable of bringing about self-development, such that spiritual perception may be achieved through people's own efforts. A new process of inner training became necessary which would be appropriate for the changes that had taken place in the I. This new path is inherent in Christ's life and teachings but, as humanity evolves, His works have to be interpreted into forms which the human consciousness of the time finds accessible. A form of training appropriate for the current era is contained within anthroposophy. Details are beyond the scope of this book but interested readers will find a thorough account in Steiner's *Knowledge of the Higher Worlds*. The kinds of spiritual development referred to includes greater empathy for others, greater self knowledge, clarity of thought, equanimity of mood, resolution and consistency of behaviour and action, and open-mindedness. Steiner describes a series of regular tasks to strengthen some of these capacities in a section entitled 'Subsidiary Exercises' in this book. Guidance on inner training is also provided by the School of Spiritual Science, within the Anthroposophical Society.

In ancient times, the training was conducted by a chosen few in great secrecy, and the pupil played a passive role. Nowadays, it is essential that the motivation to undertake inner training comes from the pupils themselves, who make their own decisions and take responsibility for their own self-development. They should retain their freedom at all times and on no account submit to the will of a guru. The anthroposophic training is open to anyone and does not require a withdrawal from everyday life – on the contrary, it is to be hoped that it would lead to a deeper involvement.

Those who undertake such a training should be under no illusions about direct spiritual perception, which is fully attained only at a very advanced stage. The first level of spiritual perception is consciousness in the etheric world, the realm of formative forces. Further development leads to direct perception of the astral, or soul, world. The third stage is consciousness in the world of the I itself. The barrier between consciousness of the physical and spiritual worlds may be seen as a threshold. It is crossed on birth and death, when our awareness enters and leaves the physical world.

Everyone has latent organs for spiritual perception, and their development requires the inner strengthening necessary to make it possible to cross this threshold during life without losing consciousness. Knowledge of this threshold, how it can be crossed, and the results of crossing it unprepared, is essential to the anthroposophic doctor. It provides an understanding of many psychiatric symptoms, and other behavioural problems which are becoming increasingly apparent in contemporary culture, such as anxiety, addiction and anti-social behaviour. An anthroposophic doctor must of course not only have some knowledge of this inner development but also practise it.

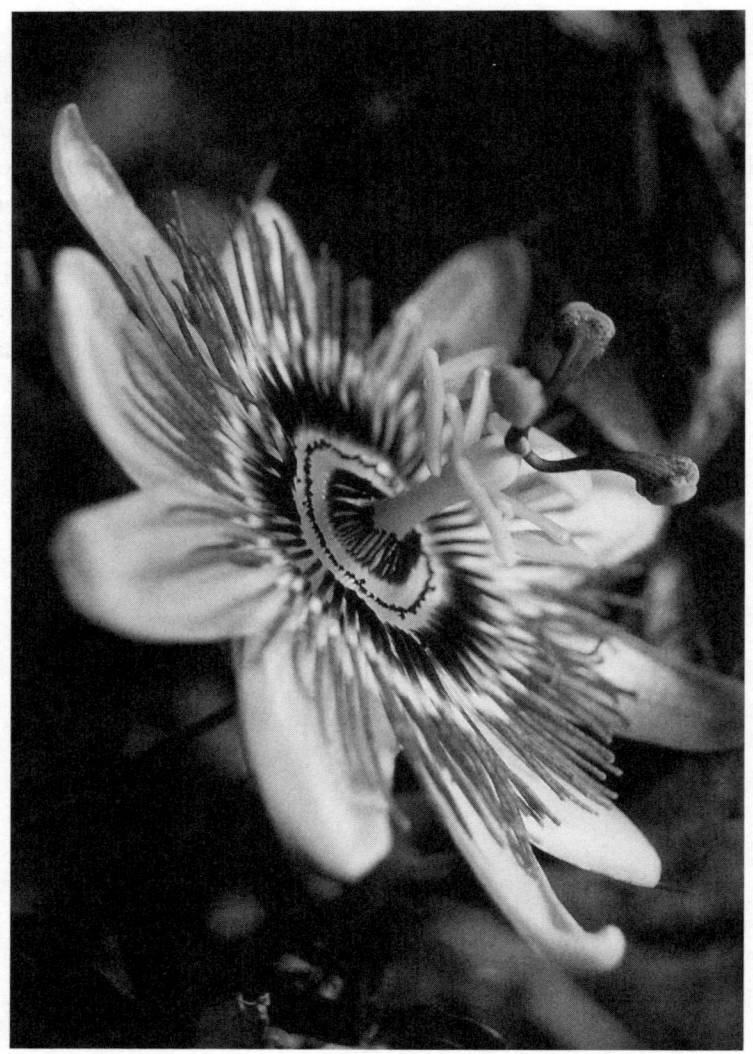

Passion flower.

12. Psychiatry

Anthroposophic doctors look beyond physical symptoms at how the I and astral body are involved in causing illness, and take these considerations into account in treatment. In mental illness, the reverse is true – causes of mental and emotional symptoms are looked for in the physical and etheric bodies. In his first course of lectures to doctors, Rudolf Steiner proposed this challenging philosophy, suggesting that psychotherapy may be most valuable when used to treat physical illnesses and that mental illnesses generally required medical treatment.

It has been seen how it is possible to develop higher forms of consciousness which enable direct perception of the spiritual realm. The first stage is perception of the etheric world – the world of formative life forces. These powerful spiritual forces drive the building and renewal of the physical body, a constant process involving the transformation of matter. In our normal, physical consciousness, we have no direct perception of these etheric processes but, when they are perceived with etheric consciousness, the impressions are more powerful and have a greater sense of reality than physical perceptions. This is sometimes found to be a feature of the experiences of patients suffering from mental illness. Some schizophrenics, in particular, find their hallucinations and delusions to be more powerful than their physical sense impressions.

Anthroposophic doctors see a connection between such experiences and spiritual perception, but consider the schizophrenic's experiences to be pathological. Someone who has developed direct perception of the spiritual realm has the inner strength to shut out such perceptions at will and concentrate exclusively on the physical world. In schizophrenia, the patient tends to be overpowered by the experiences and is often unable to relate normally to the physical world – consciousness of the two worlds, or the two sides of the threshold, is usually confused.

In conventional psychiatry, mental illnesses include psychoses and neuroses, with psychoses tending to be the more serious. Schizophrenia and manic depression are examples of psychoses, which often involve delusions and disordered thinking, although the patient may be unaware of being ill. Neuroses, on the other hand, include anxiety, certain forms of depression and obsessional, compulsive and phobic problems. These are deeply disturbing and unpleasant experiences for the patient, but generally leave thinking and understanding more or less intact. The patient is aware of the problem and, therefore, may be more concerned about it than someone with a psychosis.

Schizophrenia

The two main symptoms of schizophrenia are characteristic delusions and hearing voices. A typical delusion of schizophrenics is that their thoughts and feelings directly affect the outside world. For example, a patient might be feeling angry, then hear on the news that people have died in a rail crash and become convinced that the feelings of anger caused the crash. Alternatively, schizophrenics may feel that their thoughts are brought about by processes outside them. For example, they might believe that machinery in a nearby building causes them to think certain thoughts, or that other people are putting ideas into their heads. Another example of a typical delusion is the belief that something they may have read, say in a newspaper, refers to them, even though it is clear to everyone else that there is no connection. This symptom is closely related to what are known as paranoid delusions, when patients are convinced that others are talking secretly about them, usually negatively, and possibly plotting to do something evil against them.

An auditory hallucination usually takes the form of hearing someone who is not there talking about the patient. Typically, the voice says unpleasant things about the patient, and may even encourage self-inflicted injury. Psychiatrists usually interpret the hearing of voices as an indication that patients are experiencing their own thoughts as if they belonged to others. Normally, we feel completely independent from the outside world, with our own independent thoughts. A boundary is experienced between us and the rest of the world, which leaves our thinking free from external causes and the world free from our direct mental influence. From the symptoms described, it is clear that this boundary breaks down in schizophrenia.

When thoughts are experienced as if they belonged to others, it is as though the boundary between the inner and the outer had shifted, leaving the thoughts on the outside. The thinking processes then appear to be taken over by the laws of cause and effect of the outer, physical world and the normal sense of identity is lost. As was described in Chapter 4, self-consciousness, free will, reflective thinking and a sense of identity are characteristics of the human spirit. Although the spirit itself is eternal and cannot become ill, the loss of identity and free-thinking which takes place in schizophrenia indicates how the illness reaches right to the patient's inner core, distorting the spirit's union with the astral, etheric and physical bodies.

The etheric forces, which build and constantly maintain the physical body, obviously work into the physical realm. As was seen earlier, the sense organs and nervous system do not need the full activity of these life forces once they are fully formed, and what is then released is used in the activity of thinking. However, in the other systems of the body, particularly the metabolic region, the life forces need to be continually active in the transformation of substances in the organs. They should be engaged in this activity within the metabolic and rhythmic organs until death. Hallucinations and other symptoms of major mental illnesses occur when this breaks down – when life forces, which should be fully engaged in the activity of one of the organs of the metabolic or rhythmic systems, become free and invade the activity of thinking.

Unlike the forces released from the organs of the nerve-sense system, which provide for free thinking, the life forces from the metabolic and rhythmic systems have such power that they overwhelm the mental processes. The hallucinations they create can seem more real than the sense impressions of the physical world, such that the normal, healthy separation of the inner self from outer physical events is lost. So the relationships between the etheric and physical bodies in the organs of the metabolic and rhythmic systems should be looked at when such mental symptoms appear. Usually, changes in the etheric activity of the organ are responsible for the illness, rather than actual physical changes, although the physical changes associated with high fever can give rise to similar changes in consciousness. The toxic effects of some hallucinogenic drugs can also do so, and use of these drugs can induce schizophrenia.

Acute schizophrenia

The symptoms of schizophrenia are usually unpleasant and very disturbing although, occasionally, patients become attached to them, as might a user of hallucinogenic drugs. They are overpowered by the hallucinations to such an extent that they lose their freedom and identity and, in extreme situations, can no longer be held totally responsible for their actions. When they are unable to look after themselves, the psychiatrist has to be responsible for them until they are well enough to return to a more normal life. This is the basis for assessing the need for compulsory admissions and treatment, if patients appear to be putting themselves or others in danger.

Acute schizophrenia illustrates the need for an emphasis on medical rather than psychological forms of treatment, at least in the first instance. During an acute attack, the value of counselling or psychotherapy is usually very limited, doing little more than helping the patient to feel to some extent understood and supported. Attempts to analyse the delusions, or to show that they are not real, are usually futile and only cause further upset. In this situation, anthroposophic practice is able to offer a variety of medicines, which help to reconnect the life forces with the organs in which they should be fully active. For example, stibium (antimony) has this effect and may be given by injection in a homeopathic potency selected by the doctor. It is often necessary to use conventional psychiatric drugs as well, at least for a limited period. The initial treatment may be followed by the use of artistic therapies, eurythmy therapy and sculpture therapy, which help to calm the patient and further assist in reuniting the life forces with their proper organs.

During an acute attack, a patient may have dramatic experiences, and may well be in a highly excitable state. However, those who have suffered from severe forms of schizophrenia for some years are often left in a 'flattened' emotional state, with very little motivation. It is as if the life forces which produced the dramatic symptoms had been burnt up and were no longer available, leaving the sufferer depleted of emotional and mental vitality. Such patients used to be referred to as 'burnt-out schizophrenics'. Although the initial therapeutic emphasis is medical, artistic therapies can make a useful contribution to treating this stage by bringing colour back to the patient's inner life, which has become dulled and grey. Also, after acute attacks, it is often valuable to discuss with patients what they have been through, thereby helping them to gain some insight into the nature of the illness and what they can do to make further attacks less likely.

Just as the physical body consists of various organs, the etheric body is differentiated into various parts, and these are intimately connected with the physical organs. The different characteristics of the mental illnesses can be used to identify the organ associated with the illness, because the characteristics point to the etheric forces connected with that organ. Steiner identified the heart and lung from the rhythmic system, and the liver and kidney from the metabolic system, as the four organs principally involved in mental illness.

The I, astral body and etheric body are active in every organ of the body, but their relative activity varies from organ to organ. It has already been described how the I is particularly expressed through warmth (element of fire), the astral body through gases (air), the etheric body through fluids (water), and the physical body through solids (earth). So, if an organ has characteristics that relate it particularly to, say, the watery element, this points to a predominance of etheric activity in that organ.

Depression and the liver

The liver, for example, has a striking fluidity, indicating just such a centre of etheric activity. It is itself semi-fluid, its shape being governed by the surrounding structure, and through it there passes a constant stream of different fluids. There are arteries and veins carrying blood, and channels for lymph and bile. It is also one of only two organs in the body having a vein (carrying blood which is rich in carbon dioxide and low in oxygen) entering as well as leaving it. Such concentrations of carbon dioxide and low levels of oxygen are associated with vegetative growth. Plants use carbon dioxide to create sugars, which they store as starches, and it is the liver that is the body's prime store of sugar – in the form of glycogen, also known as animal starch. Like plants, the liver is dominated by upbuilding, anabolic activity in its vast catalogue of biochemical processes. Even in its role as neutraliser of poisons, it generally renders them harmless by adding a substance (usually a sugar) to them so that they can be safely excreted, rather than breaking them down in what would be a catabolic process.

The production of bile and its collection in the gall bladder is a quite distinct exception to the liver's mainly anabolic processes. Bile is created by the breaking down of the blood pigment, haemoglobin, and is then used to digest fats by emulsifying them prior to assimilation into the body. This catabolic activity is related to the fiery element and the activity of the I (the absorbed fats have the highest calorific value of any substances in the body and can be described as *concentrated heat*). Even so, the liver is the centre of anabolism and vitality in the body, as demonstrated by its remarkable regenerative ability. If three-quarters of the liver is removed, the remaining quarter is capable of adapting to the task of the whole organ and, in time, of growing back to full size.

Health is not merely an expression of strong upbuilding forces but a balance between anabolic and catabolic processes. The pathological danger from an excess of anabolism is that it leads to the storing of more substances than can be broken down for use by the body. If not checked by the catabolic activity of the I and astral body, the anabolic liver processes can cause a certain heaviness more akin to the earth element. On a very subtle level, this is the basis of depression, when a heavy sluggishness enters into the *watery* processes of the liver. There would not necessarily be any measurable changes in the liver or any physical liver disease – the changes are within the etheric liver rather than the physical organ. However, severe liver diseases such as hepatitis are often followed by depression.

During the regenerative time of sleep, up to about three o'clock in the morning, the liver stores more sugar in the form of glycogen than it breaks down. From three onwards, the balance shifts back in favour of breaking down glycogen, making glucose available to the muscles for bodily activity during the day. It is around this time that many depressives wake up and experience severe mental anguish and restlessness, often finding it impossible to get back to sleep. It is interesting that many of the treatments for depression considered successful by conventional medicine, involve a strengthening of the body's catabolic processes. For example, most antidepressant drugs have a stimulating effect on catabolic amines. In the same vein, depriving people of sleep can, at least temporarily, relieve depression by stopping the building-up processes becoming excessive. Similarly, very strenuous exercise, which increases the burning of glucose in the muscles, can also bring relief.

The other aspect of the liver, the production of bile, is associated with the opposite psychiatric state of mania. This is less common than depression but, when it occurs, often follows it. Whereas the depressive is weighed down, lacking motivation and inactive, the manic has an inner lightness and is bursting with motivation and excessive activity – life seems without boundaries. In the depressive, the normal flow of thoughts becomes sluggish; in the manic, it is accelerated. The mood of the depressive is like stagnant water; that of the manic is overheated.

Obsessions and the lungs

Obsessional and compulsive illnesses are characterised by a fixed idea or recurrent action that dominates the patient's life. Commonly, these obsessional thoughts are associated with being dirty. For example, the idea that the hands must be dirty after touching something, and that an illness might be passed on to someone, may lead to a compulsion to wash continually. Often the idea is not completely groundless, but is exaggerated out of all proportion. In most cases, patients know that the idea is absurd but are unable to free themselves from it, as if the idea itself had become something solid and could not be dissolved. The fixity of the idea and the patient's inability to escape from it suggests that the solidity of the earthly element is expressed in such a condition.

It might at first appear unlikely that the earth element should have a special connection with the lung, which it would seem natural to link to the element of air. However, although the organ contains air, in its structure we find hard cartilage in the larynx and rings of cartilage forming the air passages. The air breathed into the lungs is separated from the blood by the thinnest of membranes. In this sense, the lung is the one organ where the physical (earth) environment virtually touches the interior of the body. The air breathed in has a cooling effect on the lung, keeping it at a lower temperature than most of the body, and this quality of coolness is also a characteristic of the earth element. Like the heart, the lung is in constant movement but, unlike the heart, its movement is passive. Breathing in is brought about by the expansion of the chest wall and flattening of the diaphragm – the lung's elastic fibres see to it that it passively contracts again to breathe out.

Many illnesses illustrate the lung's particular relationship to the mineral world and its associated susceptibility to hardening processes. They include silicosis, which is caused by inhaling rock dust containing silica, and the miners' lung disease pneumoconiosis. Hardening of the lung often accompanies long-term infections such as recurrent bronchitis or tuberculosis, which brings about the formation of calcified areas. The lung is the key to a healthy relationship between the soul and the earth element. An excessive mineral influence in the soul leads to the fixity of obsessive ideas and compulsive behaviour, whereas a lack gives rise to flights of fancy and a tendency to be *up in the clouds* rather than *down to earth.* Tuberculosis of the lung can produce the latter symptoms. Hospitals which specialised in tuberculosis in the days when it was more common, were known for their euphoric atmospheres, and the illness was a common affliction of gifted artists.

One patient who was treated at Park Attwood Clinic for obsessional, compulsive problems was a forty-six-year-old man who had first developed symptoms in his late teens. He was obsessively preoccupied with the ageing of his body and would compulsively clean his teeth for hours for fear that they might decay. His obsession with his teeth was part of a general fear that his body was beginning to age and degenerate. He had had psychoanalysis for many years, and could discuss at length his theories on what the symptoms meant and why he had the problem, but this didn't seem to make him any more able to deal with it. He felt that he had never had fun or allowed himself to behave spontaneously in his teens and twenties and thought it was vital to make up for lost time, which he saw in terms of having affairs with younger women. But, in the presence of attractive young women, he found he became very anxious and inhibited. A striking feature of his symptoms, which was not very typical of obsessive behaviour, was that he would become stuck or frozen in the middle of doing something, such as cleaning his teeth or eating in the presence of others, and would be unable to continue. When he had these inhibited phases, he would often withdraw to bed for a day at a time.

He was thin, with a large head and a rather gaunt, bony appearance. His skin was pale and wrinkled, and his temperature often as low as 35.5 °C (95.5 °F). He had a cold laugh, was rather cynical and had a tendency to talk at length about his problems. The coldness, pallor, over-intellectuality, large head and premature ageing point strongly to a preponderant activity of the nerve-sense pole, and his desire for spontaneity and sexual encounters could be seen as an attempt to compensate for this.

With this picture in mind, the aim of treatment was to bring about movement and warmth in his soul to counteract the fixity and coldness. Initially, there was very little counselling or psychotherapy and the emphasis was on physical treatments and artistic therapies. He was given a number of medicines which have a particular relationship to the lung or to the rhythmic system in general, eurythmy therapy and painting therapy. For the deep-seated coldness, he was given viscum treatment (see Chapter 13) and pyrogenic baths (see Chapter 8), a combination which had a dramatic effect. Immediately after the baths, when he appeared flushed, he was markedly less fixed in his behaviour, and his social contacts became more relaxed and natural. He began to notice that his feet and hands were generally warmer and his body temperature rose to about 36 °C (97 °F). Although his obsessional problems did not disappear, they became less frequent and less severe. Despite having found it very difficult at first to relate to the painting therapy, he later decided to pursue it as a long-term therapy. Ten years after the initial treatment, he was largely free from his obsessive problems and, looking back, felt that the medicines and baths had been especially beneficial.

Anxiety and the kidneys

The organ which has a special relationship to the airy element and the astral body is the kidney. The outer layer of the kidney contains minute, cup-shaped structures called glomeruli which begin the process of urine production. They are remarkable in that they not only have an oxygen-rich blood supply entering them via an artery, but also oxygen-rich blood leaving them again through a small artery. This double arterial connection is the opposite of the double venous connection found in the liver. The venous blood has a relatively low pressure and is slower moving. It is also rich in carbon dioxides indicating its association with the etheric body and the plant realm. The arterial supply has a powerful pulse and is rich in the oxygen needed for the combustion of sugars, indicating its association with the astral body and the animal realm. This association is reinforced by the effects of the two hormones produced by the kidney; erythropoietin and renin. The former increases the oxygen-carrying capacity of the blood, and renin stimulates the production of angiotensin, which is thought to maintain arterial blood pressure. The kidney function is dependent on a certain blood pressure being maintained, and kidney failure is one of the consequences if it falls below the minimum, as it can in cases of prolonged shock.

The strong relationship of the kidney to the astral body, and to psychiatric disorders, is even more apparent if the adrenal gland, which sits on the kidney, is brought into the picture. The central part of this gland comprises cells that are derived from nervous tissue. They produce adrenaline at times of stress, resulting in many of the symptoms of fear, such as a racing heart, trembling, and coolness in the peripheral parts of the body. The outer part of the adrenal gland produces steroids, which also have a relationship to stress in that part of their function appears to be protecting the body from the excesses of stress reactions. The sex hormones are chemically related to steroids, and the reproductive organs are themselves embryologically related to the kidney system. The anthroposophic concept of the kidney goes far beyond the physical organ and includes the spiritual activity associated with it, the adrenal glands and, to some extent, the reproductive organs as well. Similarly, the concept of the liver encompasses the totality of the anabolic processes in the body which, though concentrated in the liver, are by no means limited to that physical organ.

The kidney's association with the astral body makes it come to mind when a patient presents severe symptoms of anxiety and agitation. Anxiety, a psychiatric problem in its own right, is a very common disorder which often colours depression and is frequently found to be an element in schizophrenia. The patient in her mid-thirties described in Chapter 4 was suffering from depression and had marked symptoms of anxiety. She had great difficulty sleeping and the lower half of her body was extremely cold. With the kidney specifically in mind, copper ointment was applied over the kidney region and a homeopathic preparation of naturally occurring copper oxide, Cuprite D6, was given orally.[1] She also had mustard footbaths and oil-dispersion baths with lavender and arnica for the coldness. To strengthen the reproductive organs, she was given a mixture of herbs called Menodoron (see Chapter 14) and injections of Argentite D10 (silver ore) under the skin. Her depression was treated with a liver medicine, Stannum per Taraxicum (tin potentised using dandelion).

At first, the main emphasis was on these medical treatments, although her anxiety was initially so extreme that, for a time, she also needed conventional sedatives. Later, she progressed to therapies such as eurythmy and painting. In the latter, she had an experience which she found to be very therapeutic when working on a series of paintings consisting of sunset, night sky and various stages of sunrise. The transition from light to darkness was accompanied by a letting go of her fixed ideas about herself. The gradual return to light through the stages of sunrise brought with it an increasing sense of identity and self-worth. Her recovery from the severe anxiety and depression proved to be an important turning-point in her life.

Rage, guilt and the heart

Just as the astral body has a special connection with the kidney, the I is associated with the heart. The I often has to resolve inner conflicts when, for example, instinctive drives are found to be incompatible with personal ideals. In this sense, the I tries to harmonise the opposing elements in the soul – the instinctive drives associated with the unconscious metabolic pole, and the ideals associated with the conscious reasoning of the head pole. The heart has the comparable role of harmonising the physical activity of the two poles in the body.

The heart is the central organ of the rhythmic system and is positioned within the chest cavity, where the head and metabolic poles meet. It fills on expansion (diastole) and empties on contraction (systole), setting up a rhythmic pulse. It is also the central point of the circulation – blood flows from the whole body towards the heart, then to the lungs and back to the heart, before flowing out to all parts of the body again. The rhythmic system as a whole is associated with feelings, and the heart is the traditional symbol of love.

The natural element associated with the I and the heart is fire. The I gives us a continuing sense of identity, despite the soul's changing thoughts, emotions and urges. It carries responsibility for our actions and steers our course through life, and in this sense is responsible for both the past and future. Two faculties that are characteristic of the human I reflect this – conscience and courage. In so far as we are aware of a responsibility for the past, this is carried within us as conscience, while it takes moral courage to face the future.

It is perhaps connected with the fact that the spirit itself cannot be ill that the heart does not give rise to a specific psychiatric illness, as do the

Human element	Natural element	Organ	Psychiatric symptom
I	Fire	Heart (and gall bladder)	Rage, guilt (and mania)
Astral body	Air	Kidney	Anxiety
Etheric body	Water	Liver	Depression
Physical body	Earth	Lung	Obsession

Figure 10.

kidney, liver and lung. Rather, it colours the illnesses of the other three organs, when the two faculties of conscience and courage become distorted. Conscience should be a spur to learn from past mistakes but, if someone is totally weighed down by guilt over past actions, this becomes harmful. Guilt can be seen as pathological distortion of conscience and, although it is not recognised as a psychiatric illness in its own right, it can be a major factor in illnesses such as depression.

The other faculty, courage, which gives us the strength to strive onward into the future, is lost in severe depression when patients can be so bound up with the past that they cannot relate to the future at all. Courage may then be expressed in a distorted, destructive way in rage, when the will to act is overpowering and beyond the control of the I. Rage and violent outbursts sometimes feature in mania and catatonic schizophrenia, but they can also be a problem in everyday life without being symptoms of a psychiatric illness. Some people are prone to swing between rage and deep guilt for what they have done, and this points particularly to a need for the moderating and harmonising qualities of the I and the heart.

Treatment of psychiatric symptoms which point to the heart includes medicines such as homeopathically prepared gold (aurum) and Onopordon comp., a mixture of *Onopordon acanthium* (cotton thistle), *Hyoscyamus niger* (henbane), and *Primula officinalis* (cowslip). This combination represents a harmonious balance of catabolic and anabolic forces. Artistic therapies can also be used to support the rhythmic system and to help restore a proper balance between the two poles. Therapeutic massage, too, may be used to reinforce the heart's harmonising activity. Such therapies would accompany treatment aimed at the other main organ involved. For example, if severe guilt formed part of a patient's depression, the heart would be treated as well as the liver.

Drug addiction

Some drugs are able to produce dramatic psychological effects through their direct biochemical action on the physical organs. The effects vary with different drugs but anthroposophic doctors consider that they all affect the total constitution – I, astral body, etheric body and physical body. Amphetamines (or speed) produce rapid thinking and hyperactivity but damage the etheric body, leading to a lack of vitality and will power. LSD gives rise to powerful hallucinations which are caused by a slight separation of the etheric body from the physical body. Marijuana has a similar but less extreme effect. Heroin completely blocks out any sense of guilt or shame. It dislocates the I from the rest of the constitution, causing the astral body to be dominated by instinctive desires. Addiction can remove any sense of conscience, with the whole life revolving around getting the next 'fix'.

A healthy path of inner development eventually leads to powerful experiences of the spiritual realms, including perception of the etheric and astral forces at work within oneself. In this sense, deeper self-knowledge is a prerequisite for true spiritual perception, however painful it might be. Becoming conscious of the astral forces within one's soul is usually a frightening experience, even for someone who is well-prepared. If it is brought about without proper preparation, it can be shattering. Initially, the experiences produced by taking LSD can seem wonderful but, sooner or later, a 'bad trip' occurs, when these inner astral forces are directly confronted.

There are anthroposophic centres for treating drug addiction, one in Germany called Siebenzwerge, and some in the Netherlands (see 'Anthroposophic hospitals, clinics and general practitioners' in the Appendix). Co-workers at Arta, a former centre in the Netherlands, have found that it is rare for addicts to take the decision to 'kick the habit' before the age of twenty-one, roughly the age at which the forces of the I become partially freed from their unconscious activity. Treatment is based on the conception that the addict's whole constitution is damaged by the drug abuse. The phases of childhood described in Chapter 10 show how the etheric body, astral body and I are emancipated at the end of each of the seven-year periods.

At Arta, the treatment programme was based on a recapitulation of these phases in order to rebuild each of the constitutional elements. Also, it was found that the medical and therapeutic work must be combined with social support to be successful – neither approach is sufficient on its own.

The first phase of treatment focused on the physical body with the physical withdrawal from use of the drugs. This was undertaken on small farms or small-holdings where five co-workers lived and worked with seven addicts, referred to as residents. They had a strict, rhythmic timetable and there was an emphasis on physical nutrition and work. They had a balanced wholefood diet and regular times when they did gardening or worked with animals. This phase usually lasted about seven weeks, during which they were given a great deal of guidance and support by the co-workers.

The second phase put the emphasis on emotional nutrition. The residents moved into the main building at Arta where they lived as a community, again with a number of co-workers. They were still prevented from leaving the centre or obtaining drugs. There was a strong emphasis on all kinds of artistic activity, group discussions and much personal conversation. All residents were involved in the household chores to reawaken an awareness of the practical necessities of everyday life. There was an environment of cultural nutrition similar to that which should be provided by school for children in the seven to fourteen phase, and there was still plenty of guidance from co-workers.

Having spent some time without drugs, the residents found that they became more emotionally vulnerable, as their feelings were no longer suppressed by the drug taking. Very often, it turned out that they were emotionally and culturally deprived in childhood, and this period could be of great benefit to them by providing the cultural enrichment and emotional support that they had always lacked. Although they were likely to be receiving anthroposophic medication and therapies during this stage, the main emphasis was on group experience. Most of the therapeutic artistic and practical activities were performed all together.

In the next stage, which relates to the fourteen to twenty-one phase, the emphasis shifted to individual responsibility and independence. Each resident now had weekly conversations with a counsellor, and the therapies used become directed to their individual needs. Having to make decisions again, residents often felt they were back where they were before they started to take drugs.

The fourth stage, relating to the twenty-one to twenty-eight phase, was entered only after the resident had been at the centre for at least twelve months. Leaving the premises unescorted was now allowed and residents handled their money for themselves. They took work or training placements outside Arta and assumed a certain amount of responsibility for newcomers at the centre.

While the various stages formed a framework for the programme at Arta, they were not a fixed, rigid structure. The programme tried to take account of the individual needs of the resident as a person with a soul and a spirit, rather than treating the problem purely as inappropriate behaviour, as do addiction centres based on behavioural therapy. Typically, behavioural therapy centres have success rates of between ten and fifteen per cent, whereas Arta, with its more comprehensive approach, was able to report a fifty-two per cent success rate.

As has been seen, when treating illnesses with physical symptoms, anthroposophic doctors look for the cause in the astral body and I so that they may deal with that as well as the physical symptoms themselves. In the same way, treatment of illnesses with mental and emotional symptoms is based on an understanding of the related disorders of the physical and etheric bodily processes.

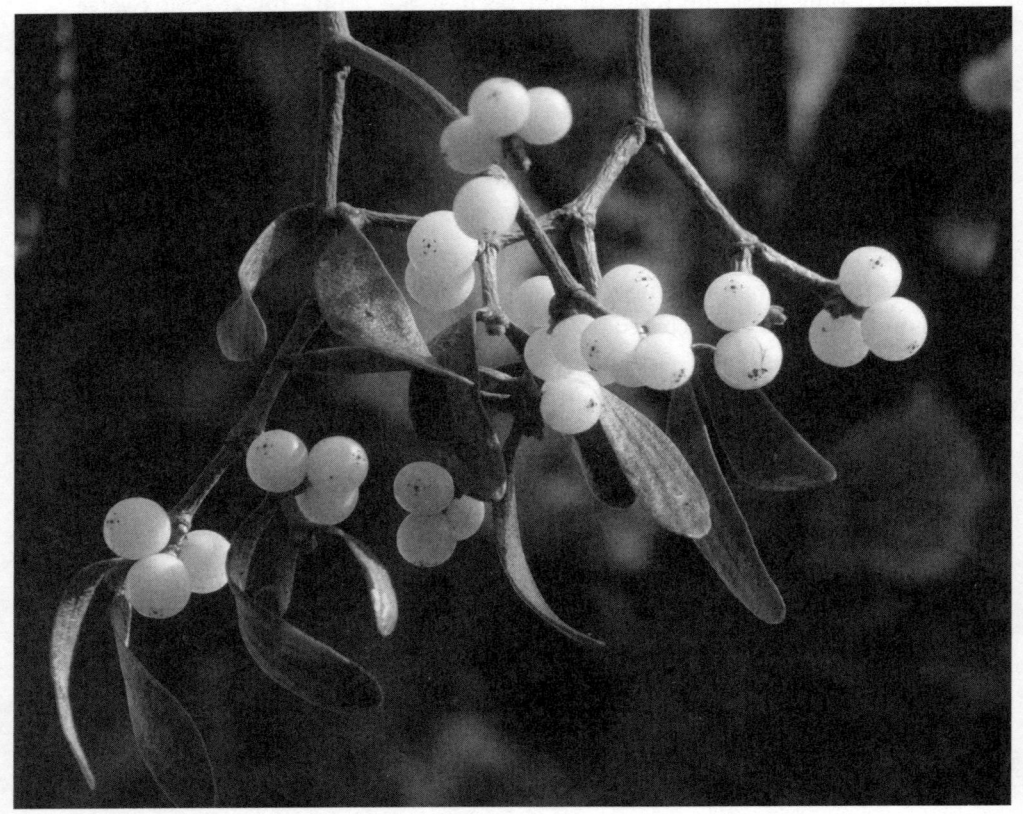

Mistletoe.

13. Immunity, Cancer and Mistletoe

The immune system protects the physical body from invading organisms and harmful substances. It helps to ensure that the body's life processes remain dominant and are not hindered by the foreign processes of other organisms. The most obvious barrier to the outside world is the skin, but the lining of the gut and the airways of the nose and lungs also act as barriers when food or air are taken into the body. These are complemented by the immune system, which recognises foreign substances inside the body and activates processes to render them harmless or destroy them.

The recognition of what is *foreign* to the body requires the ability to distinguish between human and animal, plant or mineral substances, and also between its own body and other human material. The immune processes are not only guardians of the human organism, but also an expression of the unique identity of each person. In this sense, they are connected with the activity of the I. Two major illnesses are related to the immune system – Aids (acquired immune deficiency syndrome) and cancer. In Aids, immunity breaks down, leaving the body vulnerable to massive infections of a sort not usually experienced by humans. In cancer, normal cells start behaving as if they were foreign to the organism and undermine the body from within.

The skin

Of the outer barriers to foreign substances, the skin is very effective against viruses and bacteria and is breached only when an area has been damaged or weakened. Even the human immunodeficiency virus (HIV), which causes Aids, cannot invade the body if the skin and related boundary structures remain intact. Although it does not need to be able to sense foreign forms of life, the skin has many qualities related to the nerve-sense processes of the body. It is sensitive to temperature, touch and pain, and for this reason is rightly regarded as an extensive sense organ. It also expresses the individual's identity in the sense that its markings, such as fingerprints, are unique to each person.

The breaking-down effect of nerve-sense activity and its opposite, the upbuilding of the metabolic system, form a duality which can be described as the death forces (nerve-sense) on the one hand, and the life forces (metabolic) on the other. The deadening physical effect of nerve-sense activity plays an essential part in the function of the skin. In the deeper layers, which are in close contact with the blood capillaries, skin cells rapidly reproduce. The new cells migrate upwards, gradually losing their rounded shape and their capacity to divide. They become flattened and the cytoplasm (the part of the cell surrounding the nucleus) fills with a protein called keratin. This hardens the cells and, as they die on reaching the outermost layers, they remain hard, with the keratin within them. These cells provide a tough barrier to the outer world and the dead, keratin-filled layers become particularly thick where the skin is exposed to constant abrasion, such as on the soles of the feet.

The health of the skin depends on the maintenance of a proper balance between the vital reproductive activity of the deeper layers and the deadening nearer the surface. Many skin problems, such as eczema, result from these two processes falling out of balance. When the metabolic (life) processes predominate, the inflammatory, wet phase of eczema occurs. It is in this phase that the skin can become infected because there is no longer a protective layer of hardened cells. In the dry, scaly phase of eczema, the nerve-sense (death) processes are predominant. Other moist, protective surfaces, such as those lining the gut and parts of the genitals, also have a reproductive layer and a progressive differentiation of the cells as they migrate towards the surface, but without the production of a final horny, keratinised outer layer. When this deadening process fails to occur, and the migrating cells retain their ability to reproduce, there is an increased risk of cancer. It is the detection of a loss of this differentiation in the outer layers of cells that underlies cervical smear screening, enabling treatment to be given before malignant changes take place.

The skin provides what is called a non-specific defence against substances outside. Another aspect of non-specific immunity is the ability to develop high fevers. An increase in body temperature from 37 to 39 °C (98.5 to 102 °F) is sufficient to kill a number of foreign micro-organisms and also stimulates the rest of the immune system. The white blood cells, capable of engulfing and digesting bacteria and viruses, add a third line of defence. These cells (neutrophils and macrophages) are able to migrate out of the blood vessels and are often found close to the skin and other protective surfaces. They are capable of attacking micro-organisms whether they have encountered them before or not, but they are not as effective at killing viruses as a fourth element of the immune system, called acquired immunity, which has to be developed to combat specific viruses.

Blood cells

Several types of white blood cells called lymphocytes are particularly involved in acquired immunity. For example, B-lymphocytes produce antibodies against specific micro-organisms and the poisons they create, whereas T-lymphocytes (named thus because they mature in the thymus) kill foreign organisms directly and also stimulate the production of more B-lymphocytes. The responses of these cells are geared to the unique chemical composition of the invading micro-organisms. Once the infection has been dealt with, a small number of cells specifically adapted to fight that type of micro-organism remain as a kind of memory. On further infection, they help to produce specific T-cells much more quickly, and the body is then said to be immune to that particular illness.

The way the white blood cells engulf and digest the foreign micro-organisms is closely related to the catabolic processes in the digestion of food. Similar enzymes are produced to do the breaking down in each case. The white cells' ability to 'sense' foreign substances also relates their activity to the catabolic nerve-sense system. Recent discoveries have shown that the immune system can be stimulated or inhibited by the nervous system, and the relationship can also work the other way. The lymphocytes can themselves influence the nervous system by, for example, inducing sleep.

The immune and nervous systems and the production of hormones are now seen to be so closely interrelated that they are often referred to as the neuro-immuno-endocrine system.

HIV

The white blood cells with the central function of searching for invading micro-organisms and initiating the development of cells to produce antibodies are the T-lymphocytes, and they are the key to overcoming new types of infection. It is these T-cells that are attacked and destroyed by the human immunodeficiency virus (HIV). The virus insinuates itself into a host cell's genetic material and remains dormant until another virus stimulates the infected T-cell to multiply itself. Instead of reproducing itself, it creates large numbers of new HIVs which are released into the blood as the T-cell dies. They are attracted to T-cells, and also to other white blood cells and nerve cells, so the process is then repeated on a larger scale. Another effect of the HIV is to cause as many as fifty T-cells to fuse together, rendering them inactive. The virus avoids complete destruction by antibodies by regularly changing the chemical composition of its protein coat. This makes a second HIV infection invulnerable to the large numbers of antibodies produced in response to the first infection. Not only is it therefore impossible to become immune to the HIV, but a latent tendency to develop Aids may be triggered in an infected patient when the T-cells attempt to multiply to deal with a later infection, leading to the production of further HIVs.

Outside the body, the HIV is quite fragile and is easily destroyed. It cannot penetrate the skin, and infection is transmitted only by an exchange of body fluids. At the time of writing, it was known that it could be passed on by infected blood, semen or vaginal fluid. The main ways this has happened are through sexual intercourse, when body fluids have passed from one person to another via small cuts or abrasions, through the sharing of needles by addicts injecting drugs intravenously, from the blood of an infected mother to her unborn baby, and through blood transfusions, which took place before it was known that this could transmit the virus.

The main result of HIV infection is a marked depletion in the number of T-cells. In an attempt to compensate, the B-cells become hyperactive, but the antibodies they make are incapable of destroying the HIV. Antibodies are produced which would defend the body against all the infections previously encountered but, because of the deficiency of T-cells, the body remains vulnerable to new infections. This means that HIV-positive adults keep their immunity to common human infections but become susceptible to animal viruses. They might get pneumonia from *Pneumocystis carinii,* which normally infects rats, or another form of pneumonia from *Mycobacterium avium,* which causes tuberculosis in birds. They are also vulnerable to parasitic micro-organisms that normally live on cats, dogs and cattle. In addition to this, infections which are normally localised, such as thrush (a common infection of the mouth in children and the vagina in adults), can become rampant throughout the gastro-intestinal tract.

Aids

HIV infection may remain dormant for some time, but when it progresses to the point when the immune system breaks down the patient is said to have developed Aids. Rampant infections can then have a very debilitating effect on the body. The areas that may become infected include the mouth, the gut, the lungs with various forms of pneumonia, and the skin – in other words, all the boundaries of the body are attacked. In its interference with the genetic material of T-cells, the HIV attacks perhaps the most physical expression of human individuality. An Aids patient has short periods of fever, which are quite different from the sustained high fevers of other infections. Unlike the sustained fever, which is part of a healing process, they are chaotic, indicating the inability of the I to bring about a healing effect through the medium of warmth. Perhaps as a result of the infection of the nervous system, or perhaps because of exhaustion, in the latter stages of the illness, Aids patients have poor concentration and weakened short-term memory. This again indicates interference with the activity of the I, as does the inability of patients to express themselves through gestures or facial expressions, which tend to become blank.

These phenomena indicate that the HIV destroys the body's ability to be a suitable vehicle for the I, or spirit. It is expressed most acutely in the killing of the T-cells, which normally play the key role in distinguishing self from non-self when encountering new infections. This marks out the HIV as a destroyer of the physical guardian of the human identity – the immune system. Not only does it interfere with the activity of the I in the body, but it also makes the body vulnerable to attack by a multitude of diseases that would normally be found only in animals.

Cancer

As described in Chapter 2, cancer occurs when cells in a part of the body stop limiting their growth in accordance with the normal behaviour of the tissue concerned. When the growth reaches the point when it breaks through the boundaries of the tissues in which it originated, this is taken as a sign of malignancy. It may then leave the organ of origin and travel around the body via the blood or other fluids to form further tumours called metastases. In remaining relatively undifferentiated and reproducing without restraint, the cancerous cells behave more like isolated cells living in a nutrient medium outside the body than as integrated parts of a complex organism.

About ninety-five per cent of all malignant tumours arise in surface tissue, such as the skin, the lining of the gut, and the linings of glands like the breasts. The remaining five per cent mainly originate in the muscles, bones and blood vessels. Much research has been done into cellular changes in the surface tissues, which may be intermediate stages between healthy tissues and malignant growths. In the case of the cervix (the neck of the womb) the tissue layers are similar to those in skin, except that the uppermost layers do not become as hard, although the cells do flatten and stop reproducing as they migrate upwards. Under normal circumstances, the nuclei gradually shrink as the cells migrate. By the time they reach the surface, the nuclei have disappeared and the cells are completely flat.

When this process breaks down, the cells retain their large nuclei and their ability to divide as they migrate. While these cells remain in the original tissue, it is not yet cancer, but there is a far greater risk of cancer developing. The basal layer of cells rests on a thin membrane. If this membrane is breached by the cells, this is an indication that cancer has developed. Similar changes to these are thought to take place prior to malignant tumours arising in other tissues, such as the lining of the large bowel, which is a common site of cancer.

It can be seen that a first stage leading to the possible development of cancer occurs when cells retain their reproductive ability and do not undergo a process of differentiation as they migrate through the layers of protective tissue. They retain their vitality and do not undergo a death process. In the next stage, when the tumour becomes malignant, it has to develop its own blood circulation to continue living and growing beyond a few millimetres across. It has been found that the tumours are able to attract the development of blood capillaries from outside the tissue of origin so that these grow into the tumour. This process of developing new blood vessels is called neoangiogenesis and is another characteristic of malignant growths. This enables further, much larger growth to take place and, later, cells from the tumour might break away and give rise to further growths elsewhere in the body.

Anthroposophic medicine sees the life processes originating in the etheric body as expansive, undifferentiated growth activity. But the human form is imposed upon that activity by the I, working through the astral body into the etheric body. This exerts a limiting effect on what would otherwise be formless growth. Differentiated growth – in which the cells change form as they divide to follow the human template – requires that the tendency of the cells to reproduce towards formless growth is held in check.

In the pre-cancerous stage, the form-giving death process breaks down. Cancer arises when the tumour breaches the boundaries of the original tissue. So, from an anthroposophic view, cancer represents the autonomous working of the etheric and physical bodies, without the controlling influence of the I, which bears the human image. The therapeutic aim, therefore, is to find ways of stimulating the form-giving activity of the I so that it regains mastery over the growth processes. The plant mistletoe *(Viscum album)* displays certain unique features which indicate its suitability for this task.

Mistletoe is semi-parasitic, growing on trees and drawing water and minerals from its host. Like other green plants, it is capable of photosynthesis but, in contrast, it is unable to transport sugars and has chlorophyll spread throughout its tissues, enabling it to synthesise sugars wherever they are needed. Its leaves have a simple form which changes very little during growth, and, unlike most leaves, have no difference between their upper and lower surfaces. These characteristics suggest a relatively undifferentiated nature, and this is found again in the flowers, which are so uninteresting that it is difficult to imagine how insects are attracted to pollinate the plant. Even the seeds within the familiar white translucent berries are relatively undifferentiated and, deprived of the light which passes through the berries, the seeds die within a few days.

The majority of plants respond to gravity by the upper part growing vertically into a main stem, with branches growing from it. This is evident from the first shoots, with the primary leaf always growing upwards, and the first root downwards, irrespective of how the seed lies in the ground. The mistletoe grows spherically from where it is attached to the host tree. Initially the stems grow vertically but, once established, they spread in all directions, as if the plant withdraws from any relationship to gravity. Mistletoe is also inhibited with respect to time. Unlike most plants, it begins to develop the organs of its flowers at the same time as its leaves, but the flower itself does not appear until the third year. Its cycles of activity are so slowed that the rhythm of the seasons has little influence on it. These rather primitive qualities and the way the mistletoe holds back from taking on a more specialised form are reminiscent of the way the human formative forces also hold back from specialisation to retain versatility (see Chapter 2). It is this human formative principle that is weakened in cancer. The fact that mistletoe holds back its own development so strongly suggests that it may strengthen this characteristically human formative principle, and offer an effective treatment for cancer.

Medicinal preparations of mistletoe *(Viscum album)* for treating cancer were first made in the 1920s following suggestions by Steiner. They have since been developed by six different companies. The most well known of the current remedies is Iscador, manufactured by the Hiscia Institute at Arlesheim, in Switzerland. Other mistletoe preparations include Viscum Abnoba, Helixor and Iscusin. A considerable body of scientific literature exists documenting its laboratory testing and clinical use in treating cancer patients. Research has shown that mistletoe preparations stimulate the growth of the thymus gland, where the T-cells develop. It has also been shown to stimulate the production of antibodies when the organism faces injected foreign material. More recently it has been shown in the laboratory to suppress the influence of cancer genes and render tumour cells less aggressive. It has also be shown to have some toxic properties to living cells and enhance atoptosis. (Apoptosis is the process by which body cells die in a way that their content is recycled by neighbouring cells. It is considered to be a normal activity of healthy tissues and is very different from cell death due to damage which is usually accompanied by local inflammatory reactions.)

Cancer cells show less tendency to apoptosis which is part of their biologically dominating characteristics. Mistletoe has also be demonstrated to inhibit neoangiogenesis one of the fundamental behaviours of cancer tissues described above. It has been repeated shown to be a powerful immunostimulant affecting many aspects of the immune system. It is administered by injection under the skin as it is considered less active taken by mouth. It can particularly at the start of treatment cause a moderate fever. This is welcomed as an additional stimulus to the immune system.

In the past there were many clinical studies of the use of mistletoe preparations in the treatment of many types of malignant tumour. These initial studies, although encouraging, were not double-blind trials, the standard method used by conventional medicine. More recently there have been a number of randomised controlled clinical trials with positive results. The most recent positive trial was with patients with advanced pancreas cancer who had a very poor prognosis. Patients usually only live a matter of months after the diagnosis. The patients in the mistletoe-treated group lived on average around twice as long as those randomised to the group which did not receive mistletoe. In a parallel study of the quality of life, mistletoe-treated patients also showed a reduction in symptoms and improved quality of life compared to the control group.[1]

One very large controlled trial with a positive outcome was run by Professor Grossarth-Maticek of Heidelberg University. He not only demonstrated an improved survival over a large range of cancers with patients advised to take mistletoe but also positive psychological changes.[2]

As a psychologist as well as a public health researcher, Grossarth-Maticek has done extensive research in what keeps people healthy – *salutogenesis*. One of his psychological measurements associated with better health is a 'sense of coherence'. By this he means a person's sense of meaning in life and their belief that they can affect positive life changes themselves. It could be thought of as the opposite of feeling a victim of life. People with a high sense of coherence are less likely to be addicted to nicotine or alcohol and so the positive effect of their attitude and feeling is multiplied by their healthier lifestyle. As anthroposophic medicine is concerned with healing for the body, soul and spirit, Grossarth-Maticek found it of great interest that not only did this treatment improve physical survival, but the sense of coherence of patients treated with mistletoe significantly improved. As the sense of coherence measures both feelings and fundamental attitudes to life it can be seen as a measure of soul and spiritual wellbeing.

A number of anthroposophic cancer specialists use a combination of remedies at the start of mistletoe treatment with the aim of inducing a fever. They consider that this is likely to contribute to greater efficacy. They also inject viscum directly into more superficial tumours such as breast cancers before the lump has been surgically removed. The theory behind this is that the immune system does not recognise the cancer. The cancer cells avoid the body's healthy immune surveillance. Treatment into the tumour itself when it is still present, may 'alert' the immune system to tumour cells.

Although there are some cases of tumours completely resolving with mistletoe treatment, this is not generally the case. There is no suggestion that the current viscum treatments are miracle cures, however, there is growing evidence that they can prolong life and reduce the risk of the cancer spreading. They are also free from the very unpleasant side effects of most conventional cancer drugs.

Although there is some evidence of a unique anti-tumour action, their main effect is to mobilise and strengthen aspects of the patient's immune system so that it is better able to oppose the cancer itself. They strengthen the form-giving activity of the I, and this can be further supported by eurythmy therapy, artistic therapies and counselling. They can be used alongside conventional treatments such as surgery, radiotherapy and chemotherapy, and there is growing evidence that they help patients to withstand the damaging effects of these forms of treatment and generally improve quality of life. They can help patients with the emotional challenge of what still remains an understandably frightening diagnosis.

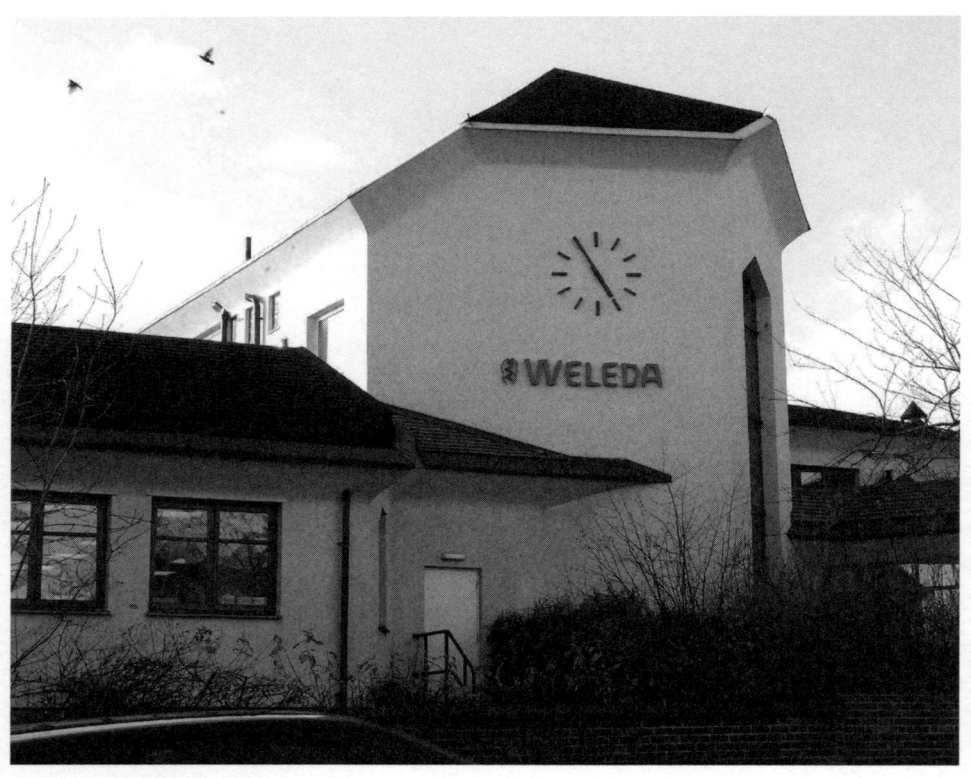

Weleda, UK, Ilkeston.

14. The Medicines

At the heart of anthroposophic medicine lies the doctor's extended view of illness, and the natural substances which can be used as remedies. The preparation of a medicine is just as important as the choice of the substance itself. Methods of preparation are used which are designed to accentuate the substance's therapeutic properties, and anthroposophic doctors work in close collaboration with pharmacists to develop appropriate methods. Traditional pharmaceutical and homeopathic techniques are used, but new methods have also been introduced as a result of this collaboration.

Great care is always taken in collecting and harvesting raw materials – whether animal, plant or mineral. When plants need to be cultivated, rather than gathered from the wild, they are grown using the methods of biodynamic farming and gardening. This is a development of organic practice which uses anthroposophic knowledge of the relationship between spirit and matter to strengthen the growth of plants and animals. Biodynamic farming and gardening is free from additives, hormones and chemicals, and makes beneficial use of the effects of the natural cycles of the sun, the moon and the seasons.[1]

Potentisation

One of the new pharmaceutical processes is a development of the homeopathic principle of potentisation, through which the non-physical qualities of a substance are released to be used therapeutically. In homeopathic potentisation, a small quantity of the material is repeatedly dissolved in water, or alcohol and water, and is succussed (vigorously shaken) for a prescribed period at each stage of the dilution. Steiner suggested that the process could be aided by having plants absorb the materials to be potentised. The substance is introduced into the soil in which given plants are growing. These are later harvested and composted, and a second generation of plants is grown on the composted material. The process is repeated, and the third generation is used to prepare a medicine.

Anthroposophic pharmacy also makes use of selected temperatures in the preparation of medicines. In classical homeopathic pharmacy, medicines are made from plants by finely chopping the material and mixing it with alcohol and water. The mixture is allowed to stand in temperatures below 20 °C (68 °F) for at least five days before being filtered. This produces the mother tincture which is used to start the process of potentisation.

In anthroposophic practice, the temperature of preparation is varied according to the particular medicine. Aconite, which bears qualities of coldness allied to the head forces, is prepared at a cool temperature. By contrast, birch leaves, which are used to overcome hardening and sclerosis, are prepared at around 90 °C (195 °F). Medicines with a particular affinity to the middle, rhythmic system – such as Crataegus, which strengthens the heart – are prepared at the mean human temperature of about 37 °C (98.5 °F). The link between warmth and the I has already been described and, in this sense, the attention paid to the temperature of preparation can be seen as helping to relate the medicines specifically to humans. Cooking food and using fire are exclusively human activities, and cooked food is considered to be more fit for humans to eat.

As was seen in the previous chapter, the special qualities of mistletoe make it suitable for treating illnesses in which the stamp of human identity is lost, such as cancer and Aids. But a very complex method of preparation is required, involving mixing winter and summer sap by adding drops of one to a fine film of the other on a rapidly spinning disc. There is also a controlled fermentation process. At least three research institutes are working independently on optimising a method of preparing mistletoe extracts for treating cancer, based on indications given in 1920 by Steiner. At least one method produced a medicine containing lectins, a group of substances which are thought by immunologists to stimulate the appropriate immune responses in the body. There is also some evidence that lectins are found in relatively higher concentrations in the higher potencies of mistletoe (i.e. more diluted). It is thought that they are less stable in the lower potencies and degenerate more rapidly. Although the special techniques for preparing mistletoe involve considerable technology, most of the methods of anthroposophic pharmacy are more akin to those of traditional pharmacy, and are often done by hand.

The development of anthroposophic pharmacy began with a single pharmacist, Otto Schmiedel, working in Arlesheim, Switzerland, next door to the clinic where Ita Wegman and Rudolf Steiner were collaborating on the founding of anthroposophic medicine. The laboratory he set up grew into the medicines manufacturer, Weleda, which now has branches in over forty countries around the world. Many of these branches make the medicines from plants gathered in their own countries. For example, Weleda (UK) Ltd, at Ilkeston in England, has its own extensive herb gardens where many of the medicinal substances are grown.

The work of Rudolf Hauschka, who developed methods of preparation of medicines which avoided the use of alcohol, led to the establishment of a second anthroposophic pharmaceutical company, Wala. This is based at Bad Boll, in southern Germany, and its products are distributed worldwide. The development of mistletoe preparations for the treatment of cancer was pioneered by the Hiscia Institute in Switzerland, which makes the most widely known medicine, Iscador. At the time of writing, Iscador was the only mistletoe preparation licensed in the UK (though this licence may soon be lost). Two newer research institutes, Abnoba and Helixor, have developed their own cancer medicines from mistletoe. These are licensed in Germany and marketed as Viscum Abnoba and Helixor. They are prescribed by doctors in the UK (and imported) on a named patient basis.

Home remedies

Often, an anthroposophic doctor's prescription is highly individualised to reflect the particular spiritual and physical constitution of the patient. This is particularly likely to be the case when homeopathically potentised metals are given. However, in certain disorders, the prescription is specific to the particular illness or symptoms. For example, Combudoron is a combination of arnica and urtica designed for the treatment of burns, and Avena Sativa comp. is a mixture of herbal and homeopathically prepared ingredients put together specifically to help in cases of sleeplessness. A number of the medicines designed for specific illnesses and symptoms could be prescribed by any doctor, without detailed knowledge of anthroposophic medicine. In Central Europe, where doctors are more open to the use of natural medicines, many do just that. Some of these medicines are also safe to be sold over the counter to patients who treat themselves without consulting a doctor.

Many small accidents and minor illnesses can be treated that way. Patients are encouraged by conventional doctors and drug companies to use aspirins or cough medicines on their own, and anthroposophic physicians can similarly recommend a number of medicines as household remedies. The following is a selection of such remedies, which could make up a very useful home medicine chest.

Unless otherwise stated, the medicines should be taken at least twenty minutes before or after meals or drinks, if possible. Pills should be dissolved in the mouth rather than swallowed whole.

Amara drops

Mixture of herbal bitters, including gentian (*Gentiana lutea*), chicory (*Chicorium intybus*), wormwood (*Artemisia absinthium*) and yarrow (*Achillea millefolium*).

Use to treat nausea and to improve poor appetite. Take fifteen drops in very little water every few hours (nausea), or about twenty minutes before food (lack of appetite).

Arnica

Homeopathic potency of leopard's bane (*Arnica montana*).

Use in potency D6 (also called 6x) following shock, either physical or emotional. One tablet every hour.

Arnica lotion

For external use, one dessertspoon in 250 ml (2 cups) of water to make compresses for treating sprains and bruises.

Arnica ointment

Can also be used externally for sprains and bruises. Massage well into the affected area twice daily or as required.

Avena Sativa comp.

Mixture of common valerian (*Valeriana officinalis*), passion flower (*Passiflora incarnata*), hops, oats and a high homeopathic potency of coffee.

Use for insomnia, particularly when caused by nervous restlessness. Twenty to thirty drops in a little water, half an hour before bed.

Balsamicum ointment

Contains marigold (*Calendula*), dog's mercury (*Mercurialis perennis*), Peru balsam-tree (*Myroxylon peruiferum*) and antimony (*stibium*).

A general ointment for wounds. Particularly useful for poorly-healing wounds and infected spots and boils. Can also be used for treating certain forms of eczema and dermatitis. Apply to the affected area directly, or on a dry dressing, two or three times a day.

Bidor

Iron sulphate (ferrous sulphate) and quartz (silica).

For the prevention or treatment of migraine and tension headaches, and the nausea that may accompany them. Bidor's action is directed at harmonising the fundamental imbalance of the nervous and metabolic systems, which is at the root of the headache, rather than acting as a painkiller. It has none of the side effects which can accompany the use of painkillers and other conventional anti-migraine medication. Treatment is often required to continue for some time to be fully effective.

To prevent migraine attacks, Bidor 1%, one tablet daily for three months. During an attack, Bidor 5%, one or two tablets every half-hour or hour until symptoms are relieved, up to a maximum of twenty tablets in a twelve-hour period. The tablets are swallowed whole with water.

Calendula ointment and lotion

Prepared from an alcoholic extract of marigold (*Calendula*).

Useful for minor abrasions, nappy rash, sore nipples and dry eczema. The ointment is applied at least twice a day, either directly to the skin or on a dry dressing. The lotion is diluted in boiled water which has cooled, one teaspoon to a glass of water. It is useful as a soak for skin infections and poorly-healing wounds. May also be used as a compress on a dressing for wet or infected eczema, or for other areas of infected skin which cannot easily be held under water.

Camomile root

A homeopathic potency of camomile root (*Matricaria chamomilla*).

Particularly useful for treating children's teething pains. Use in potency D3 (also called 3x), two drops in a little water, or two pills, hourly as required. For babies, the pills may be dissolved in a teaspoon of water. Also useful for abdominal cramps, whether associated with stomach upsets and diarrhoea or with cramp-like period pains. Ten drops in a little water, or five pills, every two to three hours until symptoms subside.

Camomile tea

Dried camomile flowers.

For cramp-like pains, from upset stomach or from period pains. Also useful in supporting the treatment of cystitis, when it can be very soothing as well as helping to provide the necessary large fluid intake. Add a half-teaspoon of flowers to 250 ml (2 cups) of boiling water and strain after three minutes. Drink a mugful every few hours, without milk or sugar.

Carvon tablets

Mixture of birch charcoal (*Carbo betulae*) and caraway seed oil.

For flatulence. Take one to two tablets straight after meals.

Cinnabar/Pyrites

A naturally occurring oxide of mercury (cinnabar) in homeopathic potency D20 and iron sulphide (pyrites) in potency D3.

For sore throats. Dissolve one tablet in the mouth, up to five times a day.

Combudoron ointment and lotion

Combination of leopard's bane (*Arnica montana*) and the small nettle (*Urtica urens*).

Designed for the treatment of burns. Has been found to be most valuable for first and second-degree burns, scalds, sunburn, inflamed insect bites and wasp stings. The lotion is diluted in water, approximately one part to ten, for bathing or compresses. It should be applied as soon as possible after a burn and regularly thereafter for a few days. In minor cases, the ointment applied locally may be more convenient.

Copper ointment

Promotes the circulation in hands and feet when coldness is noted. Massage well in, twice a day. Care should be taken as the ointment can mark fabrics – an old pair of socks might prove useful when treating the feet.

Cough elixir

Contains extracts of aniseed (*Pimpinella anisum*), marsh-mallow root (*Althaea officinalis*), white horehound (*Marrubium vulgare*) and thyme (*Thymus vulgaris*), and homeopathic potencies of sundew (*Drosera*), Brazil root (*Cephaelis ipecacuanha*) and pasque flower (*Pulsatilla vulgaris*).

Soothing expectorant for coughs, especially when caused by head colds. One teaspoon every three hours, either neat or in a little water.

Massage balm

Contains leopard's bane (*Arnica montana*), lavender, rosemary and an extract of birch leaf.

Useful in the treatment of a wide range of conditions involving muscular pains and cramps. Massage well into the affected area twice daily or as required.

Plantago comp. ointment

Contains an extract of great plantain (*Plantago*) and camphor.

For treating coughs and bronchitis, especially in children. Massage onto the chest in the morning and last thing at night. Not suitable for children under three without medical advice because of the camphor content.

Sage pastilles

Contain extracts of sage and other herbs.

For mild sore throats and dryness and irritation of the throat. Dissolve one in the mouth every one to two hours while symptoms persist.

Silicea comp.

Contains homeopathic potencies of silica (quartz), deadly nightshade (*Atropa belladonna*) and silver nitrate (argentum nitricum).

For sinusitis, both acute and chronic. May be used in conjunction with inhalations such as eucalyptus oil in hot water. Five pills should be taken, four times a day. If symptoms persist, medical supervision may be necessary.

The above medicines can be prescribed by any doctor, including general practitioners if they are open to using remedies other than conventional drugs. The medicines can also be used safely as home remedies.

Prescription remedies

Medicines in the following list can also be prescribed by any doctor, but they are not suitable as home remedies because they are for conditions that must be treated by a doctor, or because, under existing regulations in the UK, they are available only on a doctor's prescription (indicated by POM – Prescription-Only Medicine).

Apis/Belladonna

Also called Erysidoron I. Contains homeopathic potencies of honey-bee poison (*Apis mellifica*) and deadly nightshade (*Atropa belladonna*).

For acute local infections, particularly when there is redness and fever, as in acute tonsillitis, boils and mastitis. The dosage is five drops in water every two to three hours during the acute phase. It is sometimes given in hourly alternations with Carbo Betulae 5% / Sulfur 1% tablets (formerly known as Erysidoron II). Prescribed together, they can be particularly helpful in treating long-standing local infections which are not resolving.

Apis/Levisticum

Homeopathic potencies of honey-bee poison (*Apis mellifica*) and lovage (*Levisticum officinalis*).

Useful in treating earache, particularly middle-ear infections, under the supervision of a doctor. Up to five pills every two to three hours. For babies, they can be dissolved first in a teaspoon of water.

Carbo Betulae comp. (POM)

Also known as Birkenkohle comp., it contains birch charcoal (*Carbo betulae*), an extract of camomile root (*Matricaria chamomilla*) and a homeopathic potency of antimony (stibium).

For diarrhoea. One capsule every two to three hours in acute cases, otherwise three times a day.

Disci comp. c. Argentum or Disci comp. c. Stanno (POM)

Mixture of homeopathically potentised substances including red-ant juice (formica) and bamboo nodes (*Bambusa e nodo*), with either argentum (silver) or stannum (tin).

Indicated for a variety of acute or chronic back and neck conditions, including sciatica and lumbago, and other neuralgic symptoms originating in the spine. Usually, a one millilitre ampoule is injected under the skin near the area where the symptoms originate. May be given daily or three times a week, depending on the severity of the condition. Unlike customary painkillers, which tend to be the mainstay of conventional medicine in such conditions, they are aimed at speeding the natural healing process. Very often, if conventional painkillers are also needed, they can be quickly withdrawn as the symptoms resolve.

Ferrum Phos. comp. (POM)

Contains homeopathic potencies of monkshood (*Aconitum napellus*), white bryony (*Bryonia alba*), gum-tree leaves (*Eucalyptus*), hemp agrimony (*Eupatorium*), iron phosphate (ferrum phosphoricum) and sabadilla seeds (*Schoenocaulon officinalis*).

For colds and flu-like conditions, particularly in children. Five pills dissolved under the tongue every two to three hours at the first sign of a cold may be sufficient to prevent its further development. For babies, two pills dissolved in a teaspoon of water should be given with the same frequency.

Gencydo (POM)

Contains an extract of lemon (*Citrus medica*) and quince (*Cydonia*).

For hayfever and allergic rhinitis, a one-millilitre ampoule is injected two to three times a week. To prevent the onset of hayfever, it may be given in a three to six-week course in January or February. This can radically reduce the severity of any attack later in the year, and achieves a more long-lasting effect than just suppression of the symptoms.

Infludo (POM)

Same ingredients as Ferrum Phos. comp. except, instead of ferrum phosphoricum, a homeopathic potency of phosphorus is used, and it contains alcohol.

For flu, flu-like illnesses and feverish colds. The inclusion of phosphorus and alcohol makes Infludo unsuitable for children (who should be given Ferrum Phos. comp.). Five to eight drops in a little lukewarm water every hour in the acute phase of the illness then, as it resolves, two to four times a day. This dose should be continued until recovery is complete to help prevent secondary infection and post-flu debility.

Iscador (POM)

A preparation of mistletoe (*Viscum album*) supplied in ampoules for injection. Two other preparations, Helixor and Viscum Abnoba, are also prescribed by doctors in the UK (and imported) on a named patient basis.

For all forms of cancer and pre-cancerous conditions. Found to improve the patient's general physical and mental condition. Also contributes to pain relief and helps psychological adjustment to the illness (see Chapter 13).

Menodoron

Alcoholic extract of shepherd's purse (*Capsella bursa-pastoris*), sweet marjoram (*Origanum majorana*), yarrow (*Achillea millefolium*), oak (*Quercus cortex*) and stinging nettle (*Urtica dioica*) in herbal preparations.

For a variety of menstrual problems, including irregular periods, the absence of periods (amenorrhoea), painful periods (dysmenorrhoea), heavy periods (menorrhagia) and premenstrual tension. It is the first line of treatment for all abnormalities of the menstrual cycle and is usually prescribed as ten to twenty drops, three times a day in a little water.

Silicea comp. (POM)

See also entry in home remedies list.

When treating acute or chronic sinusitis, injected ampoules tend to have a more powerful effect than the pills, and are used under the supervision of a doctor in severe cases.

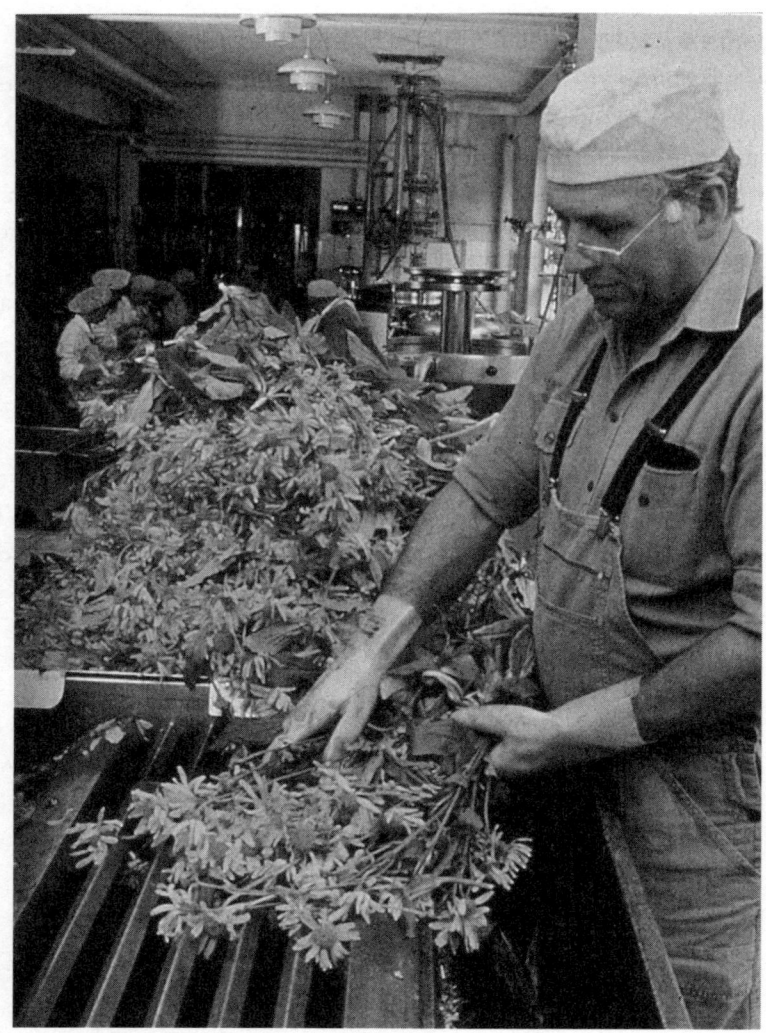

Medicine preparation.

15. Medicines and Legislation

The current detailed regulation of medicines by governments worldwide was initially prompted by the Thalidomide disaster in the 1960s. Regulations in most countries demand proofs of safety, quality and efficacy medicines. The nature of the evidence needed is the kind that conventional drug companies generate when they research and market new chemical drugs. Documentation of quality tends to be demonstrations of the drugs' chemical identity and purity. Evidence of safety is usually based on animal testing, and documentation of efficacy is based on randomised clinical trials. These compare the results of administering a particular medication to one group of patients, randomly selected from a larger group, the rest of whom are treated with a placebo. Patients in neither group know whether they are receiving the actual drug or a placebo. Ideally those administering the drugs and then measuring the outcome also do not know which is which. The term double-blind clinical trial refers to both patients and administering doctors being blind to what a particular patient is receiving.

While this is the kind of evidence involved in finding and marketing new conventional drugs, it is not the way that herbal, homeopathic and anthroposophic medicines have been developed. The costs of such trials are enormous and generally beyond the budgets of the producers of natural medicines. It is easier to prove the efficacy of powerful conventional drugs which have very focused outcome – for instance, in lowering blood pressure – than the efficacy of natural medicines which are usually gentler and prescribed to achieve a more general improvement of health.

In the 1960s and 70s when medicines legislation was introduced in many countries, there was concern that if the regulatory framework was exclusively modelled on conventional medicines it could have the side effect of excluding natural medicines from the market. As it was the safety concerns around conventional medicines that necessitated such regulations it would be ironic if precisely those medicines which had a far greater safety profile were prohibited. Campaigning was undertaken in many countries by patient groups, doctor groups and representatives of natural medicines manufacturers seeking regulations which were appropriate for these groups of medicines.

In Europe in 1992 there was a breakthrough when a European directive on homeopathic medicines came into force, and in 2004 a directive on herbal medicinal products. The homeopathic directive made provision for a simplified registration scheme for homeopathic medicines marketed without any listed indications and provided they were for external or oral administration only and above the fourth decimal potency, equivalent to a dilution of one in ten thousand. There is also the possibility of national rules being established. Through these two European directives, the availability to the public of herbal and homeopathic medicines is fairly secure. However there is as yet no suitable licensing framework for anthroposophic medicines. Some fit the criteria and can be registered as homeopathic medicines or herbal medicines, but the vast majority of the most important anthroposophic medicines do not. Without further regulations appropriate to anthroposophic medicines, their future remains insecure in Europe.

UK regulations

In the UK national rules were established for homeopathic products and for herbal medicines with indications to treat minor or self-limiting conditions. While still needing to meet conventional quality and safety standards, efficacy does not need to be proven in the same way as conventional drugs. Instead, bibliographic evidence for the traditional use within homeopathic tradition needs to be demonstrated. The wording on the packaging of natural medicines licensed in this way has to say that the indications for this medicine are purely based on traditional use.

In the UK two specialist advisory committees were set up – the Advisory Board for the Registration of Homeopathic Medicinal Products (ABRH) and the Herbal Medicines Advisory Committee (HMAC) – to advise the licensing authority, the Medicines and Healthcare products Regulatory Authority (MHRA) on the licensing of particular products. Both committees have experts in homeopathic and herbal medicine as well as conventional doctors, toxicologists and pharmacists. Currently (2017) both committees have at least one anthroposophic doctor.

Virtually all medicines which were on the market before 1968 were granted Product Licences of Right (PLRs) and hence almost all anthroposophic medicines initially received these. It was proposed to discontinue PLRs when the new human medicines regulations that came into force in 2012 were being prepared, leaving only a handful of licensed anthroposophic medicines on the UK market. After a major campaign by the patient organisation in coordination with the Anthroposophic Medical Association and Weleda (the main manufacturer of anthroposophic medicines in the UK) this threat was temporally withdrawn.

Currently (2017) there are further moves to discontinue these PLRs. It is likely that all injectable medicines will be forced to lose their licence, although it will be possible to import them for individual patients with a doctor's prescription. Any anthroposophic medicines which cannot be classified as homeopathic or traditional herbal will also cease to be licensed. This may lead to the number of licensed anthroposophic medicines being cut to around thirty to forty rather than the two thousand or so anthroposophic medicines which initially received PLRs.

The Continent of Europe

In Germany, supporters of natural remedies forced a change in the law resulting in the plurality of medical approaches becoming legally recognised. Medical herbalism, homeopathy and anthroposophic medicine were each given their own medicines commission comprising experts nominated by the professional association of doctors in the respective fields, though this has been challenged as an infringement of the Treaty of Rome, as it goes beyond what is allowed for in existing EU directives.

In France, the position of anthroposophic medicines has been very difficult, in spite of the fact that the country is bound by EU directives. There, the majority of anthroposophic medicines can be prescribed only as *magistral* preparations, meaning medicines on a doctor's prescription in which each of the ingredients is written out, and allows a pharmacist to prepare the mixture for an individual patient. This requires arduous writing on the part of the doctor and it brings distribution problems as it precludes premanufactured remedies.

In Italy, anthroposophic medicines are all imported from Switzerland and Germany. Like France they can be prescribed as *magistral* preparations with similar difficulties.

Switzerland, a non-EU member, has the most liberal regulations for anthroposophic medicines. A public referendum voted in favour of complementary medicine being covered by all health insurance and taught in medical schools. Anthroposophic medicine is one of the six forms of complementary medicine specified. The manufacturing methods of anthroposophic medicines are included in the Swiss Pharmacopoeia and the regulations have allowed virtually all anthroposophic medicines to be licensed under various categories.

The United States

In the United States, medicines must be approved by the Food and Drug Administration (FDA) before they can be marketed. This generally means that the manufacturer has to submit extensive evidence of the drug's efficacy, safety and quality to the authority. No anthroposophic or homeopathic medicines have been approved in this way and, until 1988, when the FDA issued a compliance policy guide, their legal status was unclear. The guide laid down conditions governing the marketing of homeopathic medicines throughout the country. Shops are allowed to sell them over the counter if they are for minor ailments. Toxic substances in potentially harmful strengths and medicines for more serious complaints are restricted to prescription-only sale.

All homeopathic medicines are required to carry indications for use, unlike in Europe, where it has generally been a condition of exemption from conventional testing that no indications are given on the packaging. As homeopathic medicines can often be used to treat a variety of conditions, it can be very difficult for a manufacturer to decide on one or two ailments to print on the packaging. There simply is not room for a full list, and these limited indications can lead to a narrow view of the uses of the medicines.

The Homeopathic Pharmacopoeia of the United States is the main book of standards for homeopathic medicines. A medicinal substance has to meet the *Pharmacopoeia's* criteria for eligibility to be accepted as an official drug. The FDA's policy guide does not refer specifically to anthroposophic medicines, but as many of the potentised substances used in anthroposophic medicine are listed in the *Pharmacopoeia,* they are recognised, including medicines prepared as ampoules for injection. This means that the FDA's recognition of the *Pharmacopoeia* has made the majority of anthroposophic medicines legally available in the US. For those that are not listed, inclusion in the Pharmacopoeia requires the submission of a detailed monograph, along with extensive evidence of the medicine's therapeutic value. As there are more than a hundred substances used in anthroposophic medicine that are not yet listed, there is much work to be done before the full range of anthroposophic treatment will be available.

Many other countries take their cue for regulating medicines from what is happening in the US or Europe. For this reason, progress in these regions must be monitored with great care, as it is most likely to influence the availability of natural medicines worldwide.

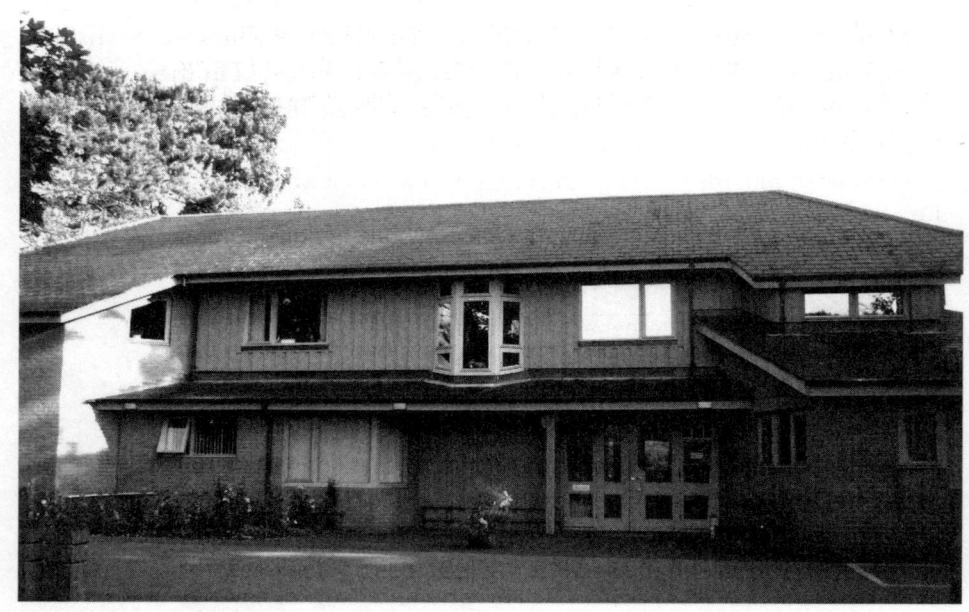

Blackthorn Centre, Maidstone.

16. Therapeutic Communities and Initiatives

The practice of anthroposophic medicine embraces the environment in which patients are treated as much as the therapies and remedies that are used. It includes the way doctors, nurses and therapists work together, the way they are paid, and how the health care is itself financially supported. In anthroposophic medicine, it is considered that the way medical staff relate to each other and make decisions can profoundly affect the outcome of treatment. In a seminal lecture on anthroposophic medicine, Rudolf Steiner emphasised the importance of establishing social institutions that could incorporate spiritual perspectives in the provision of health care if it was to make a real contribution to society over and above helping an isolated number of individuals.[1]

At the end of the 1970s, inspired by both the social ideals that Steiner outlined in that lecture and the ideas of therapeutic communities within psychiatry such as those of Maxwell Jones, Park Attwood Clinic was established in Worcestershire England.* This initiative emphasised developing the social environment so that it could become socially therapeutic as much as the specific therapies and medicines used. Unfortunately Park Attwood Clinic closed in 2003 for financial reasons.

---

* In the 1940s and 1950s, two doctors, David Clark and Maxwell Jones, developed methods of group decision-making which broke from the usual hierarchical structure to involve all the staff, and even the patients, in the running of a hospital or ward. Their notion of a therapeutic community saw the administration of the psychiatric unit as something which could be either beneficial or damaging to the health of patients, depending on how it was done. They had noted that most of the administrative decisions were made by the consultant or chief nurse, and that the hierarchical atmosphere tended to force the rest of the staff and the patients to be passive, thereby blocking their initiative and creative input. The more democratic system they recommended is still operated in a number of psychiatric units, but has remained a minority approach within psychiatry as a whole.

The work of Park Attwood Clinic

In founding Park Attwood Clinic the aim was to develop a centre where people suffering from physical illnesses or psychiatric problems would be supported in a setting which would feel like a real home, unlike the clinical atmosphere of most hospitals. The whole range of anthroposophic treatment was to be provided in a residential setting. The clinic had fourteen beds, an outpatient department, three full-time doctors and a team of nurses. It also offered therapeutic massage, hydrotherapy, eurythmy therapy and artistic therapies including painting and sculpture. Bringing all the therapies together enabled them to support each other and integrate into an intensive treatment programme. A system of regular case conferences was established where the doctors, nurses and therapists each described what they had observed about the patient, without immediately jumping to a conclusion about what they felt needed to be done.

The experience was that each profession brought a different perception of the patient to these meetings. The doctor brought the case history, aspects of the patient's biography and the results of physical examination. The therapeutic masseur described the distribution of warmth in the patient's body, and a detailed picture of the states of tension in the muscular system and the tone of the bodily tissues. The therapeutic eurythmist brought an image of how the patient moved, and artistic therapists described the patient's creative expression. Nurses added to this their view of the patient's physical and psychological condition, gained through 24-hour care. Out of this collection of observations, a diagnostic motif usually emerged.

This motif often provided a qualitative extension to the conventional diagnosis, and painted a broader picture within which to understand the patients and their illness. Its diagnostic significance pointed to the common therapeutic direction which was needed. This broad indication could then be worked out in detail by each professional, to arrive at the appropriate doctor's prescription, the type of nursing treatment required and the direction the artistic therapies should take. The therapeutic and creative initiatives of each member of the case conference was, in this way, brought into play. It was a quite different process from when a doctor makes the diagnosis alone, prescribes for the patient and gives instructions to other therapists. It is also quite different from what would be the case if each therapist made an independent diagnosis and gave treatment in isolation.

Another social aspect which can affect those working together concerns the relationship between work and remuneration. Steiner suggested that the link between the two would have to be broken, or at least loosened, if people were to develop a sense of karma and of true freedom, which involves responsibility for their actions. For example, people in the army follow orders – that is what the job demands. Therefore, their actions are largely determined by others, and it could be said that they have handed over their freedom and responsibility to the commanders. Similarly, people who are paid to work are directed by their employers, and their freedom of action is limited by those people who are prepared to pay for their labour. The extent to which they are limited varies enormously, but this often leads to an attitude of 'I'm just doing my job' – particularly to excuse an action of dubious morality. In the practice of medicine, doctors and therapists work with the intimate details of patients' lives, and can directly affect their futures. This calls for a sensitivity to, and respect for, the patients' particular paths through life, and their freedom to make their own decisions. The doctors or therapists must take this into account when deciding on treatment, while also maintaining their own therapeutic freedom and sense of responsibility.

The doctors and therapists at Park Attwood Clinic attempted to incorporate these principles into the way they worked. For example, staff remuneration was related more to the needs arising from personal circumstances than to the particular work. This meant that anyone with a large family to support was likely to receive more than an unmarried person, regardless of their respective jobs. Many professional people find that their motivation comes more from the work itself than from the salary, and an arrangement like that at Park Attwood intensified this feeling. It was a far more demanding way of working – for example, such a system tended to go hand-in-hand with a less rigid job description, and doing what needed to be done rather than just following instructions. It demanded a wider awareness of different areas of work and a responsible attitude towards the needs of others, because the level of remuneration of any one person had economic consequences for the whole community. A stronger sense of community resulted from working this way, and, together with the influence of the intensive case conferences, this was experienced by patients as a powerfully beneficial therapeutic environment.

Health care in the UK falls into two main categories: the National Health Service (NHS) and private treatment. The NHS provides free health care as of right, whereas private care is available only on payment of a set price. Private care is treated more like a commodity within the economy. It seemed to those founding Park Attwood Clinic that the positive aspect of the NHS was that treatment was available to all, regardless of means. But a drawback was that it was state-controlled, and suffered from the suppression of staff initiative which was typical of such bureaucracies. It limited the choices available to patients, and did not encourage their sense of responsibility for their own health. Patients also lost touch with the need to support the providers of health care, because a limitless amount appeared to be funded by taxation.

The positive aspect of the private system seemed to be the greater autonomy for the providers of health care and the freedom of choice and sense of responsibility engendered in patients. A major drawback, however, was that only patients with sufficient means could obtain care, and health tended to be treated as a commodity to be bought and sold. The founders of Park Attwood Clinic felt that health care should not be seen as a right or as a commodity. They considered that the best way to treat it was as a gift to patients with, ideally, the provision of such care supported in turn by contributions or gifts to the clinic.

When Park Attwood Clinic was set up as a small hospital, the doctors wanted to offer their services to anyone, regardless of their means, along the lines of NHS hospitals. A charitable trust was established, to which people who supported anthroposophic medicine could make regular donations. While undergoing treatment, patients were expected to make contributions in accordance with their means, instead of a fixed fee. It was hoped that they would become regular contributors to the trust after being discharged, if they had not been beforehand. As a registered nursing home, the clinic was also able to receive payments from private health insurance companies.

In the early years, the flow of regular donations was sufficient to meet about a third of the running costs of the clinic. Another third was covered by patients' contributions during treatment, but a third still had to be raised from charitable sources. For a time some patients from NHS anthroposophic general practices were funded by the NHS, but soon there was more dependency on patients' contributions at the time of treatment. During the recession there was a fall in the number of patients and in 2003 the clinic had to close for financial reasons.

However, in spite of existing outside NHS funding and the usual funding of private medicine, Park Attwood provided a unique service to many patients for over thirty years. Patients going through a life crisis or serious illness experienced an integrated therapeutic support in a caring human environment. For many it was a turning point in their lives. For doctors and therapists it was a confirmation of what anthroposophic medicine and therapies can offer when embedded in an innovative community context.

St Luke's Medical Practice

In keeping with its aim to be an extension of conventional medicine rather than an alternative, anthroposophic medicine has largely developed within the main health care provisions of each of the countries where it has become established. It seeks to extend and bring innovation to the conventional health care systems by working within the system, not in opposition to it. There are a small number of such practices in the UK.

One practice in Gloucestershire, St Luke's Medical Practice in Stroud, provided medical services for sixty seven years to some four thousand patients. They appreciated a general practice which offered anthroposophic medical treatment as well as all the services of a conventional general practice. Linked to the practice was a group of therapists and counsellors all housed in a purpose-built centre designed by anthroposophic architects. Through integrating the best of conventional general practice with the prescription of anthroposophic medicines and anthroposophic therapies, substantial reductions of conventional drug prescribing compared to other local practices could be achieved. In a study prepared by the National Audit Office, antibiotic prescribing at ninety per cent less than expected was demonstrated with similar reductions in the prescribing of non-steroidal anti-inflammatory drugs and painkillers. These are drugs now seen as dangerously over-prescribed in general practice and are associated with the growth of antibiotic resistant bacteria. This illustrates the potential contribution anthroposophic medicine can make to serious current medical and public health issues.

While anthroposophic medicines were paid for by the NHS – as was any medication prescribed by a general practitioner (GP) – the overall drug budget for St Luke's Medical Practice was some thirty per cent less than comparable practices, a considerable saving to the NHS. (A sceptical Public Health official suggested the GPs might be under-treating their patients resulting in more emergency hospital admissions, but a later survey of the practice's emergency admission rates showed them to be the lowest in the county, making a substantial contribution to reducing the overburdened hospital emergency admissions units.) However, none of these savings could be passed on to the practice.

NHS general practices increasingly have their income related to meeting targets for treating and reviewing chronically ill patients. St Luke's patients had less chronic illness so their 'chronic disease registers' were smaller resulting in reductions in practice income.

Together with a number of other bureaucratic quirks of NHS funding, the finances of this anthroposophic medical practice were penalised despite actually saving the NHS substantial amounts of money and alleviating some of its pressing problems. This was a major impediment in being able to recruit new partners for the practice when the two partners reached retirement age, and led to the NHS practice closing in 2015.

St Luke's Therapy Centre, as it is now called, houses some twelve anthroposophic and complementary therapists, six counsellors and four part-time anthroposophic doctors who see patients on a private basis.

Other anthroposophic general practices

There are currently several other similar anthroposophic NHS general practices in the UK who have so far survived similar challenges.

The Blackthorn Centre in Maidstone, Kent is housed in the first medical centre in the UK designed by anthroposophic architects. As well as working with a group of therapists with the help of Blackthorn Trust, they have pioneered initiative to support patients with long term mental health problems as well as patients with long term pain. The NHS-funded Blackthorn Pain Management Service offers anthroposophic medicines, rhythmical massage, art therapy, biographical counselling and eurythmy therapy. Next door, the Blackthorn Garden, Café and Craft Workshop offer rehabilitation programmes for patients with either long term physical conditions, pain or mental health issues.

The administrator for the health authority responsible for services in the area described the work of the Blackthorn Trust as one of the most exciting developments in general practice. The authority has agreed to pay seventy per cent of the salaries of the therapists, with the remainder financed by the practice's income. This makes them as much a part of the NHS as practice nurses and receptionists, who have traditionally been financed in this way.

Another NHS practice inspired by Blackthorn is the Camphill Medical Practice near Aberdeen. Initially the practice was set up to provide medical care for the children and adults with learning difficulties in the Camphill School Aberdeen and Newton Dee Camphill Village, but is now open to members of the public in the Aberdeen area providing all the services of an NHS general practice.

Linked to the practice is a charity, the Camphill Wellbeing Trust, which provides extended anthroposophic-orientated therapies such as nursing with the option of anthroposophic medicines, art therapy, eurythmy, art and therapy or counselling. These additional services are not limited to local people. While maintaining many special services for individuals with learning difficulties they also offer residential based anthroposophic treatments for people suffering from a range of long-term health conditions and patients with cancer (including mistletoe treatment). Patients are offered an intense induction of mistletoe treatment with infusions and injections over one to three weeks.

In Bristol, the Helios Medical Centre also offer the full range of NHS general practice services with the possibility of anthroposophic medicines and therapies. One of the doctors also runs a special clinic for children with learning difficulties, providing a range of anthroposophic medicines and therapies for their special needs. Another of the doctors has links with Bristol Cancer Centre, and prescribes Iscador treatment and other anthroposophic therapies for cancer patients.

Independent of the NHS, the Elysia Therapeutic Centre in Stourbridge, West Midlands, offers a wide spectrum of anthroposophic therapies: rhythmical massage, eurythmy, counselling, biography, psychotherapy and therapeutic arts as well as doctors providing anthroposophic medical treatments. It also provides advice and contacts to the general public through their website *www.elysiahealth.org.*

Melanie Taylor, one of the pioneers of this centre, has also developed Oasis Group Work. This is a structured programme of weekly sessions in three pathways including art work and biographic sharing. This is designed for individuals, many of whom are faced with long term health problems that have altered their lives and sometimes lead to social isolation. These group sessions give the opportunity to accompany (and be accompanied in) the discovery of meaning in the challenging life experiences that patients face, as well as providing invaluable social support. The groups are lead by a pair of counsellors or therapists and currently such groups run in Stourbridge, Hereford and Stroud.

Netherlands and Germany

Extending general practices to include various therapists was particularly pioneered in the Netherlands, where many cities have a practice operating along these lines. Typically, a group of doctors and therapists converted a large house into what they called a 'therapeuticum'. Patient groups are formed at these centres and given courses on how to look after their own physical and mental health. The courses include such subjects as the value of wholefood nutrition, an anthroposophic approach to childcare, meditative and other exercises, and lectures on anthroposophic medicine. Active patient participation is encouraged and, together with the creativity which the artistic therapies demand, these courses contribute to counterbalancing the rather passive role associated with taking medicines and having physical treatments. These patient groups have also united to help defend the availability of natural medicines, which have faced threats in the Netherlands as they have in the UK. More than eighty anthroposophic general practitioners work within the national health system in the Netherlands.

Germany has a similar health care system to that of the Netherlands. There is a very strong tradition of natural medicine in Germany, with over half of family doctors prescribing some herbal medicines. There are many hundreds of practising anthroposophic doctors and many thousands who prescribe some of the medicines. There are several specialist hospitals with between seventy and one hundred beds, including the Klinik Öschelbronn near Pforzheim, which is linked to the Carus-Institut, one of the anthroposophic cancer research centres. All are integrated into the general health care system which, like the Dutch system, involves both state-subsidised and private insurance schemes. These fund patients in anthroposophic hospitals in the same way as in any conventional hospital. As well as these medical hospitals, there is also a psychiatric hospital with one hundred beds, the Friedrich Husemann Klinik, near Freiburg in the Black Forest.

A major development of anthroposophic health care in Germany came about with the establishment of three large district general hospitals: one in the Ruhr, the Herdecke hospital, the Filderklinik on the outskirts of Stuttgart, and the community hospital at Havelhöhe in Berlin. These provide the full range of specialities one would expect to find in any district general hospital, including accident and emergency, surgery, paediatrics, obstetrics and gynaecology, general medicine and intensive care. All the methods of conventional medicine are available, but they are also extended through the use of anthroposophic medicines, physical treatments and artistic therapies. To set up and run hospitals on this scale, a new form of financial structure was developed.

In Germany, hospitals are usually run by the city or state authority, by religious organisations such as the Lutheran or Catholic Churches, or by charities such as the Red Cross. Others are private concerns, run in the same way as private companies. The anthroposophic hospitals were established as 'community hospitals for public benefit' – non-profit-making companies similar to charities. They are run by a circle of the leading doctors, nurses and administrators, and the doctors donate to the hospital any additional income earned from treating private patients. This money has been used to fund the therapists when their costs have not been recognised and supported by the health insurance schemes. It is also used to provide training and research.

Herdecke hospital and the Filderklinik both offer state-recognised nursing training, teaching both conventional and anthroposophic skills, and at Herdecke, the larger of the two, an independent but fully recognised university offering medical training was established. While preparing students to sit the state medical exams, the university offers a relatively critical approach to conventional medicine, exposing students to its limitations as well as its strengths, and also gives the opportunity for students to be introduced to anthroposophic methods in parallel courses.

The Clinical Pharmacology Department at Herdecke University has published many academic papers and books on the problems of conventional methods of assessing drugs through clinical trials and tests on animals. The work, and the efforts of its main author, Gerhard Kienle, were major factors in forcing changes to Germany's Medicines Act, reversing the demand for such testing as the basis for the licensing of all medicines. Herdecke supports many of the specialist departments demanded by a university hospital, such as neurosurgery, and has been a leader with advanced diagnostic imaging equipment. The hospital has aimed to stay at the forefront of conventional medical practice, while maintaining an awareness of its rightful role and complementing it with the full range of opportunities offered by anthroposophic practice.

Conclusion

The aim of anthroposophic medicine as a whole is to work with conventional medicine, while extending it through the insights gained from a spiritual knowledge of the human being. In practice, it works within conventional forms of health care provision, but introduces innovations based on these insights. The range of available anthroposophic health care extends from the small health service general practice to the district general hospital and university medical school. They serve as examples of what could develop into a future mainstream medicine.

Anthroposophic medicine has a substantial contribution to make to every aspect of health care. By so doing, it helps to counterbalance the predominantly materialistic and reductionistic view of the human being which is so fundamental to conventional medical practice. Anthroposophic medicine also helps to bring a balancing influence into society as a whole, which tends to be dominated by the same materialistic and reductionistic outlook.

Notes and Further Reading

Introduction

1. Available under the title *Introducing Anthroposophical Medicine* (Steiner Books, USA, 2010).
2. *Extending Practical Medicine: Fundamental Principles Based on the Science of the Spirit*, 5th ed. (Rudolf Steiner Press, UK, 1997).
3. For details of this process of development, see Steiner's books *Knowledge of the Higher Worlds, Occult Science* and *Theosophy* (all Rudolf Steiner Press, UK).

General background: *Rudolf Steiner: Scientist of the Invisible,* A.P. Shepherd, (Floris Books, UK, 1991). An introduction to Steiner and his work.

1. Extending the Art and Science of Medicine

1. Virchow's series of twenty lectures given in 1858 was published in English in 1863 as *Cellular Pathology as based upon Physiological and Pathological Histology.*

General background: *Extending Practical Medicine: Fundamental Principles Based on the Science of the Spirit,* Ita Wegman and Rudolf Steiner, 5th ed. (Rudolf Steiner Press, UK, 1997). A foundation work on anthroposophic medicine (requires a well-developed understanding of anthroposophy).

Anthroposophy and Science: An Introduction, Peter Heuser (Peter Lang, UK, 2016). A thorough introduction into the scientific basis of anthroposophy and anthroposophic medicine in the context of academic science.

2. A New Study of Life

1. In Chapters 13 and 14, practical steps in developing a medical treatment along these lines are described.
2. D.W. Smithers, 'Cancer – an Attack on Cytologism,' *The Lancet,* 10 March 1962.
3. Soto, A.M., C. Sonnenschein, 'The tissue organisation field theory of cancer: a testable replacement for the somatic mutation theory'. *Bioessays* 2011, 33:332–40.
4. In his books, *Knowledge of the Higher Worlds* and *Occult Science,* Steiner describes how, with the help of certain exercises, the faculty of thinking can become an organ of perception in its own right.
5. This polarity of physical forces, which centre on finite points, and etheric forces, which have a planar quality, is illustrated mathematically by projective geometry. George Adams, who did much original work in this field, used projective geometry to describe sets of laws for both realms (which he called space and counterspace) in his book *Physical and Ethereal Spaces* (Rudolf Steiner Press, UK, 1978). Lawrence Edwards developed this in his book *Vortex of Life* (Floris Books, UK, 1993).

General background: *The Metamorphosis of Plants,* J.W. von Goethe, (MIT Press, USA, 2009). A collection of Goethe's writings on botany.

Towards a Phenomenology of the Etheric World, J. Bockemühl (Ed.), (Rudolf Steiner Press, UK, 1985). A collection of essays by scientists engaged in phenomenological research which introduces various aspects of the etheric world.

3. The Soul

1. It is acknowledged that plants also burn their own sugars and, particularly at night, give off carbon dioxide.

4. The Spirit

General background: *Manifestations of Karma,* Rudolf Steiner, 4th ed. (Rudolf Steiner Press, UK, 1996). A description of the laws of karma and how, for example, events in one life can influence the bodily constitution and health in subsequent lives.

6. The Use of Medicines

1. The example is largely based on the work of Margaret Colquhoun Ph.D. (cf. *Science Forum,* No. 8, Spring 1989, published by the Science Group of the Anthroposophical Society in Great Britain) and two botany workshops held in 1989 and 1990.
2. See, for instance, C.G. Jung, *Alchemical Studies* (Vol. 13 of the *Collected Works).*

General background: *The Science and Art of Healing,* Ralph Twentyman, (Floris Books, UK, 1992). Homeopathic and anthroposophic insights into the science and art of healing with a historical and mythological background.

7. Artistic Therapies

General background: *Fundamentals of Artistic Therapy,* Margarethe Hauschka, (Rudolf Steiner Press, UK, 2015). A foundation work on artistic therapy, particularly painting therapy.
Foundations of Curative Eurythmy, Margarete Kirchner-Bockholt (Floris Books, UK, 2004).

8. Therapeutic Massage and Hydrotherapy

General background: *Rhythmical Massage,* Margarethe Hauschka, (Mercury Press, USA, 1991). Written as a textbook for those interested in training to be therapeutic masseurs.
Rhythmic Einreibung: A Handbook from the Ita Wegman Clinic, Monika Fingado (Floris Books, UK, 2011).

9. The Art of Nursing

General background: *Home Nursing for Carers,* Tineke van Bentheim (Floris Books, UK, 2006). Describes basic nursing care, including details of herbal remedies and how to administer them.

10. Childhood Illnesses

1. 'Fever: Views in Anthroposophic Medicine and their Scientific Validity', unpublished review by Prof David D. Martin, University Children's Hospital, Tübingen, Germany and Filderklinik, Filderstadt, Germany in *Evidence-Based Complementary and Alternative Medicine,* 2016, Article ID 3642659.

2. *Fever in under 5s,* NICE Clinical Guidance, May 2013.
3. Tove Ronne, 'Measles Virus Infection Without Rash in Childhood Is Related to Disease in Adult Life' *The Lancet,* 5 January 1985.
4. *A Guide to Child Health,* Michaela Glöckler and Wolfgang Goebel, 4th ed. (Floris Books, UK, 2013) is recommended for a detailed description of childhood illnesses.
5. Comp. is an abbreviation of *compositum,* and means a mixture. For example, Ferrum Phos. comp. contains a number of ingredients, the main one of which is ferrum phosphoricum.

General background: *Phases of Childhood,* Bernard Lievegoed, 3rd ed. (Floris Books, UK, 2005). A detailed description of the physical and psychological development which takes place during the seven-year phases of childhood.

11. Inner Development

General background: *Phases: Crisis and Development in the Individual,* Bernard Lievegoed, (Rudolf Steiner Press, UK, 1977). A Dutch psychiatrist writes about the challenges of the different seven-year phases of life, from childhood to old age.
Man on the Threshold, Bernard Lievegoed, (Hawthorn Press, UK, 1985). A detailed account of the threshold of consciousness between the physical and spiritual worlds.
Knowledge of Higher Worlds, Rudolf Steiner, new ed., (Rudolf Steiner Press, UK, 2011).

12. Psychiatry

1. In anthroposophic medicine, certain metals are considered to be related to particular organs. For example, copper to the kidneys, tin to the liver, and silver to the reproductive organs. For details, see Wilhelm Pelikan, *The Secrets of Metals* (Lindisfarne Books, USA, 1973).

General background: *Soulways,* Rudolf Treichler, (Hawthorn Press, UK, 1990). A psychiatrist's insights into personal development and disorders of the soul. Includes addiction, neurosis, premature ageing, psychosis, anorexia, schizophrenia, depression and mania.
Rock Bottom: Beyond Drug Addiction, by members of Arta Rehabilitation Centre in the Netherlands (Hawthorn Press, UK, 1990). Describes the work of the centre in treating and rehabilitating drug addicts.

13. Immunity, Cancer and Mistletoe

1. W. Tröger, D. Galun, M. Reif, A. Schumann, N. Stankovic, M. Milicevic, '*Viscum album* [L.] extract therapy in patients with locally advanced or metastatic pancreatic cancer: a randomised clinical trial on overall survival', *European Journal of Cancer,* 2013, 49:3788–97; and 'Quality of life of patients with advanced pancreatic cancer during treatment with mistletoe', *Deutsches Ärzteblatt International,* 2014, 111:493–502.
2. S.M. Baumgartner, R. Grossarth-Maticek, H. Kiene, R. Ziegler, 'Use of Iscador, an extract of European mistletoe *(Viscum album),* in cancer treatment', *Alternative Therapies in Health and Medicine,* May 2001, 7.3. Grossarth-Maticek, R., R. Ziegler, 'Prospective controlled cohort studies on long-term therapy of breast-cancer patients with a mistletoe preparation (Iscador)', *Forschende Komplementärmedizin,* 2006 13: 285–92.

General background: *Aids,* Arie Bos, (Hawthorn Press, UK, 1989), A practical approach to the understanding and treatment of Aids based on anthroposophic medicine.

14 & 15. Medicines

1. Further information may be obtained from the Biodynamic Agricultural Association, *www.biodynamic.org.uk* in the UK, or *www.biodynamics.com* in North America.

General background: *Biodynamic Agriculture: An Introduction,* H.H. Koepf, B.D, Pettersson, W. Schaumann, (Rudolf Steiner Press, UK, 1990). Detailed discussion of biodynamic farming and gardening, including explanation of the differences between organic, natural and biodynamic methods.

16. Therapeutic Communities and Initiatives

1. Steiner, 'The Invisible Man Within Us' in *Earthly Knowledge and Heavenly Wisdom* (Anthroposophic Press, USA, 1991).

Photographic Acknowledgments

p.14   *Calendula (marigold) flower.* (Credit: http://maxpixel.freegreatpicture.com/Blossom-Orange-Flower-Bloom-Marigold-Calendula-2023150)

p.48   *Fire* (Credit: Wikicommons)

p.60   *Arnica flower* (Credit: https://www.flickr.com/photos/59161444@N05/16421053145)

p.68   *Winter aconite* (Credit: https://commons.wikimedia.org/wiki/File:Winter_Aconite_Flower_5135.jpg)

p.84   *Music eurythmy therapy* (Credit: Ursula Browning)

p.92   *Massage* (Credit: Park Attwood Clinic)

p.100 *Preparing a compress* (Credit: Michael Evans)

p.108 *Mother and son* (Credit: istockphoto/malerapaso)

p.150 *Weleda, UK, Ilkeston* (Credit: Michael Evans)

p.162 *Medicine preparation* (Credit: Weleda, UK)

p.168 *Blackthorn Centre, Maidstone* (Credit: Michael Evans)

Appendix

Anthroposophical societies

International

General Anthroposophical Society
Goetheanum
4143 Dornach, Switzerland
www.goetheanum.org/en/aag/anthroposophical-society

Great Britain

Anthroposophical Society in Great Britain
35 Park Road, London NW1 6XT
www.anthroposophy.org.uk

United States of America

Anthroposophical Society in America
1923 Geddes Avenue
Ann Arbor MI 48104-1797
www.anthroposophy.org

Other countries

The Anthroposophical Society exists in about 60 countries worldwide.
   Details: *www.goetheanum.org/en/aag/adressen/*

Anthroposophic hospitals, clinics and general practitioners

Great Britain

Information of registered anthroposophic physicians can be found from the Council for Anthroposophic Health and Social Care, *www.cahsc.org*

Further information may be available from the Patients and Friends of Anthroposophic Medicine, *www.PAFAM.org.uk*

Some general practitioners with associated therapists

Blackthorn Medical Centre (NHS doctors and therapists) St Andrews Road, Maidstone ME16 9AN, *www.blackthorn.org.uk*

Camphill Medical Practice (NHS doctors) and Camphill Wellbeing Trust (therapies, etc.) St John's, Murtle Estate, Bieldside, Aberdeen AB1 9EP. *www.camphillwellbeing.org.uk*

Helios Medical Centre (NHS doctors) 17 Stoke Hill, Bristol BS9 1JN, *www.heliosbristol.co.uk*

Elysia Therapeutic Centre (therapies and doctor) 52 Bowling Green Road, Stourbridge DY8 3RZ, *www.elysiacentre.org*

Oasis Group Work (art and biographic therapies, run in various places), *www.elysiacentre.org/therapies/oasis_group_work.php*

Raphael Medical Centre (neuro-rehabilitation and nursing home) Hollanden Park, Coldharbour Lane, Hildenborough, Tonbridge TN11 9LE, *www.raphaelmedicalcentre.co.uk*

St Luke's Therapy Centre (therapies and part-time private doctors) 53 Cainscross Road, Stroud, GL5 4EX, *www.stlukestherapycentre.co.uk*

United States

Information from Physicians Association for Anthroposophical Medicine, 4801 Yellowwood Ave, Baltimore, MD 21209, *www.paam.wildapricot.org*

Canada

Canadian Anthroposophic Medical Association, Kenneth McAlister MD, Hesperus Community, 201-1 Hesperus Road, Thornhill, Ontario L4J 0G9. Email: *dr.k.mca@rogers.com.*

Australia

Australian Anthroposophical Medical Association, *www.aamaanthro.com*

New Zealand

New Zealand Association of Anthroposophical Doctors (NZAAD). Dr Roger Leitch, Email: *rleitch@titan.co.nz www.anthroposophy.org.nz/initiatives/health-and-wellbeing/*

Philippines

Philippine Association of Anthroposophic Health Practitioners Inc. (PAAHPI), Dr Rosalinda Maglana, Email: *moonmaglana@gmail.com*

South Africa

Anthroposophical Medical Association in Southern Africa, Syringa Medical and Therapeutical Centre, 4 Wembley Avenue, 7800 Plumsted, Email: *gwaymes@pharma.co.za*

Germany

Filderklinik, Im Haberschlai 7, 70794 Filderstadt, *www.filderklinik.de*

Herdecke Gemeinschaftskrankenhaus, Gerhard-Kienle-Weg 4, 58313 Herdecke, *www.gemeinschaftskrankenhaus.de*

Klinik Havelhöhe, Kladower Damm 221, 14089 Berlin, *www.havelhoehe.de*

Klinik Öschelbronn, Am Eichhof 30, 75223 Niefern-Öschelbronn, *www.klinik-oeschelbronn.de*

Friedrich Husemann Klinik (psychiatric clinic), Friedrich-Husemann-Weg 8, 79256 Buchenbach, *www.friedrich-husemann-klinik.de*

Siebenzwerge, Fachklinik für Drogenkrankheiten (drug addiction clinic), Grünwanger Str. 4, 88682 Salem, *www.siebenzwerge.info*

Switzerland

Casa di Cura Andrea Cristoforo, Via Collinetta 25, 6612 Ascona, *casa-andrea-cristoforo.ch*

Klinik Arlesheim, Pfeffingerweg 1, 4144 Arlesheim, *www.klinik-arlesheim.ch*

Paracelsus-Spital, Bergstrasse 16, 8805 Richterswil, *www.paracelsus-spital.com*

Manufacturers and distributors of anthroposophic medicines

International

Information from *www.weleda.com* and *www.wala.de/english*

Great Britain

Weleda (UK) Ltd, *www.weleda.co.uk*

USA and Canada

Weleda Inc, *www.weleda.com*

Australia

Weleda, *www.weleda.com.au*

New Zealand

Weleda, *www.weleda.co.nz*

Training for anthroposophic doctors

Postgraduate training courses in anthroposophic medicine for doctors have been established in Germany, Switzerland, the Netherlands, Brazil, Sweden, Hungary and the UK. They vary from full-time for one year to part-time over three years. Details: *www.anthroposophic-drs-training.org.*

For countries without the teaching resources to run their own courses, the Medical Section of the School of Spiritual Science at the Goetheanum in Switzerland (see Introduction) has pioneered International Postgraduate Medical Trainings (IPMTs) in (currently) eighteen different countries. These include the following English-speaking countries: Australia, USA, the Philippines and India. They involve a full week's course annually over five years with an opportunity for mentoring participants beginning to practice anthroposophic medicine in their own practices. Details: *www. medsektion-goetheanum.org/en*

Central to any anthroposophic medical training is the opportunity for new and independent ways of observing and thinking about the world. To this end, the training involves practising detailed observation of nature leading to independent thinking and contemplation. This can empower individuals to value their own observations and creative thinking rather than relying on conventional teaching and following protocols that can drown independent thought and practice.

Another element of the training is the study of some of Rudolf Steiner's writings. He repeatedly asks his readers not to believe him, but to come to their own thoughts stimulated by his writing, and emphasised the crucial importance of each individual thinking independently as well as deepening their powers of observation and empathy. As such, texts studied are treated more as a stimulus to exercise thinking and contemplation than for absorbing and memorising information. Additionally, there are sessions specifically devoted to the participants' own personal and spiritual development.

For further details can be found under *Anthroposophic hospitals, clinics and general practitioners* on page 184.

Training for other health professions

Since the 1980s a multidisciplinary **Training in Mental Health** has been run. It is a three-year course comprising twelve modules of three to five days each. It provides participants with an opportunity to develop understanding and skills in the field of mental health, and covers human development from an anthroposophic perspective in a creative dialogue with psychotherapeutic theory and practice. There is opportunity to explore these themes within inter-disciplinary group work. Mutual peer group supervision work fosters self-reflective practice and ensures the training connects to participants' own work and life. Details: *www.mentalhealthseminar.org.uk*. In the USA there is an **Anthroposophic Counselling Psychology Seminar** with parallels the UK Training in Mental Health. Details: *www.AnthroposophicPsychology.org*.

The **Eurythmy Therapy Training** in Great Britain prepares eurythmists to work in all fields of eurythmy therapy with an international diploma from the Medical Section of the Goetheanum in Dornach, Switzerland. It also provides students with an internationally recognised Master of Arts in Eurythmy Therapy. The training takes place over two years and consists of five taught blocks, which total twenty-two weeks. An emphasis is placed on experiential learning, linking theme-based lectures with practical sessions. In addition to these blocks the student must complete observation and practice placement blocks under the supervision of qualified eurythmy therapists. Details: *www.eurythmytherapytraining.org.uk*.

Nursing training is provided in the Anthroposophic Health Care Course, a two-year part-time course at Emerson College, Forest Row, Sussex. It offers professional training in health care, in which theory is grounded in practice and discovery through an interactive, hands-on approach. It may be taken as a diploma, continuing professional development, or simply to extend, explore and deepen a connection to nursing and care. It includes conceptual, observational, discursive, artistic, contemplative and practical work and networking; peer support and collaboration are encouraged. Details: *www.emerson.org.uk/anthroposophic-healing*. In the US there is currently an anthroposophic nurses' training, which runs as a parallel training alongside the doctors' annual IPMT sessions. Details: *aamta.org*. In New Zealand there is training at Taruna College with a Certificate in Holistic Health. Details: *www.taruna.ac.nz/courses-and-workshops/holistic-health/*

A **Biographical Counselling** Diploma Course provides professional training in counselling with anthroposophic perspectives. Biographic counselling has an awareness of the particular challenges and potential of each phase in biography as touched on in Chapter 11. The training runs over three years, currently based at Emerson College, Forest Row, Sussex and is accredited by the British Council for Counselling and Psychotherapy. Details: *www.biographywork.org/bdst-diploma-course.php.*

Also at Emerson College, is the postgraduate **Anthroposophic Psychotherapy Course,** open to qualified and experienced counsellors, psychotherapists, counselling psychologists, clinical psychologists and psychiatrists. It involves thirteen seminars and can lead to an International Certification in Anthroposophic Perspectives on Psychotherapy, Psychiatry and Psychosomatics from the Medical Section of the School of Spiritual Science at the Goetheanum. The bio-psycho-social-spiritual orientation of anthroposophy can widen and complement other psychotherapy training. As well as lecture presentations the course involves workshop exercises which have been developed for training in anthroposophic psychotherapy and small group work, linking to participants learning to their ongoing clinical work. Details: *www.emerson.org.uk/anthroposophic-psychotherapy*

Anthroposophic artistic therapy training is offered at Tobias School of Art and Therapy in East Grinstead, Sussex. The training can lead to a City and Guilds Level 7 Award (Masters Equivalent). Alongside art work, the training includes human development from anthroposophic perspectives and the perspectives of contemporary psychology and psychiatry. Counselling skills are taught as well as how to build and maintain professional contact with people within professional boundaries. Details: *www.tobiasart.org*

A two year training in **rhythmical massage** is open to physiotherapists, nurses and those with bodywork training recognised by a regulating organisation such as the General Council for Massage Therapies. In addition to learning and practising rhythmical massage techniques the training involves medical studies, general anthroposophic orientation and artistic sessions. Between block courses trainee rhythmical masseurs need to have practical placements to begin to use their massage skills. Currently, the UK training is taking place in Stroud, Gloucestershire. Details: *www.rhythmicalmassagetherapy.co.uk.* In the United States there is training which runs as a parallel training alongside the doctors' annual IPMT sessions. Details: *www.rhythmicalmassagetherapynorthamerica.org/training.*

Therapy **training in other countries** can be found via *www.medsektion-goetheanum.org/en*

Index

A Road Ran Through It

Near The End of National Service in Britain

Tony Kreit

ISBN: 1544248296
ISBN 13: 9781544248295

This work is dedicated to one woman, Joyce, who has been, at the time of writing, my wife of nearly 54 years. We were married just three days after my discharge from the RAF. I have hardly mentioned her in the pages of this story yet she was my anchor. It was she who helped to prevent me from going mad and getting myself into deep trouble, particularly during the first few very difficult months. From the beginning, no, from well before the beginning of my national service I had decided that I wanted to keep her, and her name, well away from my period of enforced incarceration. She was to be separate, a beacon of light at the end of the dark tunnel that I saw looming ahead, for the next two years. To Joyce! Alors ma chéri, Merci Bien!

Prologue

WELL, I'VE SAID it before and I'll say it again. "The past is what we remember it to be." That's at least as valid as the saying that history is written by the victors. Like all sound-bite material these statements are only partially true. Much history seems in fact to be written by authors many hundreds or even thousands of years after the event. This being the case my own earnest statement, relating to my own memory of events, in my own life, becomes quite a strong argument.

The events outlined in the following pages relate to two years of my life. For me at the time, they were dramatic years. The fact that I have taken the trouble to write them down now is the fault of three ladies at a pub lunch about 18 months ago. These ladies were asking questions about the sometimes foolhardy antics that the military seemed to impose on recruits.

One question asked was; "Could it be true that soldiers sometimes had to paint stones white." They were astonished when I, the only person present who had seen military service, advised them that that was one of the more useful chores imposed on recruits, when the military mind really got itself into gear. The tone of my response reflected the extreme resentment I felt at the call up. I had no objection to military service but the practice of the 'press gang' treatment

of young men appalled and angered me, particularly when it applied to me.

This work is as true as I can remember it to be. All the characters are real characters although I have changed their names to avoid any embarrassment.

Tony Kreit.

02-March-2017

1
Beginnings, The Invitation Arrives

THE PAST IS what we remember it to be; See! I've said it yet again just in case you skipped the Prologue.

I received my first brown envelope in 1957, just before my 18th birthday, as I remember it. It contained no money however. It was from the war office and contained my 'invitation' from the Queen to join the British Armed Forces as a national serviceman. For the first time in my life I realized that there was a power greater than my parents, and that they were powerless to intervene to help me to avoid this catastrophe, which is absolutely the way I saw it at the time. That stark realisation forced me to review my relationship with the world and my parents in particular.

I want to say at the outset that I have never been a conscientious objector. I just don't like being told what to do and I reacted badly at the thought that my government wanted to steal two years of my life and, moreover, for very little money!

In those days, you might recall, a British person did not reach majority until the age of 21. You were, therefore, under the protective umbrella; some would say the overpowering shadow, of your parents for those extra three years between 18 and 21. Luckily I

was still studying at school when I received the kind invite. For that reason I was able to postpone my entry into service by the legitimate means of a deferment on the grounds of education. One lived in the dream world that once deferred it might go away forever. In fact, as it turned out, I very nearly made it to everlasting freedom through the means of having successfully obtained several deferments. The main hole in my bucket, though, was that my success in claiming deferments was not matched by any success in subsequent exams.

There was, naturally, a lengthy form to fill in order to be enabled to complete one's involuntary inclusion into HM forces. On this form I was also able, ostensibly, to make a choice as to which of the armed services I would prefer. My order of preference was first the Navy, my second choice was the RAF and my third choice was the Army. I also had to indicate my religion. I am Jewish, although in those days I was much more of a political animal than a religious one.

My dad had emerged from his period of serving King and Country during the war as an ardent communist. Some of his ardour had rubbed off on me. I never did join the Party although my own reading at the time did include books by Maxim Gorky, Mikhail Sholokhov and the magazine, the Soviet Weekly, although I never read Karl Marx nor, in any depth, the Daily Worker. Friday evenings in our house only too frequently heralded the arrival of members of the Edmonton Communist Party for their regular meetings, rather than any celebration of the arrival of 'Queen Shabbat'.

There had been some family significance in my choice of which box to tick because my dad had served in the R.A.S.C. during the war and had registered as C. of E. as a matter of possible self-preservation had he been captured by the Nazis. That may have been a serious concern for him at that time, although even a cursory medical examination by a very incompetent doctor would have shed some doubt as to the truth of Dad's deception and claim. Nonetheless I ticked the relevant box and registered myself as Jewish.

Strictly speaking I was not Jewish because my mother was not Jewish. I had, however, decided for myself, many years earlier, that I would regard myself as Jewish as a mark of respect for all those Jews, some members of my own family, who had perished during the Holocaust. It was my own personal "fingers up" to the Nazis; a small gesture but mine and one that I guard to this day, with no thought of need to defend it to anyone. I had made the decision when quite young, when the message had begun to sink in of the depths of organised bestiality to which the German nation had sunk during those long dark years of Nazi rule. The decision to tick the 'Jewish box' on that form had little significance for me at the time, but it was, however, to prove greatly beneficial during my service for reasons as then unknown, but which I shall divulge later.

By various means I was able to continue deferring my entry into the armed services until the beginning of 1960. I stayed on at school later than my peers in the vain hope of attaining a good batch of 'A' levels in subjects that would gain me a place in a good medical college. That did not materialise, much to the chagrin of my parents. I was actually offered a place at Charing Cross Teaching Hospital after interview there. My interview skills were, however, far better honed than my exam skills and so that came to nothing because I failed the necessary exams.

My parents would not support me in my personal desire to study languages at university and insisted that science subjects were the only way forward towards a decent career. I really could not commit to this course; the result being that my study for 'A' level science and maths exams never achieved the heights that were necessary to reflect their ambitions.

I left school and had another try at my 'A' levels by signing on at Enfield Polytechnic, with the result that yet another year was wasted although my bridge game was beefed up. I then worked for a year at Chase Farm Hospital as an Operating Theatre Technician until early in 1960. This was a very interesting job but one which was, in itself,

going no-where for me. In the intervening time between then and the first brown envelope I had received a series of such missives all serving to remind me that the War Office had, unfortunately, not forgotten about me.

In March of 1960 I received a final brown envelope, the contents of which were quite blunt. The letter gave me a date for a medical examination which was to take place at the beginning of June and informed me that I was being drafted into the RAF. The letter was couched in terms that suggested very strongly that if I did not attend this medical they would come and get me! By this time I was 21 and things were not going too well at home between me and my parents.

I began to realise that the inevitable was upon me. I felt that as I would have to do my national service I might as well go and get it over with, albeit without good grace. I returned the reply slip stating that I would attend the medical. In my heart I was happy that I was being directed to the RAF rather than the Army. I have to say that, although it was convenient to me on one level at that time, I did resent the whole idea of national service very deeply and fundamentally. I regarded it as a theft of two years of my life and as a waste of my time. I was also courting my future wife, Joyce, and my impending military service produced some anxiety due to the uncertainty of not knowing where I would end up having to serve the two years.

The day of my medical was a lovely, warm, day in early summer. It was one of those 'soft' English summer days when just walking along the street can make you feel at ease with the world. I took the bus and tube to High Holborn. As it was a warm day I decided, to my mother's disgust, to wear sandals and shorts. I think that she regarded this choice as depicting a lack of respect to the doctor. This was in an era when people of a certain generation felt that due deference had to be given to the very title 'doctor'. I have to say that, to a large extent, my own views ran on the same lines. On this occasion however my choice of footwear was predicated on my own comfort

rather than the good opinion of a military doctor, who I did not want to see in any event.

I do not live in London these days and for those who do not know the place, I would claim that it was then, and still is, a wonderful city. It bustles with a myriad of sounds. In the words of Neil Diamond, it makes a "beautiful noise". It has theatres that are the envy of the world. There is a depth of theatre culture, as well as a history that serves those theatres. You can feel the hustle of a million strangers as they push past you, bent hurriedly on their own business, with no care for you, but each with the earnest intent to achieve unknown goals.

Everybody has his or her own story. You have on tap an encyclopaedia of languages brushing past; this even more true now than then. Even the traffic has its own tune, and the underground railway, the tube, will often resonate with the music of buskers through the sometimes long transfer tunnels between route interchanges. London is my town and I love it, although Joyce and I have not lived there for many years. When we were young the price of housing in London was much greater than outside London and inflation rates have more than matched this difference over the years. We were forced by price to move out of that great city when we were ready to buy a house.

It was quite hot when I left the tube station at high Holborn. I purchased an ice lolly from a kiosk at the station, a Lyons 'Orange Maid' and very refreshing it was. I walked, licking it like a schoolboy, from Holborn Station along High Holborn in the direction of the office where the proposed medical was to take place. I arrived both reluctant and earlier than I had anticipated and decided to finish my lolly on the pavement before entering the building. As one grows older one enters the doctor's surgery with more and more feelings of trepidation and fingers crossed in case he or she has further tit bits of bad news for you, more miseries for you to worry about. This was not the case however in the full brashness

of youth. One was confident in one's fitness and strength. As I walked into the building though, I could not help but think that it would be really convenient if the doctor could discover some easily curable minor misery that would prevent me from being able to do my national service.

I did not have too long to wait, however. It was only a few minutes before I was called into the 'presence'. That doctor had an aura of surliness about him which was about to be deepened dramatically. It was as if his thin smile of welcome appeared to be a 'stick on' and would quickly fade, die and slide away from his craggy face at the slightest possible provocation, which he was about to receive. He clearly wanted to get this business over as quickly as possible. He directed me gruffly towards a tall screen with an oriental design apparently painted on it.

Doctor 'gruff' told me to remove my outer garments and my socks and sandals. As I removed these items I became aware immediately that my feet would never come up to muster in this environment. They appeared to have taken on all the summer dust of London in the form of dark stripes, where the holes of the sandals had allowed it to penetrate, to darken my feet with the addition of deep, zebra-like stripes. I looked up at the doctor and viewed him with an accumulating mixture of dismay and amusement; the resultant look of angry disgust and real irritation that, somehow, quickly eclipsed the slippery smile on his face, appeared as if by magic.

He strode the few paces towards me and prepared to examine my chest with what turned out to be a very cold stethoscope. "Put your tongue out" he ordered abruptly. I did so and felt instantly a further cold shiver of deepening embarrassment as I caught a glance, in the mirror behind his head, of the same apparition that confronted him. My tongue was glowing bright, luminous and orange, from the recent applied enjoyment of the ice lolly. I had never heard a doctor swear before! "Didn't you know that you were coming for a bloody medical today?" His expletive vocabulary went far beyond 'bloody', words he

definitely did not learn at medical school! He exploded into a long and very accomplished rage.

My newly found admirer added finally, when he had recovered a modicum of composure. "You young man, are clearly fit enough, with no sign or evidence of ill health, to get yourself into such a bloody awful state when attending a medical. "As far as I'm concerned you're A1. You can dammed well prove otherwise if you want to try it. Clear off! I've seen quite enough of you. You'll hear from the RAF shortly". He chuntered on, in this vein, for some very long seconds and continued all the while that I prepared my escape by getting back into my clothes. I remember thinking that you're always at a disadvantage when undressed. Once dressed, I did think of protesting but noted the glint in his eye and decided that discretion was by far the better part of valour on this occasion. A few days later I received the final brown envelope in my singularly long series of such missives. That one, however, contained a rail warrant and instructions to report for basic training at RAF Bridgnorth, in beautiful Shropshire, just north of Birmingham, on Monday, 4th July 1960. How bloody ironic, I thought, 'What a day on which to lose my own independence!'

I was about to be absorbed into the RAF against my will. I reacted badly to this for several reasons. Firstly, I had been the recipient of many adverse tales of military life from both my Dad and my future father in law. These tales had focussed largely on the low pay, the poor conditions, and above all the poor quality food they had both experienced during their service during the War. Then there was my own strong disinclination to be ordered into giving up two years of my life. Finally, about two years earlier my Mum had shown me a letter she had received from Dad during the War, a few months prior to the D. Day landings. She had had a miscarriage and had written to Dad asking for him to come home for a while. Dad's C.O. had refused him a compassionate leave and had accused him of arranging for Mum to have an illegal abortion whilst he was on active service. I had vowed that I wanted nothing to do with people who could think like that.

2
RAF Bridgnorth

AS I WRITE this I remember that, as I travelled to Bridgnorth that day in early July 1960, the various warnings about military service, from my dad and future father in law, had occupied a great deal of my thinking. There was a mixture of emotions, a little anxiety, but mostly an enduring anger, at what I saw as the deep injustice of it all... The anger surged to a new level however when I thought of that letter written by Dad to my mother re his C.O. He had been devastated at the accusation made against him by his that officer. He had also been wracked with guilt that he could not get home to comfort Mum, at a time when she had clearly needed him. To me, that situation represented the very worst of what I saw as the ingrained class difference between officers and the 'other ranks' in the British military, during those years. I made myself a promise that I would try to keep Joyce at arm's length, from my military experience, as far as possible. This was not always possible of course, but the intention was there.

In 1960 RAF Bridgnorth, The Number 7 School of Recruit Training was an R.A.F. basic training camp in Shropshire, and lay just outside of the town of Bridgnorth. It seemed huge to me. It was only as I got down from the train, that I realized, for the first time, just how many more of the young men who had been on that train were on the same mission as me. The grey RAF bus that waited for us at the station was

soon full to bursting point, with many of our number having to stand for the short journey to the camp.

On our arrival there the bus drove on into the camp, once the barrier had been raised, and the bus had been checked in by the guard corporal. We stopped alongside a row of long wooden huts, one of which we soon learned would be our living quarters, for the next eight weeks or so. Voices from outside the bus shouted coarsely for us to get out. The scene that developed was exactly like the arrival at training camp seen in the film 'Carry-on Sergeant,' except that the language of the three NCOs was far worse than in the film. There were no euphemisms to lighten the weight of the superfluous invective. I am convinced that the aim of those N.C.Os was to create a sense of panic and confusion in their newly arrived recruits. I apologise now for some of the language that appears in the following pages. I have tempered some of it and kept some because that was the way it was.

After a short few moments of respite there was more unnecessary shouting, during which the two corporals and the sergeant managed to use more 'Fs' and B's in those few seconds than a person might reasonably use or even hear in a whole lifetime. We were apparently the scum and dregs of the earth and had no right whatsoever to be in a 'revered' service such as the RAF. I would have been quite happy, as it happens, to exit right away and relieve them of the necessity of bothering with me. Wisely, though, I kept that gem to myself.

Their impossible duty, it seemed, was to turn us from the "Fucking" scruffy individuals that we were into young men fit to wear the Queen's uniform in public. That would take all of their attention, apparently, and at least four weeks hard work on their part. This I translated to mean 'our part'. We would not be allowed outside of the camp until they, the NCOs, felt that we were up to scratch. My heart sank at this. I could not bear the thought that I would not see my Joyce for at least four weeks. I resolved there and then, by hook or by crook, to do my best to thwart that arrangement. Four weeks was an impossible time to wait but at that point it was not easy to see

a way around the order. In fact I could see little beyond the next ten minutes or so.

We were lined up alongside the bus and the sergeant called the role of the names on his list, whilst we had to respond "here Sergeant." as he called each one of us in turn, those who were paying attention, those who were not, those who were fully aware of what was happening to them, those who were not. When he was finally satisfied the sergeant instructed the corporals to take us off to stores to be kitted out.

The scene in stores proved to be a good insight into the way that the RAF intended to treat us, its new recruits. It represented a scene of disorganised chaos in which each of a long series of victims was tormented in his turn by an experienced team of inquisitors. The stores building was a long one with a counter on one side that ran almost the length of the building. There were half a dozen or so airmen standing behind the counter waiting to 'issue' our kit to us. Behind these airmen were racks of assorted equipment that was destined to come our way. We, the identified victims and would-be recipients of that soon to be forthcoming bounty, simply milled around as a disorganised crowd. We were finally told to line up in some semblance of order and to move along the counter as in a cafeteria. As we did so a confusing and growing pile of items was thrown across the counter at us and 'Growed like Topsy' in front of each of us, as we proceeded, confusedly, along. Peremptory questions such as; "Hat size? Neck-size? Chest? Waist? - Feet?" were being thrown at us in no apparently logical order as the pile of assorted items grew ever larger and, seemingly, more unmanageable. When the 'foot' question came to pass, I helpfully answered "two". A pair of boots were thrown at me with such force that I immediately regretted my witticism and decided to close the 'funny' book at once. The airman dishing out the 'clobber' had obviously had a hard day and was in no mood for newbies taking the wee-wee.

The pile included; blankets, sheets, two hats, (one peaked one beret), one pair of boots, one pair of shoes, two uniforms, (one dress,

one every day), one greatcoat [very useful on cold winter nights] one belt (webbing), black polish, Blanco-(one tin), Brasso- (one tin), a tin mug, and a set of needles and cottons together with a wooden mushroom, laughingly referred to, by the NCOs as the "housewife"! Finally we were issued with an R.A.F. blue kitbag and a blue holdall into which some of the pile could be quickly stuffed.

Once we had all received this huge pile of equipment we were marched off to our billet, the place we were now destined to refer to as 'home' for the next 8 or so weeks. I say we were marched but most of us simply staggered as best we could, under the weight and bulk of the huge pile of equipment from stores. That pile was now our personal responsibility: for when the confusing rain of equipment ceased to pour down we were required to sign our names to the appropriate form and take ownership of it.

The billet was a long; double fronted, single-story building of wooden construction. It was one of a row of such structures, all aligned alongside an internal road of the camp and about fifteen feet or so apart. Behind us, as we had left the bus, was a large square of tarmac, the significance of which, for us, we would become only too well aware, over the next days and weeks.

We quickly discovered that there were two dormitories in the hut, each containing 11 beds. These were arranged as separate rooms, one on either side of a central section that contained loos, showers and two single rooms; one for each of the two corporals. Amid a great deal of shouting and swearing these two NCOs allocated beds, henceforth referred to as our 'pits', and pointed out the charts at each end of the room that introduced us to the twin joys of bed packs and inspection layout plans.

We speedily discovered that our 'pits' were not for sleeping in so much as they were the focus of morning inspections of our equipment. These were carried out by the sergeant, often together with the Officer in Charge of both our billet and our 'flight'; (Flight being the R.A.F. equivalent of an army platoon). The bed pack was an

interesting concept designed as one component in a range of carefully prepared military miseries, each designed to make an airman's
life as uncomfortable and full of unbelievable hurdles as possible. It
resembled a large Battenberg cake arrangement to be constructed
from the blankets and sheets topped by the two pillows with which
we had been issued. This construction was then positioned at the
head end of the bed with one remaining blanket being spread neatly
over the mattress. Once the Battenberg was placed in position, specified items of our equipment had to be arranged, as required, on the
blanket. The exact order of this arrangement being stipulated in the
charts displayed at each end of the billet.

On one side of each bed stood a wardrobe and on the other there
was a locker, half the height of the wardrobe. Each man's RAF issue
mug had to be placed centrally on top of the locker together with
shaving equipment. During our first inspection the next morning it
quickly became clear that there was an absolute necessity that all
mug handles had to be pointing in the same direction. There were
two corporals in charge of our flight and, naturally, each of these preferred that the mug handles should point in a different direction. The
game that they managed to play over mug handles does not need
much brain power to work out. The corporals themselves certainly
did not demonstrate any personal attributes by way of quantity or
quality of grey matter. They seemed to find the subsequent waste
of our time and taxpayers money most amusing, but then they were
highly trained junior NCOs at the peak of their powers!

When I was asked, on that recent occasion, if servicemen were
really ordered to paint stones white, my reply did not do justice to
the question. That particular task was indeed one of the more sensible of the seemingly nonsensical tasks imposed on young adults,
who were often quite well educated, at the whim of the sometimes
obscure military objective. White stones were, after all, used as road-
side markers in camp and thereby served a useful purpose on dark
nights and evenings.

I am fully convinced, though, that some of the time wasting tasks had been devised with the sole purpose of keeping large numbers of men quietly busy, by a system that had no better mental resources at its disposal and, in reality, did not want large numbers of conscripts cluttering its otherwise well-ordered regime. Such a task was one that now entered into our unsuspecting, small minded, 'new recruit' world. It involved all the copper pipe work in the loos in the central section of the billet hut. As a necessary part of our 'bulling' of the building, we had to paint all of this pipe work with shiny black lacquer paint. It became clear, however, that soppy as this idea was, we had the better end of the task, because the 'flight' before us had had to scrape off the black lacquer paint applied by the 'flight' before them; and so on, turn and turn about as 'flights' had been ordered. One to paint pipes black, the next to clean off the black paint so that the pipe work could, on each change over, become fit for inspection again as shiny copper metal. Such is the eternal madness of men! There was a lot of piping in those loos. It was a damned miracle that there was any actual pipe-work left, as it must have gradually wore thinner, after all the changes of state that had been applied over the years!

Nor were we allowed to walk directly on the lino floors of the billet except in socks for, when wearing shoes or boots; we had to glide around on small sections of blankets known as 'pads'. The officer and N.C.Os of course did not recognise this rule for themselves. It was simply another device wherein the establishment saw, as its continuing role "to make men of us". This was a phrase that the sergeant, Sergeant H., in particular, used quite frequently. From his mouth this seemed to me to become a particularly ironic use of the English language. He made a sad figure who I could not take seriously, neither physically nor intellectually. A man in his mid-forties, he was at the height of his lifetime's achievement. He was a drill sergeant in an organisation that his paymasters were in the process of deconstructing. His main accomplishment appeared to be his ability to shout. Sergeant. H. was the most-shouting man that I ever did meet. His

voice could be heard right across the parade ground at a decibel level
that was phenomenal. That was it though. That was the one and only
real attribute the man had, as far as I could tell. His poor intelligence
was linked directly into the RAF drill manual with very little by way of
osmosis into it from the real world. To Sergeant H. the model of an
ideal airman was imprinted on his psyche. He used phrases such as,
"We are going to take you to pieces and put you back together the
RAF way". I am convinced that he truly believed these homilies, and
that was the sadness of the man. The sergeant had two corporals to
assist him in his chosen task. They were both national servicemen,
each of whom had shown a particular lack of personal intelligence
and initiative. Each one did have, though, a high aptitude for 'bull' and
'drill'. They were, therefore, quite suitable to be selected to become
junior drill NCOs. They had shown promise as 'smart' airmen during
their own basic training. They had been chosen to train as drill corporals and had returned to Bridgnorth in that capacity. The smarter
and more acerbic of the two was Corporal Gavin. When he was not
shouting orders words rolled from his mouth like acid from a glass
spoon. I cannot remember the name of the other corporal nor do I
pine for that knowledge. These two, then, became the bane of our
lives because they lived in our billet and could, therefore, devote as
much time as they chose to making our lives a misery.

There are two more of the many indignities inflicted upon us,
in the name of the God of greater discipline, to which I must refer.
These are the loo cabins and the "piss house rose" as it was affection-
ately named. There were, ostensibly, a number of loo cabins available
for our use. It came to pass, however, that all but one had to be roped
off, this because they were needed to be in 'pristine' condition, so as
to pass inspection requirements. The same applied to a long stretch
of the pee channel, which left only a short length available for the
necessary needs of some 26 airmen. The "rose" was inevitably in this
section and became my responsibility through a mysterious and complicated lottery process. The rose, a brass, perforated bowl, sat at

the end of the channel. It was there in order to prevent unwanted detritus, such as 'fag' ends, from disappearing into the bowels of the plumbing system. It was up to me to keep it spick, span and shiny, for the above mentioned inspections. I quickly came to the conclusion that the only way a nice Jewish boy could deal with this problem, without coming far too close to the pee of the nation, was to hide the rose where no others could find it, but from whence it could be produced, solely when required for scrutiny in its proper position. In that way I became the protector of the cleanest "piss house rose" in the history of the RAF, and sod the plumbing!

I first heard what has become a very unfortunate phrase at this point in my very unwelcome military career. It was addressed to all of us, new recruits and captive audience by our newly-acquired mega-shouting three-striper. "This is where you do all your morning ablutions. This is where you shit, shower, shave and shampoo". He let us have this pearl of information with such a superior attitude that one got the impression that he had issued the advice thousands of times previously and had been greeted by the same dull reception, notwithstanding which he continued to try his tired old gem. The problem inflicted on me, tragically, is that, even now, decades later, I cannot have a shower without the damned phrase going through my head. I curse that ill-begotten sergeant each and every time.

At the head of this small team of would be 'makers of men' resided the officer, the Flight Lieutenant. He was a red faced man, also in his mid-forties. Unlike his junior staff he did not have even a semblance of physical fitness to his credit. Again I cannot remember his name nor, as before, do I care. His red face, I judged, had been acquired from years of self-indulgence at the bar of the officers' mess. He wore a moustache which, on some men, can be an adornment of which to be proud. His, though, did nothing for him. It simply sat on his face as if embarrassed for itself, not knowing why it was there. As far as I could tell, the Flight Lieutenant was in a similar situation to that of the sergeant, worse if at all possible. His only role seemed to be

that of daily inspector of the work of his N.C.Os, and our 'progress'. He was a commissioned officer without a real job, in an air force that had been, not many years before, the hero and envy of the world. This officer had never been a flying type; he wore no insignia. He had, apparently, been deployed from another 'desk' position as a going-nowhere management symbol of a system of National Service that was in its death throes. At that stage of my RAF career I resented every moment that I had to spend in the company of such people. I found it very difficult to have respect for them, other than that which was enforced on me by their rank and by the military service to which we all now belonged. I was determined to get through my time by applying myself to doing as little as possible of any military value and by waging small 'wars' against the system wherever I could and wherever it was compatible with my own well-being.

Our days began with reveille, ablutions and inspections, which could be relied upon to bring abuse and even more work for us to do later that evening. This aspect of inspections became par for the course to such effect that the impact and anticipation of these daily events soon wore off. When there was so little possibility of achieving a 'well done' there was no sense in putting in the greater effort, other than that required to stave off further acrimony.

Inspections, with the concomitant negativity, were followed by breakfast. Food was plentiful and of universally good quality in the R.A.F. To my great surprise I found this to be the case during the whole of my two years and my experience of four different camps. This was quite contrary to the horrific tales told both by my dad and my future father-in-law, Joy's dad, from their own admittedly hard and bitter wartime experiences.

The miseries of inspection complete, we were then required to muster outside our billet to discover what range of further miseries our team of captors had in store for us that day. The possible range included all the well-known favourites, for example, rifle drill, marching or running whatever unreasonable distances that our tormentors

might decide. There were other forms of physical exercise, even occasionally, games. This would invariably be on a Wednesday afternoon, the time set aside in all of the services for competitive games. We could also be required to attend class based lessons on the history of the R.A.F. or how to recognise the varying ranks of officers and N.C.Os in all of the services by their ranges of insignia. Our evenings were invariably taken up with preparing our uniforms and billets, ready for the inevitable inspections that would follow the next morning. This all took place amid much noise, sometimes bad temper and, of course, the seemingly inevitable range of swearing and coarse humour. During all of this service-based activity we were subject to periodic tests, both physical and written, to assess progress towards a final passing out parade.

Finally, however, came the one day to which I had truly been looking forward. We were going to be shown how to use our rifles for that purpose for which they had been designed. We were going to begin to learn to shoot them instead of marching them around the drill square in bizarre patterns. I cannot begin to explain how eagerly I had anticipated the day. For years I had had an almost morbid fascination for the idea of shooting a rifle and now it was going to happen.

I intend to explain the happenings of those eventful days in more detail later on in my story. Suffice it to say that, much to my joy and satisfaction, I passed the standard that entitled me to a 'marksman's' badge at the very first possible opportunity. This even earned me a few kind words of praise from the R.A.F. Regiment Flight Sergeant who was the instructor for the session and who had witnessed, only a few minutes previously, a very unpleasant professional and alarming experience. I shall tell more of that later, though, as I say. Nonetheless I can say that I wore my badge with some pride and that even my dad had a few complimentary words to say when he saw my new acquisition, neatly sewn by yours truly at the bottom of my left sleeve on the next weekend when, as usual, I went home, unofficially of course.

Another day, not so welcome, came when we were to be introduced to the 'gas chamber'. Tear gas that is. My own guess is that the RAF and possibly other forces were still living in fear of the times of the First World War when men in trenches were horribly gassed by the Germans. The Gas Training Building, where we were due to experience the gassing seemed to be, as far as I can remember it, nothing more impressive than a rectangular concrete block with what looked like a square chimney tower stuck to one side of it. There was an entrance door to a small anteroom across from which was an observation window into the 'gas-room' where we were due to have our unwelcome and unwanted experience.

A sergeant sat by the observation window, at a small desk on which were situated some control buttons. I can remember nothing about this NCO other than that he gathered us around him, in the anteroom, to give us each a gas-mask and some instructions. He instructed us, just how and when, to don the gas masks and advised us that in a few short moments he would tell us to go into the chamber. He further advised us that, once in the chamber, he would give us a few minutes to sit down on the wooden benches in order to get used to breathing through the gas masks. He would then release tear-gas into the chamber so that we could experience breathing safely through the gas mask. After a few minutes he would tell us to remove the gas masks and for a few seconds only we would experience the extreme discomfort of trying to breathe in a room full of teargas. He said that we should replace the gas mask as soon as breathing became too uncomfortable without it.

My memory is that breathing became far too uncomfortable to bear in a very few seconds. My eyes welled with tears, my nose and mouth choked up, so that I was very, very quickly gasping for breath and needed to replace the mask almost at once, as did everyone else. After what seemed an eternity we were allowed to escape. On our way out we were told to run around the nearby sports field. "Without rubbing your eyes or you will be on a charge for self-injury,"

he shouted. The idiot apparently regarded himself as something of a parade ground wit.

I cannot imagine why or how the service regarded this training as a useful exercise, because I could not, at that time, imagine any circumstances whereby an enemy would spray us with teargas. I have to say, though, that I would not have liked to have been in that chamber without the gas mask and so, on reflection at a later date, I had to admit that there may have been some benefits that resulted from the exercise, those in terms of making one understand that when gas masks are issued they need to be kept well to hand, because if teargas can render one so ill, so very quickly, other gases would be much worse, even impossible, to bear or survive. One just had to hope that the masks issued, under those future circumstances, would be capable of dealing with gases more potent than tear gas.

I have to admit reluctantly, but honestly, that one change took place in my own behaviour during my years in the RAF and which began to take ground firmly during basic training. It was my use of what, many years later, a work colleague referred to as my use of 'street' language. It is a feature of which I am not at all proud. I have tried very hard, particularly in recent years, to curb my use of this unpleasant aspect of my behaviour. I have had some success for I do not think that my grandchildren would regard it as a major failing of mine. Sometimes though, even now, in a moment of stress, there will be an explosion of a word or two that I will always regret too late. Usually and thankfully it is when I am alone. I am still working on it. It is, as they say, a work in progress.

Three events of some significance to me took place during my first week of basic training. The first was instigated by the sergeant at our post breakfast morning parade. One of the joys of each evening was to clean our webbing belts. These were composed of white webbing that needed to be 'blancoed'. This belt was interspersed and held together by brass spacers and buckles which in their turn had to be 'brassoed'. The admixture of these two, cleaning and shining,

applications rendered the belt cleaning task into a very fiddly operation. One was continually removing Blanco from the brass or covering up Brasso that had escaped onto the white webbing. I hated my belt!

On the morning in question, the sergeant had inspected my belt and had proclaimed it to be the worst example of a parade-ready webbing belt that he had ever seen. I hated my belt so much that I was very ready to believe him. As a punishment he ordered me to report to the cookhouse that evening for extra duties after the day's tasks. At the end of the day I decided that I just had time for a short nap before reporting to the cookhouse. "Wrong!" I did not wake up until I heard the others getting ready to go to the mess for our evening meal, the one, even, that I had been ordered to help to prepare.

I felt unusually nervous the next morning as we waited for the sergeant to appear on parade. I was nervous as to what further punishment he would order, as a result of my failure to comply with his previous one. I had disobeyed an order and surely that would be dealt with quite severely. As it turned out, however, I need not have worried. The sergeant was oblivious to the fact that I had not gone, as required, to the cookhouse. I quickly realised that my webbing belt had not necessarily been the issue. It had merely been a device for him to send a few extra hands to his mate, the cookhouse sergeant, to help with the evening meal. It was a pattern that became clear during the weeks that followed and I never once complied with such an order after that first time, although I was one of the 'selected few' on several subsequent occasions. The accident of falling asleep stood me in good stead throughout my basic training. I have to confess that I did not share my discovery with any of my companions. I had won another little war with the system that I loathed. I had no intention of passing this successful ammunition on to anyone else, thereby encouraging wider 'punishment' avoidance which might have scuppered my own situation. No indeed, this was a time to keep one's cards close to one's chest.

The second significant event took place at morning parade when the sergeant called our names to check that we were present. He came to my name and, suddenly, seemingly, a propos of nothing, he barked at me, "You're Jewish". "I know that Sarge" was all I could think to say by way of reply. I was amazed though, as I quickly realised that the information must have followed me to that place from the form that I had completed those several years before. "You don't have to attend church parade this Sunday." That was fortuitous, because I would not have attended a church parade under any circumstances that the R.A.F. might devise.

"There is a Jewish faith chapel that you can use on Friday evenings and Saturdays if you want to." This was, in the event, an exaggeration. The faith chapel alluded to was actually a multi-faith chapel used apparently solely by Jews at that time and there was only a small group of us to use it. It was nonetheless very welcome. He went on to advise the others that they were required to attend church parade every Sunday whilst they were on basic training. Yet another way of occupying hundreds of young men was my cynical view of this arrangement. It was also a means of assuring that they could not leave the camp, for there would certainly be a roll call at the time of the parade. This, though, all suited me very well. I was beginning to formulate a possible plan of my own, that plan needed just one more cog to tumble into place to be as complete as I could make it, under the circumstances in which I found myself.

The twists and turns of a benevolent fate permitted the fall of the final cog into place on the second or third day of my first week at Bridgnorth. It was evening time, after dinner, on a beautiful summer's evening. It was still quite light and I had set out for a walk around the inside perimeter of the camp. I was really only interested in looking at the size of the place on that occasion. Walking around the camp made me realise just how huge it really was. A quick count of barrack huts realised a rough figure of accommodation for well over three thousand men, not counting permanent staff.

As I walked alongside a large football pitch; to my left and ahead of me, I noticed a small group of permanent staff who seemed to be walking directly towards what I had taken to be the perimeter hedge around the camp. They seemed to be chatting aimlessly as one does when walking together with friends. I was not interested in them at all at first, except that as they got closer and closer to the hedge they appeared to be unconcerned about its' looming presence. They seemed not to notice it until finally, from my perspective, they disappeared right into it. I was amazed and somewhat amused as I hurried towards the spot where this dematerialisation had taken place. The hedge had seemed to be impenetrable from my, then, vantage point. That long hedge had formed much of that leg of the perimeter.

I became more and more intrigued as I hurried to approach the point where I had last seen the vanished ones. To my complete amazement there was a substantial gap in the hedge quite wide enough for several persons to step through comfortably. I moved through the hedge onto a narrow 'made up' road. Across the road I found myself confronted by a small housing estate of what appeared to be 'council' type housing. It was, I quickly realized, the junior ranks' married quarters. They clearly used this gap in the hedge as a shortcut home, rather than walk the long way around via the guard room each time they needed to leave the camp to get to their quarters. More to the point though, as far as I was concerned, the gap gave out directly onto a public road and, to my left, a short way along the narrow road on which I was now standing, I could see occasional traffic moving. What a find! I felt that it must be the road that ran past the guard room on the outside of the camp. Possibilities began to tumble into place. My dream plan began to finalise. That weekend I said to myself, I would be going home!

To a civilian it must seem incredible, as it did to me at that time, that there should be such a breach in the secure perimeter of a military establishment. All I can say is that I served on four R.A.F. camps during my two years of National Service and just one of the four had

a fully secure perimeter. On a second one it was necessary to exit the camp via the guard room but the checks were perfunctory. One might make the argument that the two remaining totally insecure camps, both being training camps, were therefore not strategically sensitive. My response to that argument is uncomplicated – nuts! Each of those camps had an armoury containing a mixture of deadly weapons. Those weapons were at the mercy of criminals or terrorists alike, due to the lack of security that I have just identified. More of this later, though, when I get to my final RAF destination in Norfolk.

I planned my escape for that Saturday as soon as parade had ended. I decided to leave the camp via my route through the hedge and out onto the open road, turning left at the gap, and then a short walk to the A254. I had little money so had decided to try my hand at hitch hiking home. I had not tried this since my early teenage years, when I had always used this means of locomotion when travelling and camping around the country with, my old school friend Bill.

This is an ideal time to outline the difference between hitch hiking, in uniform, then and now. Nowadays service men and women are instructed not to leave their camps in uniform, due to the serious possibility that they might be attacked, whether by terrorists, or despicably, by gangs of indigenous thugs, with scant regard or respect for the uniform of the country in which they live.

In 1960 there were very few service women, none of whom were national service women. On the other hand the majority of men had known military service one way or another. Most of those over about forty years of age had been in uniform during the war. Those under that age, again the majority of them, had been required to do national service.

As soon as I began to hitch hike I realised that my uniform was as good as a ticket home. I only had my uniform available in any case, because my civilian clothing had been taken away, to be returned when I was allowed home after my basic training was completed. At 12.10 pm or so, on the forthcoming Saturday, I walked through

my gap in the hedge, along the road past the married quarters and out on to the main public road. I turned right and walked along a bit so that I could not be seen from the guard room and began to hitch.

It was a bit tricky as I did not know the area, and between me and London lay the vast conurbations of Wolverhampton and Birmingham. I need not have worried, though, because the great majority of drivers who stopped were both sympathetic to the needs of a national serviceman, and as helpful as they could possibly be. I reached home by 4pm. My dad, to my surprise, was furious and very worried. He was totally convinced, at first, that I had gone AWOL and that I would be in trouble. As I had every intention of returning to camp the next day that thought had not occurred to me. It caused me some concern for a few minutes but that quickly dispersed at the thought of going round to see Joy. I was also quite rebellious with respect to the Air Force at the time. As far as I was concerned they were not my best friends, and the thought of what punishment might be imposed did not really concern me so very much, other than the wild thought that it might separate me from Joyce for a while. After all was said and done, they couldn't shoot me. Could they?

The weekend passed only too quickly. I remember the usual negative refrain from my mum, ably endorsed by my dad, that I was only using them as a convenience. I was able, though, to spend some time with Joy which made the agro worth-while. I spent Saturday evening and Sunday morning with Joy, sleeping at home on Saturday night. No other arrangement being possible before marriage in those days. After lunch at Joy's home I returned to spend the afternoon with my parents and my young sister Denise.

I set out to return to camp after tea on the Sunday. Dad softened in his aggravation over my illicit absence from camp once he realised that I fully intended to return there. He gave me a lift out of Enfield to a convenient roundabout from which to begin my return journey. During that short drive Dad and I spoke privately for the

first time for a long while. It was clear to me that he was missing me and needed to chat. In the short while that I had been away from home I had selfishly dismissed from my mind the tensions that my mum and dad constantly inflicted on each other and, more importantly, on my sister.

I let him know some of my feelings towards the RAF and also made it clear that I would get away from camp on each and every occasion that I could. I was not intending to desert but I had no intention of sticking around any-more than I needed to. I also let him know in no uncertain terms that I intended to be as uncooperative as possible towards the authority of the RAF. I told him about the cookhouse incident which did amuse him. He gave me some money and a hug before he left me. I said that I hoped to see him next weekend if I managed to get back into my billet without being caught.

I arrived back at camp quite late, but, as I had no intention of entering camp via the Guard Room, the time was not an issue. I did begin to have concerns that I might have been missed on the Saturday night but, as it turned out, I had no need to worry. I wandered into camp through my hedge entrance and managed to get into the billet without either of the corporals noticing or even, seemingly, caring that I had only just 'come home'. I did not even know if they were in their rooms. With as little noise as possible I changed my clothes and got into bed. On reflection later, I came to the conclusion that the corporals would not have considered the possibility that a new recruit would have had the 'balls' to leave camp without permission, let alone for the weekend.

Monday morning came and went as expected, with nothing said. I did not discuss my adventure with any of my peers, although a few of them knew about my escapade but chose not to try the temporary absence for themselves. Most of them were tied to Church Parade on Sunday mornings in any case. It was all to the good as I did not want to open up an escape route for anyone else. That might have nobbled things for me in the future. One empty bed had gone unnoticed,

six or seven might be a 'breach too far'. As far as I was concerned, moreover, that weekend fell into the very same category as my non-compliance with parade ground punishments. It was a secret that I hugged determinedly to my chest.

I went home every weekend after that with one exception. That was the fourth weekend, when we had been promised 'Town Leave', but the cynical b*******s chose to give us a full set of injections on the Friday. We were fit for nothing all weekend. I felt, though, that, on balance, I had very much won the battle of the weekends. I used my side exit from the camp and hitched home each and every week-end, other than on that sole occasion. I can add that the only time that I exited via the Guard Room was on the day that I cleared camp to go off to R.A.F. Kirton-in-Lindsey, finally, to undertake my trade training.

As I went through the process of clearing camp via the stores and the admin block I reflected on my time at RAF Bridgnorth. It had been, in my view, a period of eight wasted weeks; of press ups, of early morning runs, of rounds of drilling with a rifle, of learning to shoot the Lee Enfield 303 rifle and a Bren gun, although these last two were the real stars in my firmament! There were other time wasting activities, though, like painting perfectly good copper pipes black, of digging ditches and making rope bridges over them; of shouting, swearing NCO's who's only ambition was to get the flight through the eight weeks of training and successfully achieve a reasonable perfor-mance in the final passing out parade.

It was also a time of small victories; like never doing extra duties at the cookhouse, and not attending church parades; also there were bigger victories like never leaving the camp by the guardroom and never staying on camp over a weekend, other than the one where we were all laid low by multiple injections. That thought made me feel good. I felt that I had won my first real battle with H.M. forces and that I had also learned some valuable lessons regarding hitchhiking in England in uniform in 1960. Most drivers in those days were men

and most men had known some form of military service but it was not unknown, even for unaccompanied women, to give lifts to men in the trusted uniform of British Serving Forces. As I said before, it was almost like having a ticket home!

3
Coming to Lincolnshire

I DID NOT want to move to Lincolnshire. More importantly, I did not like the reason for the move, nor the very abrupt way it was arranged. A short while before we were all due to leave RAF Bridgnorth, we were each asked to complete a form to indicate our preferences for trade training options. I had requested to be sent to RAF Melksham, in Wiltshire, for trade training as an RAF electronics fitter. My sole qualification at 'A' level GCSE being a fairly decent pass in applied maths, which I thought would be useful for an electronics fitter. My request was originally given the thumbs up, which pleased me no end. Firstly I saw this trade as being one that could offer opportunities after my national service, secondly, RAF Melksham is sited in Wiltshire which is a pleasant and beautiful County and which seemed also to offer good direct hitchhiking opportunities back to London for my weekends. This was always of prime importance to me. I had not ceased to regard my compulsory national service both as a challenge and a real imposition in my life. In view of that I was determined, as far as possible, to force my life in the RAF to conform to my own requirements and be as pleasant and beneficial to me as I could make it.

On the very morning that I was due to get on the bus for the station to catch the train to Melksham, however, I was commanded to go to the admin office because the admin officer needed to see me

urgently. When I heard what he had to say I was furious, because, apparently, my orders to go to Melksham for technical training had been rescinded. I was now required to go to RAF Kirton in Lindsey for trade training as a pay accounts clerk! This did not fit my image of myself at all. It was a huge disappointment and one that I could not disguise in my voice, as I responded to the admin officer's announcement. As far as I can remember I was quite rude to him although, to be fair, he was only the messenger. I was not in a mood to be fair at that moment, however. Looking back on the scene, I can only feel that I got away with it through my own ignorance and naivety, and that the officer took pity on me because of that. As an RAF officer he was not used to being spoken to in the way that I responded to his unwelcome news. He did, moreover, advise me very clearly after my first outburst that if I uttered one more angry word I would be charged with insubordination and that that matter, he reminded me, would have to be heard by the station commander. He added that the consequences might be quite serious.

My anger at the disappointment continued to boil away inside my heaving chest but I managed to bite my tongue to disguise the inner turmoil as best I could. I realized, angrily, that I would have to try to tackle this situation in another way. As I left the admin office I began, slowly, to realise that the officer could have taken much more drastic action and that he had let me off very lightly. I also began to formulate a plan whereby I would sabotage the accounts clerk proposal. After all, I thought, 'you can take a horse to water but.....etc.'

The change in direction of my trade training required me to remain at RAF Bridgnorth for a further few days, during which time the inevitable paperwork had to be reorganized. I never did know or find out why the change had needed to be made, although my dad had an unshakeable idea that he knew.

A year or so prior to my final entry into National Service I had applied to enter the RAF as an aircrew officer. I had survived the three days at RAF Hornchurch where I undertook and passed a series

of tests, both physical and mental. I was very pleased with my ability to endure and survive the three days because a high proportion of young men had been de-selected during each of various stages that took place during that period. Those of us, a very small minority, who were left at the end of this intensive selection process, were told that we would hear from the selection board in due course. I waited several anxious months before I received a letter stating that, after long consideration, I would not be offered a place on the aircrew training programme. At that point my dad told me that he was not at all surprised at the final outcome, which, as far as he was concerned, was entirely political. He reminded me that he was a registered member of the Communist Party and that that, in his view, would certainly have precluded my selection to such a sensitive programme at that time, the year being 1957 or 58.

It was that rejection, together with my dad's explanation for it that made me all the more resentful of my eventual 'call up'. I would have been very happy to enter the RAF when it was my choice but resented bitterly the compulsion that forced me into National Service. Dad took care to remind me of this episode when he heard my news of the switch in my trade training prospects. His reasoning was that they had switched me from a sensitive trade area to one that was much less sensitive. I had been sceptical of this explanation when dad had first proposed it after my attempt to become RAF aircrew. Following the sudden switch of trade training regime, however, I was more inclined to think that he could well have been right.

The mere thought of this, now probable reasoning for this my latest failure, merely strengthened my anger and resolve against my new military masters. It was at that point that I decided to arrange to have the Soviet Weekly delivered to me when I finally arrived at a permanent camp. As a socialist I was already well versed in the works of such Soviet writers as Maxim Gorky and Mikhail Sholokhov, although I was never a member of the Communist Party, nor had I, nor have I ever wanted to be. The rebel in me, however, decided that if they

were going to treat me as a security risk then I would act as if I might just possibly appear to be one after all.

The truth of that, however, was quite different for, unlike my dad, I hated Joe Stalin and all his communist cronies around Europe as well as what they stood for. As time has passed, though, I have realised that, although I resented those Friday night meetings of the Edmonton Communist Party that took place in our house during the whole of my childhood, I did benefit hugely from the contact that they gave me with political dialectic, and with an experience-broadening contact with party members from all over the country and, even, the world.

I have gradually realised that my dad was very well known and respected hugely by his peers. He was a man of both great integrity as well as intense loyalty to his friends. He was a very strong minded man, who had emerged from six years of war with fierce ambitions to fight the battles of the working classes and to promote their causes with all his strength, and in any way that he could think to do so. My own thoughts became much more centred on the specific and continuing battle against people like Oswald Mosley and Colin Jordon, the British Fascists, together with the various neo Nazi movements that emerged from under their stones, as soon as they dared, after the years of War that had been intended to eradicate them.

I spent an irritable extra couple of days at RAF Bridgnorth. There was little to do on camp and not being certain of my departure date, there was not enough time to return home and come back to make sure of catching the required train to get across country to Lincolnshire. I did, however, have time to explore the pretty town of Bridgnorth that I had so deliberately avoided during my eight weeks of Basic training.

Bridgnorth was once one of the busiest river ports in Europe, but nowadays, the Severn, clear and unpolluted, is a quiet haven for anglers, walkers and wildlife. The river presents the town as a backdrop of High Town and Low Town; the two are linked by seven sets of

ancient donkey steps and a Victorian funicular, the Bridgnorth Cliff Railway. As I walked the town those late summer days of 1960, I was able to enjoy the views described by Charles 1 as *"The finest view in my entire Kingdom"*.

Whether you admire the view over the king's shoulder from the sandstone cliff of Bridgnorth, or stand on the bridge below, (at the height of summer the Severn is almost covered by the flowers of water crowfoot), you won't have to look far to find a superlative in the Severn Valley. The beauty of the Town by the river Severn helped me ditch my foul mood during those few inactive days at RAF Bridgnorth. I was left entirely alone during that time. My only duty was to report to the admin officer each morning, to see if my movement orders had arrived.

When all the documentation was cleared and completed I was issued with a one-way travel warrant to my new camp. The journey took place just over fifty years ago, when train timetables, and the lines on which to complete journeys by rail were quite different than they are now. For these reasons I do not remember the details of the journey, other than the fact that it was tedious, boring, and that I hated every part of it, including the continuing realisation that I was going somewhere that was not of my choice; where I did not want to go, to train for something the thought of which I hated. I do remember, however, that the train took me through a Birmingham main line railway station from where I was able to take a second train across country direct to the station at Kirton-in-Lindsey itself.

It will surprise no-one to read that I took an instant dislike to RAF Kirton in Lindsey, as soon as I arrived there. The staff seemed friendly enough but I have to admit that I was determined to dislike the place and that feeling never fully left me. This pit of anger did not auger well for me to get the best out of my time there. The trade training was due to last six weeks but my intended strategy was that I would fail to qualify as a pay clerk. This intention hatched directly from my thoughts about horses and water etc.!

The mere thought of undertaking training as an accounts clerk drove me to distraction and so I did look around for ways to ameliorate the impending boredom. My first attempt at ingratiating myself into an attractive looking activity went embarrassingly badly for me. I spent my first weekend after my transfer to Kirton at home in Enfield as usual. I had managed to scrounge a lift home from an airman, permanently based at the camp but whose family actually lived in Palmers Green, not far from where I lived. I passed some of the time with my parents, exchanging news and so on but, as usual, the majority of my time was spent with Joyce.

For the return journey, Geoff, my airman friend with the car, picked me up in the centre of Enfield Town. He had another couple of pick-ups to make on our way out to the A1 and our journey back to camp. We were, therefore, four of us in the car for the majority of the journey. It was early September as I remember. The days were still quite warm and had not shortened too much. We still had some quietened twilight to enjoy as we left Enfield Town but it was quite dark by the time we had moved up towards East Anglia.

It was harvest time and the evening was quite warm. The only air conditioning in cars in those days was to open windows. With four of us in the car we had opened the two front windows from early on in the journey. The smells of the countryside blew an evening welcome into the car. I remember still the strong sweet smell from passing beat Lorries taking the sugary root crop to the refineries.

The scent of mown wheat and the hay newly harvested and stacked are all reminiscent of England at the time of year, a period that moulds the end of summer into the beginning of autumn. We had entered Lincolnshire when I began to dig the hole from which there was no escape. Up till that time the discussion in the car had been benign, of the weekend and plans for next week and the like.

Geoff was a decent man but one of whom I was quite envious, as he was nearing the end of his National Service; neither could he stop himself from reminding others of this fact at every opportunity.

I was far more envious of Geoff, however, over the car he owned and in which we were driving. That car was a beautiful 1955 Armstrong Siddeley Sapphire 236. It had the full spec; a 2300 cc engine, leather upholstery, which smelt so very rich as you got into the car that it fair made your taste buds dance. It was, moreover, finished in pure white and it even had the winged Armstrong Siddeley upright sphinx motif mounted at the top of the V shaped radiator. The powerful engine just seemed to purr along the dark ribbon of the moonlit country roads, the stars and moon reflected in the ghostly, seemingly, half acre of bonnet stretching out from the windscreen. Geoff did not need to tell us that he loved his car; he always referred to it in the third person as 'she' or 'her'. He also let us know that he had inherited 'her' from an elderly aunt, who had passed, away two years before without having put much mileage 'on the clock'. I have to confess that I was more envious of Geoff, because of that car, than I have ever been of anyone since that time. For reasons that follow, however, I only rode in it for that one return journey!

I remember Geoff as a big man, size one, built like the proverbial b**** s*** h**** He also bore the scars of a person who, man and boy, had fought his battles in the second row of several tasty rugby union clubs. Now I fancied myself as a would-be player of rugby union, although I knew very little about the game. I had never played it but, when the conversation in the car inevitably came to the subject of RAF rugby opportunities and, in particular, opportunities in The RAF Kirton-in-Lindsey team, I heard myself saying that I was quite a good player and that I played as a second row forward. This was believable on the face of it, because I did look the part of a second row man. Geoff was immediately interested in me and eagerly demanded to know who I had played for. Now, I was not ready for that one and it is where my train came off the rails big time! In my eagerness to press my case I had put myself in a position of answering a question to which I did not have any true answers and for which I could not think of any convincing lies. I could not concentrate well enough to

save myself. It felt as if my brain had suddenly shrunk to the size of a walnut. My mind was in a state of numbness, through blind panic, as I searched for an appropriate name to give him, as well as the other two passengers in the car, who had suddenly grown their interest in the conversation, as they sensed my impending difficulty. Through the haze I heard myself say..."Oh - the Harlequins."...I had suddenly dug myself a hole so deep that I could no longer even glimpse the sky! Geoff, on the other hand, became so excited at the thought of having such an eminent player suddenly fall into his grasp that he failed to ask himself the question of "how many Tony Kreits have you heard of at that level in the Game?"

I was digging the hole ever deeper. As I dug, the weight of the embarrassing ammunition that I needed to use, to try to extricate myself, made it finally impossible for me to associate ever again with poor Geoff. I had quite forgotten the maxim that, "if you're in a hole stop digging!" In fact I had gone far too far along the path of digging that the idea 'stop digging' was now of little use to me. As it was I was extremely glad to get out of that beautiful car that night. I had, though, learned some valuable lessons for the future; mainly not to lie about my abilities, or experience, in an effort to show off or to ingratiate myself. I have never ever been able to watch the famous Harlequins play on TV without cringing over that night in the car. I am still embarrassed at the thought of the impossible hole that I had dug for myself during that journey back to Lincolnshire, just by trying to show off. It was not one of my better moments!

A few days' later things improved for me, when I noticed that the camp boasted a boxing club. This was run by an RAF- PT instructor. As a teenager I had done some judo and had enjoyed it very much, as it afforded an interesting way to keep fit. I decided to give boxing a try.

The boxing trainer at RAF Kirton in Lindsey, Flight Sergeant Groome, was also the senior PT instructor. There was an officer in charge of station physical health but he hardly ever put in an appearance 'on the ground' so to speak. The flight sergeant seemed to be

left alone to construct and conduct his world to his own satisfaction. He was afforded a greater level of personal autonomy than I ever witnessed for any other NCO, below the rank of warrant officer, during my two years of service. He was a tall man, broad and exuded a high level of physical fitness with every movement. Simply walking across the floor he displayed an arrogant self-confidence, charm and a grace that many of us would not, or could not; aspire to at any time in our lives.

There was a tale about Flight Sergeant Groome that persisted in the camp's rumour mill that, when he was a PT instructor at RAF Bridgnorth, he had been attacked by two young men, whilst walking, one evening, across the bridge that enables traffic over the River Severn in the town itself. The story glorified him by concluding that both of his attackers ended up in the river. Whatever the truth or otherwise of the story, there is no argument that he was a physically impressive man. In the argot of the Old West "He walked tall!"

I sought the flight sergeant out in the station boxing club a couple of evenings after my debacle over the Rugby. I needed something, very quickly, to begin to erase that particular memory. The boxing club had been established at one end of a hangar that was no longer needed to house airplanes of any sort. The other end of the hangar being used as a five a side football pitch. The two sports worked well, side by side, because Groome took an interest in all sporting activity on the station. He was irritatingly good, as well as knowledgeable, at all sports that were a part of the RAF curriculum. He had clearly made it his business to be so.

As I approached the flight sergeant it became clearer that the boxing ring was a more impressive construction than I had anticipated. He had been standing next to the ring talking to another airman as I approached. I stood close by and waited as they finished their conversation, not so much a conversation, however, as a monologue by Groome.

"Now you listen to me..." as he poked the other man in the chest.

"If you want to stay with the team you will do the training, NO Ifs, NO BUTS!" This as the airman tried to interject something back into the mix. The flight sergeant turned to me in a move that told it all. That particular discussion had ended. The airman wandered off to join a group busily engaged with a selection of training equipment.

"Yes?" he enquired of me, rather brusquely I thought at the time. "Some people don't like getting up early in the morning for their training runs." He looked over his shoulder at his previous interlocutor and continued "Do you?" In fact the one life-long change that came about due to my RAF service was the ability to get up early in the morning. I now rise regularly between 5-5.30 am.

"Don't know Sarge, err Flight." I added the last very quickly as he began to point towards the crown above his three stripes.

"I would like to try for the boxing team though." He did not seem impressed.

"What are you doing here, at Kirton?"

"Trade training". "How long?" "About six weeks."

"Well son, you won't get into the team in six weeks. You any good?"

"I've never done any boxing flight." Total honesty being my recently adopted policy.

"Bloody good! At that rate we might not even be able to use you for sparring."

"I have done quite a bit of Judo; err, a few years ago."

"Cissy sport Judo." This being his abrupt reply and my only reward for that gem of information. I was determined, though, to improve on the fiasco of the 'Harlequins' debacle.

"I want to join the boxing club whilst I am here Flight".

"What billet are you in?" he asked gruffly. "I'm not promising anything but you can come on the training run tomorrow. We'll see what you're made of."

I groaned inwardly. Running was never my thing. I had always felt that if the good lord had wanted me to run he would have given me

four legs and shaped me like a deer. Still, here was my first opportunity to join the boxing group and my chance to put the Rugby nightmare behind me. I was not prepared, however, for the mini nightmare that the flight sergeant had in store for his simpleton volunteers the following morning. I should have known better, I thought wryly, as our small group greeted the early dawn air and the chattering of noisy birds, by setting off on a projected six mile run at 5.15 a.m.

My dad had warned me enough times about volunteering. I had not listened to much of his advice re the RAF, mostly because these were different times and circumstances to those in which he had served. I began to doubt this strategy very quickly that morning, however. It began at 5a.m. when the flight sergeant woke me from a very cosy dream about Joyce and the forthcoming weekend. 5 o'clock! Only shift workers get up at 5 o'clock I thought to myself. People don't volunteer to do it. My protestations to the flight sergeant fell on very stony ground. Moreover, it became very clear, very soon, that he regarded himself as something of a wit.

"Get up you lazy sod." He grinned at me. "Tiny birds have been up and singing in their nests for ages. It won't hurt you to get up from yours. Get your boots on and shorts and a vest and you'll be just right for our little run. 5 minutes!" and that's all he gave me!

The flight sergeant's 'short' run proved to be a real hard slog for me. As I say, I have never appreciated the joy of running and this, my first real experience of the art, was just a torture. What made it worse was the fact that the flight sergeant actually did seem to enjoy it. It also became very apparent that he found it easy. This was, no doubt, from much practice but that did not make it any easier or better for the rest of us. What was worse was the fact that he was able to run back and forth along and around our small group to chivvy us up. In this way he must have covered at least twice the distance that we did. It was all quite galling and very disheartening. The thought of doing these runs every morning did not appeal. It did not appeal at all! I did, though, continue to cooperate for the sake of being allowed to join

the boxing group. I ran with the flight sergeant's training group for three mornings. It did not get any easier!

On the evening after my first run with the group, I had gone to the gym fully expecting that I would take a turn in the ring for some real life sparring. No such luck! The flight sergeant put me onto a circuit training programme for that night. That was switched to a weights programme for the second evening and back again to circuits for the third evening session. I was becoming really fed up because I had hoped that at least some of the time would be spent in the ring. I badgered the flight sergeant but he was bluntly obdurate. "You'll get in the ring when I say you're ready!" was all that he would say to me. "I might get you started next week" was his final concession after I had battered his ear for the umpteenth time.

I went home that weekend with my exciting news that I had joined the boxing group at Kirton. That too went down like a lead balloon. My dad was against it on grounds that were somewhat too vague to me. I could not understand his reasons nor his wish to object. He had always spoken warmly about his own prowess as a wrestler and a boxer when younger and in the Jewish Lads Brigade. I got the impression that he was simply against it because it was an RAF activity and that that was enough for him to come down against it. As for Joyce, her reasons were more direct and very clear. She felt that I might get hurt and she did not want me to continue boxing under any circumstances. My protestations that I was getting fitter by the day cut no ice at all. She was against it. I went back to camp that Sunday night quite deflated but determined to continue, at least for the time that I was at Kirton. Cheesed off though! Two weekends of deflation in a row!

The situation was about to take its own path towards a final outcome, however. It was not until the Wednesday that I was allowed into the ring. I was to spar with another of the training group, a big guy, bigger than me, but flabby and even more unfit than I. The first couple of rounds, I felt, were fairly even, although he did get in some

punches that must have looked quite heavy. There was no real force in them, though, but the flight sergeant stopped the fight before the third round could begin. I was livid because I really felt that the lad was not hurting me and I dearly wanted the experience of going the three rounds.

My protestations went unheeded, as usual. I was rapidly becoming disenchanted with this flight sergeant and his notion of running the boxing group. I had put a lot of emotional effort into staying in the group, against total family opposition, and I wanted to make progress in the short time available to me at this camp. I was beginning to feel that this NCO was not going to allow that and there was no knowing what might or might not be available at my next posting.

"You were getting hurt!" was all he would say in reply to my protestation. My denial of this as a fact went completely unheard and totally ignored.

The next morning I decided that I would not get up for the 5am run. I had counted without the flight sergeant and his experience of 'malingerers' however. Through the sheer force of his presence, he did make me get up and join the group that morning. It was, though, to be the last morning that I went running against my will. The day was Friday and I did not stay on the camp that weekend. As usual I went home, hitch hiking this time. That was no real problem because the roads from Lincolnshire down to London were fairly direct and there were no great cities in the way, as Birmingham and Wolverhampton had been from Bridgnorth. I was also able to get away on the Friday night for some reason that I cannot remember.

On the Monday I was ready for him! I simply swapped huts. I moved all my bedding, quite unofficially, into the hut next door. No-one knew except for the lads in the two huts and they weren't going to admit to knowing anything. Other than that no-one cared anyway, except for the flight sergeant, who could not find me when he made his dawn call. Our conversation in the gym that evening was short and sweet. It ended with my exit from the boxing group. His

attitude was; "You'll do as you're told." My attitude was; "The War Office is already stealing...etc....etc. I'm not going to let you waste my time when I'm trying to volunteer for your group!" The language was quite a bit more flowery than that but the general flow is there. In any case I had more important fish to fry whilst I was at Kirton!

The more important issue was that of my trade training. I had been learning to be an accounts clerk for a couple of weeks by that time. It was genuinely boring in the extreme. The style of accounts was quite 'Janet and John' and I was really hating every moment of it. I was actually finding it hard to stay awake, with the warm autumn sun shining through the windows of the hut that passed as a classroom. My plan was simple; it was to fail the course in order to make it clear that I had been wrongly allocated to accounts training. The fact was, however, that I was being too simple. The forces do not work in such a quaint, logical, manner. Basically it's like this - you do as you're told until you're told to do something different.

It was all made clear to me on the Monday morning after I had failed my end of course examination. I was quite smug and self-satisfied as I was sent to see the warrant officer in charge of that training section. He seemed quite a pleasant man as he greeted me and told me to sit down. He even asked me why I thought I had failed the exam. "I don't think I'm suited to pay accounts sir." I responded. I had been practicing this interview in my head for days.

It was at that point that all the fruits of my practice went quite out of the window. I was quickly made to realise that a man does not get to the top of his tree, as a warrant officer is, by being a complete fool. "Do you think that I'm a fool?" was his second question. I did not get a chance to reply to this one. "This is the RAF and you're a national service man. I don't care if you're suited to pay accounts or not, we're not at Harrods where you can pick and choose. You are going to sit the exam next Friday and you'll pass or fail. That's up to you. I don't give a s***." He suddenly changed tack. "Do you see that man out there?" I looked through the window; there were several men out there. "It's

the one sweeping the path." He added helpfully. "What rank is he?" "He's an A/C [aircraftman] like me." He looked at me quizzically for a moment. "No, not like you, he's an A/C and he's almost done his two years. That's just how you'll be if you do not pass your exam next Friday. I'll see to that. You'll never be promoted and you'll serve your time doing menial tasks like him. That's all I have to say."

I did not even try to protest. I realised that I had been thoroughly outgunned and out manoeuvred. I did pass the exam on the next occasion and was rewarded by receiving a posting to Norfolk, to a small training station I'd never heard of. It was called RAF Bircham Newton.

4
Final home - RAF Bircham Newton

MY FINAL PERMANENT home in the RAF was to be in Norfolk at RAF Bircham Newton. It was situated in a very lovely setting, on both sides of what was then a quiet country 'B' road, hereby identified as 'The Road that ran Through It'. Its broad grass airfield, still in use at that time, backed close to the edge of the Royal Estate at Sandringham. Even at a cursory first glance, though, it was obvious that security was not high on the list of priorities for the camp.

I reported to the Guard Room but, in fact, there was no need to do so, from a security point of view. I could just as easily have stepped over any one of the very low, single stretches of linked chain that were looped in sections between a series of low wooden posts. This formed an unimpressive barrier on either side of the road and between the public road and the camp itself. This is the road, indeed, that in the title of this story did, in all truth, run through it; through the camp itself that is! These low barriers were easily surmounted by simply stepping over them. They ran the full length of the camp as far as I could see at that time. I approached the guard room tentatively, having humped my kit-bag the short distance from where the bus had stopped.

I handed my movement order to the guard corporal, Corporal James. Fred, as I later came to know him, was an NCO in the RAF regiment. This was identified by the semi-circular badges at the shoulder of each arm of his tunic. Fred was the first black man that I had seen in the RAF up to that time. I was immediately wary of him, because I had developed a theory that corporals were the most officious of all the NCO ranks in the RAF. 'Rock Ape' corporals being the worst of the species. ['Rock Ape' was and still is I believe the accepted and usual vernacular for RAF Regiment in The RAF. I have mentioned the somewhat odious title here because that was the way it was. I did not then, nor do I now, like the connotations behind the title. To my certain knowledge it held within it a level of disparagement. From now on, if I feel the need to identify an RAF regiment NCO as such, then I shall do so by using the title 'regiment' or RAF regiment plus their rank].

The RAF Regiment was formed to perform a particular and very necessary function within the Royal Air Force. Its members were and are, trained to a much higher level of military competence than their non-regiment colleagues. Their role is to defend RAF personnel, buildings, equipment and establishments from attack in time of conflict.

He was a biggish man, Fred, not size one but quite big and tending towards a bit of extra weight. We later became friends, however, after I had done a couple of guard duty shifts with him. During the first of these he had introduced me to the delights of Fitzgerald's various translations of 'The Rubayat of Omar Khayyam'. I fell so much in love with this work that Joyce gave me a present of a copy of it for Christmas 1960. I have that beloved copy to this day.

I also found out, later, that Fred had been a flight sergeant serving in Cyprus during the height of the ENOSIS crisis. As a senior NCO in the regiment, he had been required to carry a side arm. This he had refused to do on the basis that he was never going to shoot a Cypriot. For that 'offence' Fred was court marshalled and reduced to the ranks. When I knew him he was in the process of working his

way back up the ladder. This was a very tall order for a black man in the forces in those days. As I came to know him my respect for the man grew exponentially. When I first met him, however, he was just another 'regiment' corporal and I was very wary of him. He looked at my papers. Corporal James looked up from my papers at me and then, suddenly, he grinned a welcome grin.

"Good to meet you son." He offered the grin again "Bring your bags into the guard room. The SWO wants to see you in his office and you don't need to lug those all over the place."

Oh no! I thought. Not the SWO! What with the WO at Kirton in Lindsey I had had quite enough of warrant officers to last me for a good while. I would have bet that the two of them had been in communication about me.

"Don't worry about Mac!" the corporal grinned again. "He's O.K.; he's one of the best."

I left my kit bag and hold-all in the guard room and then, after receiving directions, walked the short distance down to the admin block. I say down, there really isn't much by way of either ups or downs at all in Norfolk. There was something of a gentle slope, though, as I remember it. As I approached the admin block I began to realise that there were officers in abundance coming in and out of the building. My saluting arm was working overtime. Hell! I thought, I hope it's not always like this. Bircham Newton was a small camp. I was soon to find out why there were so many officers mooching about. I poked my head into the admin office from where a helpful clerk directed me back the short distance to the SWO's office.

"His name is MacFarlane, Mr. MacFarlane," was the final piece of helpful information from this clerk, who also, later, became a very good friend but who, at that time, just saw me as a nuisance. His first name was the same as mine, Tony. Tony Haynes. He later married the daughter of a long term friend of my dad, having met her at Joyce and my wedding. I knocked on the SWO's door. It took a few moments before I received the expected "Come in!"

Station Warrant Officer MacFarlane was not as I had expected him to be! In my mind's eye I had pictured a big, impressive man, with an iron jaw and a fierce countenance. Mr MacFarlane did not fit at all into my preconception of what an SWO should look like.

"And who are you?" he looked at me quizzically.

"Kreit Sir, erm, A/C Kreit." I handed him my movement order.

"Ah... yes. We've been expecting you." He did not explain this remark any further. I was left wondering.......

Mr. MacFarlane was not an impressive man in the physical sense. I have to say, though, that the more you got to know him the more impressive he became, as a mentally strong and helpful individual. He was genial in appearance but, as I came to discover myself, one of some considerable intellectual depth, of mental strength greater than my prejudices against the military would have previously allowed, as well as kindness.

My thoughts, whenever I have had such thoughts over the years, about SWO MacFarlane, have always been of a kind, intelligent man. What was more, he smoked a pipe! This had been my own main vice since I was seventeen years old. What he smoked, though, was way beyond my own poor experience. I being, in the main and when I could afford it, a smoker of the refined Balkan Sobranie. As he talked to me he pulled what looked like a very short length of black, tarred rope from his pocket. From another pocket he produced a small smokers' knife and cut a short stub from this length of rope. Putting away both the rope and the knife he proceeded to rub the stub into the palm of his hand until it became shredded into something that did begin to look like tobacco as I knew it. I could smell the pungent, sickly sweet aroma of this material from across the room; the more as he continued to kneed it into his palm. He then began, slowly, to load his pipe with this unhealthy looking mass.

"C'mon on." He said suddenly. "I'll show you around and introduce you to everyone you need to meet today."

I was amazed that the SWO would take the time to do this. I had hardly even got to see the SWOs in the distance at my first two camps let alone having personal attention like this guided tour.

The admin block, as far as I can remember it, was in the form of a long rectangle, with the two arms of the inside corridor running away to the left and to the right as you entered the building. There was a further rectangle built onto the back and this ran away from you as you entered the front door and walked the five yards or so to the meeting of the corridors, forming the shape of a T but with an elongated top bar, thereby cutting the building into accessible sections. Offices were situated on either side of these corridors. The SWO's office was the first on the left, as one came through the front door.

"I like to see who's coming in and out of my building." Was his only explanation. His office also had a very good view of much of the rest of the camp along the main internal road through it.

We left his office and made our way back across the small square, formed by the crossing point of the two corridors, to the main admin room. Mr. MacFarlane introduced me to those of the admin staff in the office at that time, including Tony Haynes, whom I had already met.

"Well he said after a few minutes. We'd better go and meet your new partners in crime; I suppose you'd like to do that?"

I nodded doubtfully. I had no urgent desire to see the inside of a pay accounts office. I followed him back, past his own office, to the right and to the far end. We came to a very large and unexpectedly pleasant room that was flooded with light by windows on three sides. As we crossed the large room towards the sergeant at its opposite end from the door, I noticed an SAC sitting at a desk on my left. He was a national service man, which I could tell from his uniform. The desk opposite him was empty, I wondered if that was destined to be mine. On my right, sitting at desks, were an A/C and a corporal technician. Both were regular servicemen. We reached the sergeant who stood as he saw the SWO approaching.

"Sergeant Lane." The SWO began as we were part way across the room. "This is the reluctant recruit you've been waiting for." Finally it was out in the open. The two warrant officers had been talking about me. This sergeant knew I had not wanted to work for him. Bloody good! I thought to myself. This is a good start! Then there came the big surprise, the sergeant held out his hand towards me and grinned. "Welcome son. We understand you've been bucking the system at Kirton."

I must have frowned, or made some facial expression, that showed my concern at this evidence of the collusion between Kirton and Bircham. I suspected the two warrant officers. As these thoughts were emerging once again, Mr. MacFarlane had motioned me to follow him and we were on our way out of the building. The SWO spoke; and for the first time I caught just the trace of an Aussie accent.

"No worries as far as we're concerned". He explained. "WO Franks was quite impressed with your solo effort at bucking the system." He paused a moment or two to light his pipe. The angle of his head, together with the animated breathing sounds, as he drew the smoke through the pipe, breathed life into its fire, all indicating that he had not finished talking on this subject. The old pipe was finally belching smoke to his satisfaction so he continued;

"The truth is that WO Franks also got wind of your caper with the boxing club and felt that you showed a bit of gumption there. The problem that you would have had with the 'system', though, is that it generally doesn't exist in the way that you might have thought. I'm only telling you this so that you might want to think about your strategies in the future, should the need arise." He paused again, looking at me thoughtfully and puffing just a bit as we walked up the slight slope towards the main camp buildings.

"You see son. The system mostly stops with people like WO Franks and me. It's our job to make sure that everything runs smoothly and that officers aren't disturbed and don't have to become involved in disturbances to the way things have been ordained to be."

His style of speech had become a bit pompous and I began to wonder if he was taking the 'p***'. There was a basic truth hidden there, though, as I was quickly learning. HM Forces are run, on a day to day basis, by its warrant officers and NCOs. Senior officers decide and devise working strategies. Junior officers supervise these, but at arm's length. Warrant officers and NCOs carry them out. They tend to regard any would-be bucking of a strategy, or order, as a personal challenge to themselves, and as a personal slight on their ability, should the matter get as far as the officer above them. I had stood very little chance of succeeding with WO Franks for that reason. In those terms it appeared that he had dealt with me very reasonably. The SWO continued.

"Let's go have a look at some of the camp."

I could not get used to the idea that I was getting something of a guided tour by the SWO. I was no veteran but I did know by that time that this was very unusual. As we walked away from the admin building, we had to leave it by way of an oval roundabout immediately in front of it. The inside of the oval was neatly grassed over. A flag pole, with the camp's RAF Ensign gently flapping in the late summer breeze, neatly centralised within the grassy oval.

We moved on from the oval and further up the slope. I noticed something that struck me as being, quite frankly, absurd. The main internal camp road ran down towards us from the Guard Room. This camp road branched off towards and to, the public road that actually cut the camp in two and along which public access was totally unrestricted. As the camp road passed the Guard Room it became subject to security scrutiny by those on duty, by way of a security pole in front of the Guard Post itself. This self-same road ran through the camp and returned to the public road as an offshoot from the oval roundabout in front of the admin block.

The absurdity, as I saw it, was that this road re-joined the public road in a totally unrestricted manner. A lorry load of terrorists could enter the camp at that point without any physical barrier. There was

a pole gate in position there, but it was raised, and this pole was not manned. I questioned the SWO on this matter and was told that there had never been any security reason or need to lower this pole-gate. I went further and asked then, why there was a pole at the other end of the road by the Guard Room. I left the questioning for another time, though, when it became clear that the SWO was finding my sarcastic comments on the subject of camp security not a little annoying. What had always been done was the way things were going to be done in the future. I, as a new and very junior boy on the block, had no right to question this natural order of things. The SWO had, after all, treated me very well from the time of my arrival at his office door.

We proceeded up the road, past a couple of red brick two story buildings. Mr. MacFarlane stopped at the third building and signalled me to follow him inside. It became clear at once that this was a barrack block.

"This is where you'll be bunking down for a while until a room becomes vacant." He indicated a long room with about a dozen beds in it, none of them made up.

"You can choose which bed you want." He continued. "You're the only one in here at the moment." I did not hear most of this, however, as I was much more interested in his earlier remark. I thought he had said something about a room becoming vacant. I could not believe it though. I passed it off as the old chap being a bit confused. He began to explain the personnel structure of the camp. We had moved out of the barrack block and were on our way up towards the Guard Room. The situation was surreal. Here I was, a brand new A/C being given a guided tour around a camp to which I had really not wanted to come.

"This is a training camp." The SWO began to explain. "There are three types of trainee here. The youngest group is made up of about 150 boy entrants. They age from fourteen to sixteen and are often sons of servicemen. They undergo general schooling as well as RAF familiarisation and training but at a junior level. They observe a school year of three terms in the same way as normal schools."

Mac paused for breath as we moved further on up the slope of the road. He took the opportunity to point out areas of particular interest as we proceeded. The airmen's mess, for example, was situated almost opposite the barrack block where I was to sleep.

"The second group of trainees are the RAF Apprentices. They are boys of 16 to 18, who are learning trades with a view to entering men's' service' when they are old enough, provided they pass out O.K. from their training. They also observe school terms."

The SWO paused for breath again. He was clearly not used to walking, talking whilst breathing in very pungent tobacco smoke, all at the same time. He needed more oxygen with it, to paraphrase an altogether different saying.

"You will not have much to do with either the boy entrants or the apprentices." He advised me.

"They will come into your office from time to time for pay advice. When they do they must refer to you as 'staff'. I do not want to hear any of them call you by your first name, is that clear?"

I nodded. On this point, the fact is, that I have referred to the SWO here as Mac on occasion. I have only done so because everyone else did so when talking about him. Few, though, were on close enough terms to do so to his face. I never did call him anything but Sir or Mr. MacFarlane in the nearly two years that I knew him. I never felt either the need or the desire to refer to any RAF person above the rank of corporal in that familiar way. As things were then, moreover, I had not lost anything of my initial hostility towards the service and had no desire to get onto familiar terms with any of it. I was resigned to do my time in the best fashion that I could and to go home as often as possible. Mac continued once he had caught his breath.

"The third cohort of trainees does not live in this part of the camp. They have their own new quarters on the other side of the public road next to the officers' married quarters. They are officers who have been selected for re-training, often having come to the end of flying duties. You will have very little contact with them. They will

discuss their pay and allowances with the officer in charge of your section, Flight Lieutenant 'P'." Suddenly he noticed my marksman's badge.

"Do you enjoy shooting?"

"Yes sir." I answered with some enthusiasm.

"You may get a call from Squadron Leader 'B'. He runs a camp shooting team. I'll let him know that you might be a candidate." He paused as we neared the Guard Room.

"Trainees far outnumber permanent staff at Bircham." He explained. "Only permanent staff are allowed to represent the camp and so anyone keen enough or qualified to participate in any sport is very welcome. Do you play rugby?" I steered well away from that one. I simply said that I liked the game but did not play very well. The time for showing off had been confined solidly to history.

"You can get your gear over to your billet and settle in. Don't bother to get into your section today. I expect you're tired. Report for work at 8.30am sharp tomorrow and the sergeant will show you your duties. I expect your section officer will want to have a word with you at some time; Flight Lieutenant 'P' that is. You know where my office is..."

It seemed that my guided tour by the SWO was over. I was not altogether sorry about that either. I still could not believe that it had happened at all. I was very suspicious about the special treatment. I watched him as he strolled away down the slope back towards the admin block, his old pipe casting small puffs of black cloud into the late summer air. I glance over at the corporal.

"Is that normal here?" I ventured at him.

"What's that?" he replied.

"The SWO giving a new A/C a personal guided tour?"

"I wouldn't say it's normal. It has happened before though. Don't worry about it. He's a decent chap actually..........for an SWO that is."

It did not take me long to settle my gear in. I took a quick trip to stores to draw some bedding and other necessaries. This was

quite a different chore than my previous experiences at stores. It was much more relaxed. The stores corporal was actually quite chatty, even interested in my short history in the RAF, and kept asking questions about me; where I came from etc. So much so, that I used a faked appointment with my new section sergeant in order to get away.

As I walked back to the billet, though, I came to a decision that I would go to the section and re-introduce myself and try to get to know a few people there. I knew no-one on camp, other than the two corporals and the SWO. I decided that that would not get me through the evening. I made my bed up and strolled down to the admin block. The sergeant was quite surprised to see me again that day. He did not notice me until I was half way across the room towards him, as he had been working with his head down. "Nose to the grindstone!" I chuckled to myself as I approached him.

"What was that?" The sergeant looked up at me as if I were a quite unwelcome interruption to his afternoon.

"What are you doing here? I thought the SWO was going to tell you to take a couple of hours off this afternoon." His voice actually began to soften as the sentence rolled out.

"Yes Sarge, he did, but I was hoping that you might have time to introduce me to some of the others. It's going to be a bit boring in camp tonight otherwise, not knowing anyone."

He grinned. "I have the feeling that it wouldn't take you long to get to know a few people."

There was not much that I could say to this. In any case he was probably right, although I did want to get to know the people in my section. The sergeant noticed my hesitation, grinned again and got to his feet, slowly, as if stiff with pain.

"I'm suffering from over exercise of unused muscles." The grin was a bit constrained this time, probably due to the suffering!

"Played tennis yesterday evening, against Corporal James! Did you meet him at the Guard Room?" "Yeees!" he nodded to himself.

"Do not play tennis against Corporal James unless you are really good at the game. He had me running around the court like a good'un, and he won a fiver off me! I'm now suffering." These last few words were delivered with just a trace of Norfolk, like someone who is not from the county but who has lived there for a while and has absorbed a soupçon of accent as if by osmotic pressure.

He crossed the room to his left; to the desk of a corporal technician. The man had been following my progress ever since I reached the sergeant's desk. He stood up as we approached and offered his hand. The sergeant introduced him.

"Corporal Technician Tanner." "Brian will do fine" he responded. "Great." I replied. "I'm Tony."

Brian was a decent chap. Regular Air Force but O.K. nonetheless. He kept himself to himself most of the time but that was his prerogative.

NCO ranks in the RAF were created mainly from those used by the original Royal Flying Corps. After WW2 a new range of NCO ranks was introduced to differentiate between Technical and Non-Technical trades and between ground trades and NCO aircrew. Until 1950 all ground tradesmen wore the same rank badges, however in that year an additional rank structure was introduced and during this period there were two separate rank structures - 'Technical' and 'Command'. It was quite normal to move between the two structures while still being within a Technical trade. This range of technical trades and its insignia remained in force, largely unchanged from 1950 to 1964. The only real change in this system was that, in 1952, the crowns of the flight sergeant and chief technician ranks changed from King's crown to Queen's crown.

The Technician ranks indicated levels of technical qualifications and did not indicate 'command' capabilities, whilst the Command ranks indicated levels of command authority. One of the reasons that I had been so disappointed at not going to Melksham for technical trade training was that, if I had succeeded in completing the

course there I would have been awarded the rank of junior technician at the end of it, with the possibility of gaining that rank of corporal technician during my two years. I was not interested in any command authority. The increase in earnings in the technician ranks would have been significant and very useful to me and to Joyce. As it was she was earning a salary and felt an obligation to subsidise me during my trips home. I realised, of course, that she was handing me money. It was only some years later, however, that her mum told me just how much Joyce had forgone for herself, in order to do so.

Technician ranks in the Air force rose upwards from that of junior technician and ran up through the ranks to that of master technician for technicians of warrant officer rank. The ranks were pretty much the equivalent of the related NCO 'command' ranks of corporal etc. They could be easily distinguished, however, because their stripes were inverted with the point at the top. At the time of which I am writing, 1960-62, there was no 'command' NCO rank equivalent to that of junior technician. That would have been the rank of lance corporal of which there was no such animal in the Royal Air Force at the time of which I am writing. RAF NCO and technician Ranks have been revised over the years since my time, beginning in 1964. My educated guess is that the RAF had to undergo many changes from about that time, one of the largest of which being the revisions that had to accompany the ending of National Service. That, however, is another story.

Corporal Technician Brian Tanner was an interesting man but one who, as I say, kept himself to himself outside of the office. He was, though, congenial enough as a work colleague and always ready to help with a problem. He was a horse racing addict and read the 'Racing Times' avidly, in the office and outside, whenever he could. He made a great 'play' of planning a season's betting campaign in what he regarded as a scientific manner. He did, moreover, have some remarkable wins over which he crowed magnificently. We never did get to hear about any unfortunate losses, however. Corporal Tanner also organised the section's 'pools' syndicate which never did have a

significant win. I was never around when he was checking the weekly pools news. I am told, however, that this check was always conducted in highly dramatic fashion! He was also a MAN. U. Fan. There have to be some!

At the desk adjoining and opposite that of Brian Tanner sat a young LAC. He was Welsh and, as I discovered later, was Welsh speaking. He was very young and had only recently been entered into 'man's service' from being a graduate of the RAF apprentice system. Dai, as he was inevitable called, was also very unsure of himself, both at work amongst his colleagues, and with peers in the service. He was a tall, gangly lad; he was courting a young girl from a local village and tried to spend as much time as possible with her. That was a behaviour that I understood very well and with which I could empathise. Dai, though, was the object of many unseemly and uncalled for jokes and remarks over this, mostly not from within the office team though, I'm happy to report.

Across the room, facing the sergeant, but at the same distance as Dai sat an SAC who was introduced to me as Norman, Norman Planter. He was a national serviceman in his last year, I discovered later. Like me he had resented being called up for national service. Like me he regarded it as a theft of two years of his life. He also resented the loss of earnings that he was suffering. Just before his inevitable call up he had qualified as a chartered accountant, as such he would have been at the beginning of a hopefully lucrative career. Instead of which he was being forced to do 'Janet and John' account-ing for HM government. Norman's penchant was to ostentatiously read his daily copy of 'The Times' as he sat at his desk in the morning and before beginning any work. It also transpired that Norman had a motor bike and that he lived in Enfield, very close to my own home at that time. Wonderful!

My desk, I was advised, was to be the vacant one that was adjoined to and facing Norman's. Just as my tour of the office ended, a war-rant officer strode into the room. He noticed me when he was about half way across the room.

"Hello." He declared, "Stranger in the camp!"

The sergeant grinned. He was obviously used to this officer's somewhat peremptory style of speech.

"This is Tony, er Tony Kreit, A/C Kreit. " The introduction did not flow as well as it might have. Still, that did not seem to bother the warrant officer. He walked towards me, briskly, but with his hand held out.

"Welcome." He offered the greeting effusively.

"Good afternoon Sir." I replied, wondering who the hell he was. The sergeant filled this gap belatedly.

"This officer is our warrant officer...Warrant Officer Rubin. Well, I thought, I've met almost the whole team now. That'll do me for today. The W.O. continued to speak.

"My name is Maurice but to you it's Sir!" He seemed to see this as a joke but I had never had any wish or desire to call him by his first name. Nonetheless, I acknowledged the remark with an unremarkable "Yes Sir, of course." He moved away with the sergeant to the latter's desk. I tried a smile at Norman. He grinned, stood up and offered his hand. It was a limp handshake but not unfriendly.

"Where are you sleeping?" He asked me. I told him but he came back at me with a helpful "well that won't be for long. We'll soon have you in your own room like the rest of us." I could not believe that I had heard the SWO correctly. Was it really possible that ordinary airmen, in this extraordinary place, were allocated their own rooms? Norman quickly became aware of my disbelief. "Yes." He added. "We do get our own rooms here. Hot and cold running to boot! You see there are not many permanent staff here. Most of the people on camp are trainees of one form or another. Officer trainees are billeted in new officers' accommodation next to the officers' married quarters across the road. We use their old quarters in a couple of blocks next to the billet you've now got all to yourself. The SWO will certainly allocate one to you as soon as someone moves on or out." He smiled at the puzzled look that greeted this last remark of his.

"Well, you see, people do sometimes get transferred, if they can't avoid it, but mostly people leave because they are national service men coming to the end of their two years. Believe me, that's the only reason you want to leave here. It's the best posting you could have imagined. You've really fallen on your feet coming to Bircham. C'mon, I'll show you my room before dinner."

He said this as the sergeant gave us all permission to leave for the day. Just as we had nearly made it to the door a raucous barking order followed me across the room.

"A/C Kreit, I want to see you in my office, 8.30 sharp tomorrow morning. Clear?" I turned slowly towards him. "Yes sir, absolutely." I had already decided that I didn't like this warrant officer. He was the only person about whom I had felt that way since arriving at the camp earlier that day and he just happened to be the most senior NCO with whom I was likely to have the most contact......Just my ******luck! I thought bitterly.

My first impressions of Mr Rubin were therefore less than favourable. Those impressions continued to be confirmed during the first few months of my time at Bircham Newton. From the time that I had very unwillingly entered the service of the RAF I had never experienced any hard, overt, anti-Semitism. There had been a few raucous jokes but nothing I could not handle and, in any case, they were delivered by raw recruits like me, so there was no 'rank' issue to deal with. With Mr. Rubin I experienced something that, strangely, was new to me; the person who goes out of his way to prove overtly to the world that he holds no prejudices.

It was not unreasonable in military terms for a senior rank to ask a junior rank to run a small errand for him. The first time that this involved me was a few days into my work under his command. He sidled up to my desk one morning and, before I could stand up to acknowledge him, he put his hand ostentatiously on my shoulder and asked me if I would 'pop' up to the NAFFI and collect some bacon that his wife had ordered. "Don't go, though, if it offends your religion".

This was delivered with no sarcastic content, simply that air of a man who wants to demonstrate publically what a 'good egg' he is.

This happened a few times during my first few weeks at Bircham, sometimes with bacon, sometimes ham. I certainly did not mind, firstly, because the errand got me out of the office for a short time with a cast iron excuse for being away from my work place. Secondly, as I did finally explain to Mr Rubin I was quite happy to eat both ham and bacon myself. That was true in those days as, like many Jewish men, I used to make an illogical exception for both ham and bacon. My exclusion of both of these items from my diet came much later in my life. I have, however, never in my life knowingly eaten pork meat, hence the extreme illogicality of my, then, stance over bacon and ham.

"Yes, that's our warrant officer and he's a prat!" Norman explained as we made our way on that first afternoon into the camp. He turned right as we reached the second of the barrack blocks. "This is where I call home." I quickly learned that Norman was ready to use sarcasm from time to time, particularly when referring to anything RAF!

Norman showed me his room. I had to pinch myself and simply hope that I was not dreaming and that some mischievous gremlin was not just about to burst my bubble and fly me away to a 'real' RAF camp. The room was of a decent size; about 12' by 12'. He had a bed, a 'butler' sink and had personalised the room with pictures. He also had a standard RAF single wardrobe and a bedside cabinet. More home comforts than I had imagined, or could have imagined, for a simple airman. The cream on the cake was that there was a toilet and shower block just a few yards away, opposite the head of the stairs and along the corridor that gave off to the left at the top of the stairs. Talk about the comforts of home!

We chatted for a while; some about the camp, some about the surrounding area but mostly about home and the resentment we both felt at the enforced national service that had been perpetrated on us. Norman was totally in accord with me on that subject.

By now it was time for dinner, so we strolled over to the airmen's mess. This time I was not at all surprised at the quality of the food. My experience of RAF catering was reaffirmed once more at RAF Bircham Newton. In 1962 Arnold Wesker provided the world of entertainment with his very funny play 'Chips with Everything'. I made a point of going to see the play soon after my de-mob because it was a portrayal of his life, and therefore mine, as a national serviceman in the RAF. It was funny, as I say, and there was some truth to the theme that RAF catering staff often produced chips as one of the alternative potato offerings for lunch and dinner. On the other hand, there was always a selection of alternatives, both for potatoes and other vegetables. There were also alternatives of meat and or fish that gave airmen a decent range of choices at every meal. In total I served on four RAF stations and can confirm that the standard of food supplied to airmen was consistently good.

That evening I was very hungry and, in spite of the novelty and interest of meeting a good number of new acquaintances, I am happy to say that I was able to do justice to the meal. One of the most interesting new personalities for me was John Robinson, also from Kent and a fellow 'left wing' traveller, although he was just a tad further to the left than I, because he was a member of the Communist Party like my dad. He sat at the dinner table with a folded copy of the Daily Worker beside his plate. I remember that he read bits, out loud, here and there as he ate. Over the months John and I became good friends. My only criticism of him during that time was that he was such a slow eater. He could make a sausage last longer than a set of tyres! Our friendship lasted well past the time when we had completed our national service. He and his lovely wife, Nina, moved to Kent, to Cheriton, near Folkestone. Joyce and I saw quite a bit of them in those early years.

John was a three year man. That is, he had signed on for a three year period as a regular airman when he received his call-up. In this way he received a higher salary than he would have done as a national

service man. He also received a second, and more practical, uniform. As well as the standard dress tunic, he had been allocated a more convenient, shorter and more comfortable battle dress tunic. In my view, though, this was all poor reward for giving up an extra year of your life rather than serve as an ordinary airman. John was serving as a clerk typist, whereas in civilian life he had been a bricklayer. Such is the way of the Air Force trade allocation process. Although the reason for John being allocated a non-sensitive trade may well have been along the lines of which my dad was totally convinced that I had been singled out. It was all political as far as he was concerned.

Norman was the only person I ever met who had been allocated to a trade that was in any way connected to his civilian qualifications. The RAF must have made a mistake with him although, from their point of view, his politics were sound!

My brother in law went into the army just after I got called up. He had served a five year apprenticeship as an engineer. Was he selected for REME? Like hell! He was drafted into the Para Medics. It was a logical process designed by civil servants from the War Office in their baths one Sunday morning after a late night, the night before! My personal opinion was that the RAF trade training systems for national service men were so 'Janet and John' and the NCOs so poorly qualified, that they would have been shown in a very poor light, up against men who had trained for years in particular trades. The RAF and other forces could not countenance the resultant odious comparison. I have to agree, of course, that my opinion was biased but it did serve to cheer me during long winter evenings, when chewing the fat in the bars of local pubs in Docking and Heacham and other nearby villages; whereas my dad's belief seemed so far-fetched to me in those days. Experience and the passing of time have served to convince me that there could well be, however, a lot of truth in Dad's view.

My two years of living in Norfolk has made me realise that it is a county with two personalities. In winter the cold of Norfolk comes direct from the Arctic or the Russian Steppes. It gathers extra degrees

of cold as it sweeps across the North Sea and drives itself right into the bones of the poor National Service Man, standing lonely picket duty on a dark and windy grass airfield. In the summer it provides a very pleasant contrast; it is a warm and friendly place where fruit, grain and vegetable seasons come and go. Well, that's how it was in the 1960s.

As I have said previously, one of my abiding memories of the place comes from autumn and the rattle of the sugar beet Lorries as they clattered along the road that ran through the camp. The strong, sweet, smell of the newly harvested beet quite recognisable as it drifted through open windows on the warmth of an abiding summer.

Dinner that first evening passed off very well as far as I was concerned. I had a good meal, made some new friends and arranged to go off for a drink with several of them afterwards. We did not have to go far; just off to Docking, a short distance from the camp. Docking is, or was, a quite small village with just one pub. I think that it was called the Railway Inn. We had a few drinks, a few of us smoked pipes, which you were allowed to do inside the pub in those days, and we chatted. One of the lads, I simply cannot remember his name, had given a few of us a lift in his old Austin car. He was due to be de-mobbed in a few days' time, and was in the process of planning his de-mob party; tonight was something of a rehearsal for that. I gathered that there had been a number of such rehearsals over the past few weeks. This chap had a friend, a cook, in the catering section who had agreed to provide him with a range of sandwiches and other tasties for the forthcoming event. We were all invited, generously, magnanimously, whilst he was in his cups. I arrived back in my billet that night feeling well satisfied with my first day at Bircham Newton. I had even forgotten my impending meeting with Warrant Officer 'R' for the next morning. Still, drink does have an anaesthetic effect.

I did not sleep well, however. I was not used to sleeping on the ground floor, alone in a room designed for multiple-occupation. This

barrack block was empty apart from me and quite eerie in the dark. I did not sleep well, and did not linger in bed the next morning. I took a welcome shower, dressed and went over to breakfast at the first shout. Again I was to be pleasantly surprised at the breakfast arrangements here.

By the serving hatch were arranged a diverse assortment of cereals, milk, beans etc. Just off to one side, though, was a large hotplate onto which was mounted the largest frying pan I have ever seen. Next to this was a huge supply of bacon and a large tray of eggs. It was help yourself, and do it yourself time! This was all rolled into one beautiful and very welcome package! The concomitant supplies of bread, toast, fried bread as well as butter etc. all appeared to be endless. One could easily have made it through the day on the breakfast that was achievable at RAF Bircham Newton!

I made my way down to the admin block early, as soon as I had finished my very ample breakfast. In those days, as I say, I was still making an 'honourable' exception in my diet for bacon and ham, for I enjoyed both. It was, however, a quite illogical exception to make and one which I have totally revoked in the last twenty-five, or so, years. I had never eaten pork as a meat nor do I eat other 'forbidden' foods, such as seafood or rabbit, as a matter of personal choice and based upon the strictures of Exodus 23, Leviticus 11 and Deuteronomy 14. I have never observed the strict laws of Kashrut by observing the separation of milk and meat at mealtimes for a very simple reason. In my view it is a totally illogical extrapolation of the Biblical injunction "thou shalt not seethe the kid in its own mother's milk!" I have managed always to observe that injunction absolutely but to render this simple requirement, based upon laws of decent and humane animal husbandry, into the all-encompassing way of life that is imposed upon those who become committed to the full observation of Kashrut, strikes me as being a sophistry of the highest order. In the words of one of my female cousins, "it is a law made by men for the control of women." She, somewhat illogically, keeps a Kosher Home.

I arrived in the accounts section at the same time as Sergeant Lane but before the warrant officer. The sergeant had begun to outline my duties as other members of the section started to arrive, one by one, bright and ready to meet the day. After a few moments more the sergeant spotted the W.O. through the window as he made his way down the path and towards his office. The time was exactly 8.30. I was standing respectfully to attention outside his office door as he arrived. "Good morning sir." He grunted something by way of reply and signalled me to enter the room.

"Why didn't you want to come here?" The question was brusque and blunt and delivered at me the moment after he had directed me to sit down opposite him.

"That's not the case sir." I responded. "I never said to anyone that I didn't want to come here."

"Are you calling Warrant Officer 'X' a liar?" He mentioned the name of the W.O. in charge of accounts training at Kirton, WO Franks.

"No sir. I am simply saying that I never did say, neither to him nor to anyone else, that I did not want to come here to Bircham. I did not know anything about this place after all."

He grunted, obviously unsatisfied at the way the conversation was going.

"I did tell him, though, that I had not wanted to go to Kirton in Lindsey for training in pay accounts." I paused but he did not seem to want to interrupt me at that point.

"You see sir; I did apply for and was allocated to, technician training at Melksham. At the very last minute that was cancelled and I was re-allocated to pay accounts training. I was disappointed and very angry."

"Angry?" His question seemed to imply that I had been out of order to be angry.

"Yes sir. As I see it the RAF has me in a bind. I have to be in the Service against my will. The least that I could have expected is that

I would receive training in a trade of my choice and which would be useful to me when I leave."

"Accounts training is useful." He was becoming defensive but there was no way back for me now.

"Yes sir, but not for me! It's not a life that I have planned for myself. I tried to sabotage the training by failing the course. W.O. Franks realised that and gave me an ultimatum. I passed the course and was posted here......I don't think that I could have got a better posting in the RAF from what I've seen so far." I had added this last bit in order to try to placate the situation but I also meant it. Warrant officer Rubin sat for a few moments as if summing up the facts in his mind. He turned and looked out of the window behind him for a few moments as if seeking inspiration there. After several very long moments he turned back towards me and grinned.

"Shall we start over?"

"Yes sir, please." It was all that I could think of by way of reply.

"Do you have everything that you need for the moment?"

"Yes sir, thank you. I believe that I might even be allocated a room to myself in the old officer block?"

He waived a dismissive hand the size of a bunch of bananas.

"That's up to Mac." He responded quickly. "He covers the admin side of things. I don't interfere." This short interchange, though, was a further indication of how much of the general running of the service was covered by its senior NCOs. He moved into new territory.

"You're Jewish, is that right?" "Yes sir." I replied, immediately suspicious as to the reason for the question; part of my own paranoia I suppose.

"That's a relief." Was his surprise response. "I've arranged for a Jewish Rabbi to visit you here on Friday afternoon, about 14.00 hours. I've booked you a quiet room in the Sergeants' Mess where you won't be disturbed." I wasn't sure what sort of Rabbi other than a Jewish one to whom he might have spoken but, whatever the case, this turn of events came as a complete surprise and personal challenge to me.

I did not know how to respond. W.O. Rubin had obviously thought that he was acting for the best. Now that we were on better terms I was not about to throw a grenade into that pond!

"Thank you sir! Thank you very much." I heard myself saying, totally hypocritically. I stood up, ready to get back to the section but in a turmoil. What on earth would I have to discuss with a Rabbi? The last time I had seen one of those, close up, was at my cousin's Bar Mitzvah!

"Before you go back to the office," the warrant officer cleared his throat before going on, "the squadron leader wants to see you. I think that Mac has told him you might be a good candidate for the shooting team. I see you have a marksman's badge. His office is just along the corridor." He waived his hand in the general direction of the squadron leader's office. I walked the few yards along the corridor full of anticipation as to what this development might mean for me. What might it mean to be included in the team? What was the squadron leader like?

5
Threads

I AM WRITING this story more than 50 years after the actual events. I did not then, nor ever in my life, write a diary. My memories of my time in the RAF are, therefore, broad brush memories. I have good recall of particular events and days but a full account of each and every day and evening largely escapes me. In this chapter I intend to try to weave a tread through those years with a broad look at some of the characters who played a more or less important part in my life at Bircham Newton.

The first of these characters, chronologically, was Norman Planter. He worked at the desk opposite mine in the pay accounts section at RAF Bircham Newton. Norman was an S.A.C. [Senior aircraftman] by the time that I knew him and he was just about half way through his National Service. Norman had been through the 'deferment' route before the military got him, just as I had and just as it got me too, in the end. He had been spending his time more profitably than I had though because he had qualified as a chartered accountant prior to being drafted into the Air Force. His qualification had had one benefit for him, it had enabled him to move up the limited RAF promotion ladder quicker than most in pay accounts.

Norman resented having to do national service just as profoundly as I did. The main difference between us, however, was that, for him,

the missing two years meant the loss of two years of earning power and, thereby, the loss of two years of movement up that particular promotion ladder.

As far as I was concerned the picture was quite different. I had no profession to mourn, no income or money stream to worry about losing. No! My resentment was much more directly based on what I perceived as the loss of liberty at a time when the RAF did not really want me. One other major difference between Norman and me was the fact that he was about as well placed tradewise as he could have been by the R.A.F. From a trade point of view I felt like a fish out of water. The work was not difficult; it was simply that I felt bored out of my skull most of the time.

Norman, however, although we were quite different characters, did help to make life bearable for me in the pay accounts office, particularly in those first few months, when I was feeling at my most resentful towards the R.A.F. He was a quite unforgettable and strong character. Unlike me, moreover, he never did lose the full strength of his anti RAF resentment. Norman made a point of reading his copy of the 'Times', flamboyantly, and ostentatiously, every morning before he would condescend to do any work at all. The Times in those days, of course, was not a tabloid, oh no! it was a broadsheet of huge and unmistakeable proportions. It became clear to me quite soon in my tenure at Bircham, that Norman's profound knowledge of all aspects of accounting, gave him a power within the office that was not open to the rest of us. My own strategy involved being away from the office as much as could be 'legally' justified.

I can remember one occasion in particular. Norman, Brian and I were in the office before anyone else. Norman settled down to read his Times as per his norm. I had a quick glance at my rebel version of the Soviet Weekly, even though I had already read it to death. Brian, as usual, had his copy of his favourite horse racing form magazine 'The Sporting Life', under the microscope. Like all the betting folk that I have met during my life, Brian was totally convinced that, each

year, he came out on the upside with his betting. Asked why then he didn't do it for a living, he would begin to get grouchy, so we did not go down that route too often. Anyway, during this quiet interlude at the beginning of the day the sergeant entered the room. He came in as a man with a purpose and his attention quickly settled on Norman.

"Put that paper away Planter." He barked from across the room without breaking his stride. It took him just a few paces to realise that Norman had not acknowledged either his presence or the order. He repeated the order but slowed his stride. Sergeants, particularly in those days, were used to giving orders to the lower ranks and to having them obeyed without demur. He actually broke his stride to watch as his instruction was ignored for the second time. By this time, of course, his attention was all on Norman.

I am convinced that I could have continued to read my magazine without any problem. Discretion, however, overcame valour and, in any case, I wanted to see how this one played out. I opened my work ledger and pretended to begin to get down to it, to a productive day at the workface! Norman could not see me, or anyone else for that matter. The Times, in its broadsheet form, was a huge area of reading kit. The sergeant reached his desk, sat down, took a deep breath, and once more repeated the order, he almost bellowed it.

"Planter put that damned paper away!"

This time Norman did deign to acknowledge the sergeant. He lowered the paper and peered over it at our leader.

"Sorry Sarge" he responded sweetly. "Were you talking to me?" Then, slowly, oh so slowly and very carefully, he closed and folded his paper, patting it properly into good order until, finally, he put it aside on the windowsill next to his desk.

One nil to Norman I felt! I did, nonetheless, feel some charity towards the sergeant despite my own antagonism of all things military. This NCO was a decent man. It was not his fault that Norman and I were being forced to work in his office. To be frank he probably did not want us in his RAF any more than we wanted to be there.

Yes, Norman was one of the more unforgettable characters that I met during those two years. Not a big man but one with huge intent and inner strength was our Norman. We were never to be bosom buddies but did enjoy a co-domain of purpose. To this end we were friends in adversity.

Tony Haynes, however, was a friend who worked in the admin office. It was useful to have a friend in that strategic position because that was where important things happened like; the collection of post, the issuing of travel warrants and it was also where news about postings first came into the camp. Tony, like my friend John Robinson, was a three year man, the nature of which I have already explained.

Tony was a very pleasant man who hailed from Birmingham. One important positive aspect for me of being in the RAF, one that I only recognised much later, was the opportunity to meet and associate with young men from all over the British Isles. It was a broadening of my horizons that I now cherish. My two years of national service actually enabled me to absorb quite a bit of knowledge about the wider geography and cultures of Britain.

Tony and I spent many a pleasant evening in local pubs, along with others, to form a group of like-minded young men who were only waiting for the day of their discharge from the service. Tony and I lost contact very quickly after I was demobbed, although he did come to our wedding, Joyce and mine, together with a couple of others from the camp, who came down with him to spend the weekend in London. Their names are lost to me through the ravages of time. Tony, as already mentioned, met his future wife at our wedding party. Barbara was the daughter of a long term friend of my dad from the Edmonton Communist party. I have often thought of the two of them over the years in the hope, most sincerely, that they had a long and fruitful life together.

Tony's office was only 20 or so yards from my office and Tony and I were able to do each other small but important services over the nearly two years that I knew him. One such was in the organisation of guard duties over the Christmas/New Year period.

It was not, of course, possible to obtain totally illicit travel warrants, although it was occasionally possible to acquire one that was not needed, for a variety of reasons by the rightful owner. The acquisition could be made by way of a 'trade' to mutual advantage between the two parties. The potential twin flies in this ointment, however, were the RAF Form 1250, the ID card, and the possible scrutiny of the British Railway ticket clerk, when converting the warrant into a useable ticket to ride! Tony was a friend and was prepared to help wherever he could but it was just too dangerous to put the wrong name on a warrant, because they were numbered and subject to checking when they came back to source after being used at the station.

The form 1250 was a photo ID card. The BR staff had a perfect right to ask for it to be produced whenever a warrant was presented at the counter. I took the risk of being exposed on about three occasions during my two years. I was never discovered. I was not even convinced that the members of staff at King's Lynn were too bothered, as long as they had a valid warrant to process and the apparent owner was in uniform. On one occasion I even produced my 1250. The clerk glanced at it but made no comment, even if he had noticed a difference in the name. As I have already indicated, most British men had, at that time, completed military service and so there was a great deal of masculine sympathy abroad for the National Serviceman.

We have already met Mr MacFarlane. He became one of my most important threads during my time at Bircham Newton. His friends and colleagues called him Mac. I was never one of that number, due to the wide difference in rank. I came to respect him, though, in a way that I could never have anticipated when I was first hauled into the service. The rank of warrant officer is, in fact, one to be generally respected. HM forces have the great good fortune to be serviced by a well-respected band of senior NCOs and warrant officers. The services depend on them hugely, for they run the show, leaving commissioned officers to develop policy and strategy. It is a combination that has worked well over time. With specific exceptions, it is

not difficult to develop a healthy respect for men who have gained rank and experience through hard work and have worked their way to the very top of their respective trees. My unit WO, Mr Rubin, and the SWO, Mr MacFarlane, were two of these. More of Mr Rubin later!

The position of SWO [Station Warrant Officer] is an important one. He or she is the most senior non-commissioned officer in the establishment. The SWO on an RAF Station is responsible for discipline and is therefore comparable to the Garrison Sergeant Major in a British Army unit. He or she is the station commander's link to the other ranks and his or her eyes and ears on the ground for all issues that may affect the smooth running of the station.

Mr MacFarlane's office was situated only a few yards from the pay accounts office. He would often wander into our office as he strolled around the admin building. He quickly noticed that I smoked a pipe as he was a fellow pipe smoker. His pipe tobacco, though, was something else! The first time that I saw him fill his pipe and light it, I came to the instant conclusion that he was in the habit of smoking rope impregnated with tar. That was just what his tobacco looked like and is exactly the way it is marketed, as a 'rope' form of this product. He would stand quietly talking whilst he extracted his pipe knife from the depths of his pocket. Without pausing, he would then cut off a length of about an inch of 'rope' and begin to kneed it gently into the palm of his hand until it had been ground into the 'rubbed' version. These were days well before health pressures had developed policies to prevent smoking in the workplace. He then began the process of lighting his old briar. Mac was a traditionalist; he smoked 'rope', in a briar and used matches to light up, never, as I recall, a lighter. Occasionally he would offer me a 'cut' from his rope. I accepted only once. That was enough for me. I had a fit of coughing that lasted minutes and I had been smoking a pipe for several years by that time.

My first experience of Mac's humanity was during one of my weekends on guard duty. It came about one Saturday in the spring of 1961. The night had not been totally without incident, because, at

about 5.15am, just as I was about to make my last night patrol and to give the kitchen staff their early morning call, there came a loud rat-tat-tat on guard room door. The corporal signalled me to open the door as he had recognised, through the window, the originator of the noisy demand to enter our domain.

As I opened the door a pristine figure in flight sergeant's uniform strode past me, as if he owned the place. I did not recognise this apparition but the corporal obviously did.

"Morning Flight!" He opened the conversation.

The flight sergeant turned sharply on his heel towards me. "What have I done now?" I thought to myself.

"Have you done your morning calls to my kitchen staff yet, son?"

He spoke very precisely, in a sharp southern accent but the 'son' at the end of his question softened the delivery. I quickly realised that this was the Flight Sergeant Cook, newly flown in from Germany, who was about to take charge of the cuisine in the other ranks mess.

"No Flight, just about to go."

"Good, I'm going with you."

I remember thinking, as we walked the short distance to the block where the cooks were living, that this SNCO might be just what the cooks needed to roust them into a decent standard of personal cleanliness. He looked the type and, if so, his arrival would be greeted with a huge 'Hurrah!" by the other ranks. As I have always maintained, the food in the RAF and at B.N. in particular, was excellent but the one downside at Bircham had been the lack of personal hygiene and appearance of the kitchen staff per se. Their 'whites' were never so. They were grey and often stained with food. I had always hated the job of waking them. They had chosen to live in rooms on the same landing. No rooms being far from a shower, yet they never seemed to use them. Life though, was about to change big-time for those, not very lovable, rogues!

We arrived at the landing. The Ft. Sgt motioned me forward to make my usual attempts to rouse them. There were three doors to beat into submission that morning. I did my duty several times before

receiving the usual flattering responses of 'f-off' 'go wank yourself'' and such-like charming invitations. The NCO grinned at me.

"We'll see," he muttered to himself. He then began to bang on doors as if he didn't give a jot if he broke them down. He announced himself [I cannot remember his name] and made it very clear, sans swearing, that he wanted them out on the landing, NOW! Whatever state they might be in!

Three tired and miserable individuals dragged themselves out onto the cold landing. They looked dreadful and had clearly slept in whatever clothing they had been wearing the evening before. The Flt Sgt was not impressed and made his feelings very clear in very short order. The basic tenor of the message was clear and succinct. "There are going to be changes around here and you are going to like them!" "Now, get yourselves into those showers!"

Whilst they were in the shower he took a turn around their rooms. He returned to the landing with a face like thunder. He began immediately to issue orders and expectations like the fall of leaves in the autumn. It is doubtful if they could hear all of what he said due to the noise of the shower. Suddenly, though, he seemed to remember that I was still there.

"Sorry son, you can get on your way now, thanks for your help." I must have looked disappointed for I was enjoying the show. He grinned at me.

"Yes lad, I know, but this is between them and me." He motioned me away with a nod of his head. I finished my round and returned to the guardroom where, later, the real fun was about to start.

At about 11 am on that Saturday morning I was back in the guardroom after having had a freshening shower and a really good breakfast. There was little to do in the guardroom during the weekend days. The duty involved simple monitoring of the camp. There was no requirement for people leaving camp to sign in and out of the guardroom, as the place was completely open to the road that ran through the middle. I have already mentioned my feelings regarding the open pole gate at the far end of the station. I had whiled some time away

by reading some of my new copy of 'The Rubayat'. Fred and I had topped ourselves right up on several cups of coffee and tea.

After a while, in a really, really, bored frame of mind, I had even begun to read some pages of 'Command' standing orders. I could not remember anyone ever doing so before during guard duty and so this activity did begin to take on something of a pioneering dimension. Most of it was really straightforward and involved common sense behaviour about which one really felt that adults would not need instruction.

As far as guard duty was concerned it was all stuff that had become part of the ritual. Two items, however, did take my attention; the first was a general warning about IRA activity in the area. I simply cannot remember the wording of the guidance regarding this organisation but I can remember my own immediate reaction to it, it being along the lines of "Stuff you!" Taking into account the general low level of security in the place, there was no way that I was going to attempt to defend anything on the site from an armed IRA gang with my Air Force issue torch, no-matter how heavy!

The second item, though, was more interesting. It spoke of the weekly testing of the Air Raid Siren. This, apparently, was supposed to happen every Saturday at mid-day. I drew this to Fred's attention as he was the ranking individual. We were both perturbed about this order because neither of us could remember the ritual ever having been performed. In fact neither of us could even, immediately, think where the mysterious siren might be located.

"Is that it, on that pole over there?" Fred asked as if to the world in general.

"That looks like it," I replied with authority from my extensive experience of War Time sirens as a war child. I was all of six years old when the war ended.

"Hey, there's a button here that looks as if it might play the part." Fred was at the peak of his powers. The button towards which he was pointing was a grubby and faded off-white thing to the right of the desk and partially hidden by what we laughingly referred to as 'the out tray'.

"Give it a shove." I urged him.

This was a big thing and Fred was clearly in turmoil. What would happen if the siren was sounded and the whole camp thought that War had been declared? Officers would be called out and it would be Fred's fault that there was no war! Fred's dilemma was not going to resolve itself and it was already a couple of minutes past twelve.

"Turn your back!" I said to him. He did so, without thinking, and I gave the button a sharp shove. My motivation was that, no-matter who got pee'd off, it was in station orders and there should be no come back against me. Fred wasn't even looking so he couldn't be blamed for the lack of a new war. That would have to fall solely on my shoulders.

In the event nothing happened. I pushed the button more and more forcefully but, nothing! Zilch! A non-event!

We looked at each other and...

"Right!" said Fred... Yes that really did happen. Then he picked up the phone and dialled the internal number for the RAF regiment office. He spoke for a short while, some talk about the camp fire engine and, just before he put the phone down...

"Yes!" said Fred. And that really happened too. Then he put the phone down.

"What's going on?" I asked him.

"Wait a minute and you'll see. You pushed the bloody button; you can just wait a minute."

I didn't have long to wait, just a few minutes later and the fire engine appeared from behind the hangars. Another RAF Regiment corporal, who I didn't know but did recognise, jumped out of the engine and came over to the guard-room door where we were now standing,.

"Could you run the ladder up to that Air Raid Siren and see if you can find out why it isn't working?"

"Sure anything for you Fred; just before lunch, just what I wanted... running up and down ladders... mutter, mutter mutter..."

He continued in this vein all the time it took him to run the ladder out and begin the relatively short climb to the siren itself. He had barely reached the siren itself when I noticed the determined figure of the SWO striding towards the guardroom from the road linking to the officers' mess.

"Christ!" I nudged Fred. "It's Mr. MacFarlane".

"Don't worry lad. We're doing nothing wrong. We're just trying to follow orders…"

The SWO strode right up to us and demanded from Fred;

"What's going on here? Why have you got the bloody fire engine out and what's he doing up that pole?" He waived his hand towards corporal 'what's his name', who, by this time, had reached the alarm box and cone but was looking down at us and the SWO. Nothing deterred, this chap shouted down directly to the SWO. He spoke as if Mr MacFarlane knew the score whereas Fred was still trying to quickly get him up to speed.

"It's a bird's nest blocking it all up. Shall I scruff it out?"

"Just stay where you are, don't touch anything and shut up until I know what the bloody hell's going on." The SWO was sounding tetchy. The up-the –pole corporal did as he was told whilst Fred finished the tale of the section order and the reluctant AIR RAID SIREN.

Mac shouted up to the corporal.

"Anything in it?"

"What Sir?"

"In the damned bird's nest you idiot."

"Like what sir?"

Mr Mac Farlane turned on Fred with a face like thunder.

"You speak to the idiot. What does he think might be in a bloody bird's nest?"

Fred decided that it would be better to explain to his colleague face to face and summoned him down to the ground. He then, Janet and John style, asked him once more if there was anything in the nest other than twigs.

"Oh Yeh, there's some eggs."

The SWO looked as if he was about to commit murder and probably would have done if there was any chance of passing it off as an accident.

"Get your ladder down and take your fire engine back to its box." He gave the order to that corporal in a dangerously quiet voice. Before he did so, however, he turned to Fred and issued an order to him.

"That AIR RAID SIREN is not to be tested until those eggs are hatched and the birds are fledged. That's an order and I'll clear it with the CO."

That was not quite the end of the saga, however, for a few minutes after the SWO had disappeared towards the admin block, the duty officer came onto the scene from the opposite direction, the officers' mess. Word had obviously got back to him that something of interest had taken place and he felt that he needed to know what it was all about. Fred was keen to explain in full, including a mention that it was we two who had discovered the long ignored order to sound the ARS at mid-day on Saturdays. He related the whole story carefully and concluded with Mr MacFarlane's order to leave the nest alone until the eggs had hatched and the young birds had fledged.

The officer's lips tightened at this news. He was a junior officer of flying officer rank but, as a commissioned officer, he clearly outranked the SWO. We could see that he was on the horns of a dilemma and Fred allowed the tension to persist. The silent internal struggle, to countermand or not to countermand the SWO's order, was clearly visible on the officer's face...

"Well...I'm not sure about that... a Command order you say...I think that we need to review that decision."

I liked the way he used the term 'we need to review'. Perhaps though he was using the 'royal' we; for Fred and I did not feel either inclined or in a position to review an order by the SWO. He was the most powerful mojo in our world. In any case, I got the distinct impression that Fred wanted this situation to play itself out, just to see how far this young officer was prepared to go in the face of Mr.

MacFarlane's instructions. I was right in this...The officer came to a final decision; or at least he thought it was final...

"Yes, the standing order must take precedence. Get the fire engine back! We'll have the corporal clear the bird's nest away to see if that clears the siren."

He pulled himself to his full height as if quite satisfied that a proper decision had been made.

"But sir."

Fred interjected but strangely half-heartedly considering the trump card I knew he held up his sleeve.

"No corporal! I'm the duty officer and I've made my decision"

He clearly expected that this would end the matter. Fred had one more 'but' up his sleeve before delivering his coup de grace.

"But sir...Mr MacFarlane?"

The officer turned on Fred clearly angry at his persistence.

"Enough Corporal! Get the fire engine back here!"

This was a good time to end the battle before it all turned nasty.

"Sir! I've been trying to tell you, Mr MacFarlane's on his way at this moment to see the CO to clear the matter with him. It was the last thing that he said to us before he left."

If only looks could talk! Fred knew, I knew, and the officer knew very well, that Fred could have imparted this information right at the beginning of the exchange. He gave Fred a glare that said it all, the man straightened his tie and strode out of the office.

"What was that all about Fred? You could have ended that right at the beginning."

He smiled at me, a big, white, ear to ear grin.

"Small victories son; yes, that's it; small victories oil the wheels but don't ruffle too many dangerous feathers." He paused.

"That man got up my nose on his very first day on this camp," he added.

Despite my probing for more information Fred would not reveal any further details.

Mr MacFarlane demonstrated his humanity in a variety of ways. There was one occasion, in the spring or summer of 1961 I believe. Norman Planter was still in the RAF so it could not have been much later. Our valiant SWO came around the camp, set about speaking to all permanent staff, in order to ask for volunteers to take part in the Group sports event at RAF Uxbridge. Now I had been well instructed by my dad in the principle of non-volunteering when in the forces. I was initially, therefore, quite slow to take the SWO up on his kind offer or even to listen to it for that matter. Norman, however, did listen...

It transpired that the event was to be a three day one, even less attractive as far as I was concerned. I had stopped listening at that point, although Norman seemed to be surprisingly alert to Mr MacFarlane's blandishments regarding the need to have the camp represented, the CO's wishes and all that stuff. Mac left our office to continue his search for volunteers and Norman became quite excited. He grinned at me across our desks.

"Did you hear what he said?"

"Course! Load of rubbish." I was not prepared to be charitable at that point.

No! He responded abruptly. There are times when you really should listen you know." He heaved a sigh as if to indicate that he was dealing with a well-known fool.

"Mr MacFarlane was here trying to get people to attend a three day event in London, away from here, excused work, and you weren't listening? By the way, where do you live?"

The penny began to drop. I'm really quick sometimes. To be fair it was the prospect of being asked to volunteer for something, anything that had clouded my judgement and made me switch off.

"Mac also said, when you were busy not listening, that we could have free time when we were not needed to compete."

I hadn't listened properly to the SWO but I began to listen carefully to Norman.

"What could we do though? I'm no athlete nor are you!"

He took no offence at this observation.

"I've been thinking of tug-of-war. There must be at least eight guys from London or the south on camp."

I laughed out loud at this.

"Tug-of-war; Tug of bloody war? You have to be fit, strong and heavy to stand any chance of winning at that game."

"Who wants to win?"

He asked the question coyly, and in such a way as to indicate that I really wasn't catching on quick enough for him.

Another penny began to be minted and to slowly drop into place.

"You mean we might lose on purpose?"

"No, that would be really mean on the SWO. What I think is, that if the team turns out to be as I think it will, we will be able to try just as hard as we like and the end result will be the same. We'll be knocked out in the first round and we can then go home."

"How can we go home? We might be knocked out on the first afternoon."

"I bloody well hope so. The SWO has said that we can have free time when we are not needed for competition."

"I'm pretty sure that he didn't mean we could go home for an extra two and a half days home leave."

"You can't be sure if we don't ask the damned question, which is one thing I'm not going to do, are you?"

I began to realise that Norman's idea, hatched on the moment, was legally sound enough for me. I felt just a bit sorry for Mr MacFarlane but not enough to put me off the plan when I weighed plusses against minuses. I nodded.

"Fine by me; let's form a team and put it to Mr Mac."

And that's how it came about that RAF Bircham Newton was represented in the Group Sports event at RAF Uxbridge on that occasion. We did manage to round up a quorum of eight more or less

willing volunteers from the general London area as the BN tug-of-war team. Mr MacFarlane did look somewhat askance at the structure of our team. Norman, all eight stone or so of him, for example, installed himself as our 'anchor' man which did not inspire supreme confidence.

Once the word of the finer details of the plan got around the permanent staff 'other ranks', we even had offers from sudden volunteers who wanted to offer their services on our 'substitutes' bench. The SWO would not hear of this but did offer places on other sports.

There were no takers, unsurprisingly, for boxing, as you never knew who you might be up against and RAF boxing had a well-deserved reputation for quality. No-one was prepared to risk pain and suffering for the cause! A couple of devious individuals took opportunities to make their efforts in field events like discus, shot and javelin. As it turned out this was good for our group, as the tug-of-war was scheduled to begin on the first afternoon, during which we had every hope that we would be eliminated. Any field sports candidates left over to the Thursday might take Mr MAC'S eye off any notion that we had actually gone missing.

The tug-of-war, being a 'fun' event, at least as far as the spectators were concerned, was scheduled to begin right at the start of the three day gala of sporting competition. Forces sports events always began on a Wednesday afternoon. We were delighted to be competing in one of the first heats. We must have presented as a really motley crew when we put in our first appearance.

Our 'anchor' man, for example, did not possess a pair of navy shorts of his own and so had to borrow a pair that were much too long for him. He looked like an out-of-sorts 'Jimmy Greaves', tucked away at the business end of our half of the rope, when we took up our positions. I think that the other team must have been riddled with very understandable over confidence before the first pull, because we actually beat them, and so we began our afternoon, much to the SWO's surprise and joy, with a win. He was clearly overjoyed and full

of unwarranted optimism and enthusiasm when he came over to congratulate us.

It was all downhill after that though. The other team, overcome with shame, put in a huge effort and our 'anchor' man was over the line on the second pull before the last tones of the start whistle had died away. We put in a tremendous effort for the third pull. It's a never to be ignored wonder, just how pride can seek to overturn the most potent plan. Even Norman, the originator of the scheme, really put in an effort, but, in the real world, we stood little chance of beating any of the teams that had been entered with 'true intent'. We were eliminated from the Group Sports Event within 90 minutes of its opening.

The interview with a very disappointed, even hurt, SWO the next Monday morning was the first time I had felt really sorry for any senior RAF member of staff. He clearly had not expected us to disappear on him from the Wednesday afternoon until after the weekend. He was not in trouble of course but other WOs and NCOs had asked him some very challenging questions, as to why their staff had not been required to return to camp, or at least stay at the sports event until the Friday.

Our 'legal' argument was not lost on Mr Mac but he resented the interpretation we had put on his generosity. He did not propose to impose any punishment but made it very clear to all of us that ground-rules would be very explicit for any future expeditions led by him. As he dismissed us from his office I could not help feeling that, in the final analysis, the game had not been worth the candle. For my part I knew that I had offended one of the nicest men I had ever met.

My final example relating to the decent nature of the man who was our SWO came from an action of his in the early spring of 1962. I was on count-down towards the very end of my two years of national service, although I pride myself that I never did construct a 'count-down calendar' for myself, in the way that many of my peers did. I felt that that sort of activity only made the time drag more slowly, in any case, I had had plenty of outside interests and activities that helped to make the time pass more interestingly and quickly.

Joyce, of course, was always top of that list, followed by my newly acquired attachment to my paternal family in Manchester; more of that later. Finally though, and Joyce was in great part the generator of this, there was my avid following of all things 'Spurs'. Yes, just after we began to go out together, Joyce informed me that she was a fan of Tottenham Hotspur Football Club. Now, it has to be said that my own allegiance had always been for Spurs but this had been in a much more theoretical dimension than Joyce's.

For me, bearing in mind that Tottenham Hotspurs were the dominant affiliation in the part of London where I lived out my childhood, support for that team rather than any other was more of a case of getting through that period of my life unscathed. For Joyce, though, it was a true affiliation and I quickly fell into the habit of going with her to every Spurs home game, as well as some away games in London whenever I could. Her older cousin John would often accompany us.

I do realise that there are people in this world for whom football fanaticism is a complete and utter mystery. I can only counter this with the observation that, for football fans, those with the lack of any such passion are regarded as poor souls whose lives are not yet complete. Such is the way of the world and perspectives on human nature!

The beginning of my RAF career coincided, by pure chance, with Spurs' greatest achievement, the LEAGUE and CUP Double. By May 1961 they had already done enough to win the league title; they then went on to win the FA cup on May 6th by beating Leicester City 2-1. They were at the top of the football world in England, which allowed me to be quite cocky during discussions on camp, after most weekends. This was all the sweeter for me because our corporal tech. Brian Tanner was a Man.U. Fan. During the two years that I spent in the RAF I definitely held the 'bragging rights' and, you may be sure, that I took every opportunity to use them.

The ripples from my post weekend verbal jousting with rival football fans must have brought themselves up on shores more remote

than I had anticipated though, because one morning, a day or two after the last game of the season in the spring of 1962, the cup semi-finals had also been played. Spurs were due to meet Burnley at Wembley on May 6 for the final. Joyce and I were going to be able to watch the game on the new tele that her dad had just bought. Except for the fact that I had not yet secured a job, all was contentment in my world, as I anticipated that, just two months later, I was due to be demobbed and Joy and I were to be married.

I had my head down to face the array of names in my ledger; names whose pay needed to be calculated for the coming Friday pay parade. At this point in my career I was an SAC [senior aircraftman] and my duties were second nature. I had felt for some time that without the various ex officio, but always legal, pay accounts activities that I had been able to involve myself in, I would have gone slowly mad from boredom.

One 'frowned upon' pay activity that I had developed over my service period had become very popular among my fellow service men and had also relieved some of my ennui. It was not illegal but was irregular. It was predicated on a rule by the RAF that, in order to streamline pay parades, they would not pay out loose change on parade. Notes only were to be used unless the airman was leaving the station for a new posting or was leaving the service. This meant that the lowest denomination that could be paid out was a ten shilling note. Smaller amounts of money [credits] had to accumulate on the ledger until such time as a further 10s or £1 could be paid.

One evening early in my service, during a drinking session with some friends in my room, I hit upon the idea that the process could be refined and extended for those who needed a bit extra money for a future event and were happy for a couple of pounds or so to accumulate on their ledger for a few weeks. This is how we came to have a 'bumper' pay parade for selected persons just before my first Christmas at Bircham Newton.

Now, please allow me remind any reader that pay scales were not high for RAF personnel in those days; particularly national-servicemen. I think that I was receiving just about £1-12s-6p, just over £1-62p in today's money, per week during my first six months. This rose in stages, depending on time served and rank to something like £3-15s [£3-75p] per week as an SAC in my final six months.

The paying officer conducting pay parade, in that late December of 1960, was not, therefore, used to seeing national service individuals receiving pay-outs that were, on average, £2-£3 more than usual, just because they had asked me to save their 'credits' on their ledger for six weeks or so prior to the Christmas or New Year leave period. The pay accounts officer was furious with me but, as I had done nothing illegal, he simply told me angrily not to do it again. I steadfastly ignored that instruction, working on the principle that there were few perks for a draftee and that the officer might very well not remember by next year and it all helped to relieve the boredom of a job that I had never wanted to do anyway.

Anyway, getting back to the spring of 1962, I was getting my head down at the ledgers, doing a quick calculation for one of the chaps in the admin office, to see how much I could save up for him for a trip home to see his nan for her birthday in June. I became aware that there was someone standing beside me. I looked up, it was the SWO.

"Sorry Sir," I began to say as I made to stand up, I just had not seen him came into the room. He put his hand on my shoulder.

"Don't bother about all that son. I've got something for you." He handed me an envelope.

"What's this?" I asked uncertainly.

"Take a look," he replied with a grin.

Now, the SWO was a fairly genial man but he did not grin too often. I was intrigued. I opened the envelope and simply sat back in my chair to stare at the contents uncomprehendingly. Into my hand had arrived a pristine item, one of which I had never expected in my entire life to hold in my hand. It was a Cup final ticket! It portrayed the magic message, pure gold-dust!

Final Tie
Burnley
V
Tottenham Hotspur

Below which was the information that the game was to be played on Saturday May 5th 1962 at the Empire Stadium, Wembley. I looked up at Mr MacFarlane not really understanding what was going on. How was it that I was holding this jewel in my hand? He put me out of my misery with great pleasure and much smiling. It transpired that among all the concessional tickets that were awarded for the FA cup final was one for every military base in the country. He continued his explanation;

"The CO told me to dispose of the ticket as fairly as possible. I've had officers coming into my office in a stream since they knew it was here. You are the only real Spurs supporter that I know of on this camp...I know that the others only want to show off and to be seen at the match. I've told them all that I drew names out of a hat and that you won the ticket. The Group Captain sends his best wishes, hoping that you enjoy the game."

I thanked the SWO from the bottom of my heart. What a gent! I had never, ever, even dreamt about having a cup final ticket let alone one for that particular match. That though is the story of just how I managed to acquire my Spurs-Burnley cup final ticket!!!

The fourth character that I intend to include as a main thread for me during my time at Bircham Newton is my long-time friend John Robinson. We have already met him on my first day at Bircham. We stayed friends for many years after our RAF careers had ended. John was a 'three year' man who still had about the same time to 'run' as I had. We were due to be demobbed at about the same time with John going just a few weeks before me. The RAF had decided, incongruously as usual, that John should be a clerk typist. He was in fact a qualified and skilled bricklayer by trade, in the real world.

I had only been at Bircham Newton for a few days when our political paths crossed for real and for the first time. I was still living in the Barrack block. It was John, in fact, who was the leader of the group of kind souls who helped me to wreck my, soon to be, room and so incur the wrath of the SWO; usually a difficult thing to do but one that I had managed to achieve at my very first attempt.

At lunchtime though, on my second or third day, I took a seat at a table where, clearly, an argument was well in play. It was a political argument and John was in the thick of it, holding his own but well outnumbered. I took a seat at that table deliberately because I have always enjoyed such entertainments.

The argument was, of course, a 'left'-'right' rainbow war of words. John's position was well towards the left hand end of the colour spectrum. I recognised many of his arguments from my association with my dad's communist party friends. I had never wished to join the party because of its close affiliation to Soviet Russian Communism but I was staunchly anchored within the ambit of British Left Wing Socialism.

As I sat down I decided on the tactic that I was going to adopt. John was trying to argue against everyone at once. He was doing pretty well but the balance was against him. I quickly spotted that there was one man in particular who was well to the right of the others. It turned out that he was an accountant. All of his political arguments seemed to be predicated on what he saw as simple accounting principles. This may be OK when one is of the opinion that life is about every man for himself but we live in a society wherein the strands, the social layers if you like, are interdependent. I decided, too quickly I admit, that I did not like him, always an advantage I feel in an argument. I concentrated on that man and attacked every one of his points whenever he opened his mouth. He did not like this and became angry, which loaded my gun even more. I countered his somewhat narrow accounting approach with what I felt were strong socialist economics. During that meal I made one firm friend and lost

the possibility of making one other. The other erstwhile participants, except for John, lost interest during the battle between the 'accountant' and me and settled down to concentrate on their meals.

At that meal a long friendship was begun. I was never a communist because I could not get over the anti-Semitism prevalent in Soviet Russia and exemplified by its powerful leader, Joseph Stalin. John and I had to agree to disagree on this one issue. He was an affirmed communist and I remained socialist and the differences between us remained at that level; hardly a 'fag' paper between us, particularly when it came to arguments with other servicemen.

The friendship between John and I lasted for at least twenty five years after we left the RAF, because he and his wife Nina and their children came to our 25th Wedding anniversary celebration. I had long regretted that we lost that contact over the years since that time. I have recently made efforts to regain contact, inspired by these poor pages. I have finally made contact with Nina who informs me that John has suffered the onset of dementia over recent years. This news has given me greater reason to regret the loss of contact in earlier years. Nonetheless, in the words of the great Omar Khayyam – *"The moving finger writes and having writ moves on. Nor all your prayers will lure it back to cancel half a line nor all your tears wash out a part of it."* I only quote Omar because I first read him when in the RAF at Bircham Newton. My usual reading matter up to that point had been English and Russian socialist literature. I also have my much read copy of The Rubayat of Omar Khayyam that Joyce gave to me for my first Christmas at Bircham Newton.

John and I did not visit each other's homes during my two years of National Service. My home of course was in London, whilst John came from the Thanet area of Kent. Any visits home were to our respective families. We did, though, spend a lot of time together when our RAF duties allowed. Apart from our left wing politics we also had one important habit in common. We both smoked pipes! We also drank beer in quantities that were not good for us, when we could gather

the money together that is. I am ashamed to say that both Joy and my Dad supplemented my meagre RAF income and thereby supported both of these bad habits. In mitigation, though, I am able to say that I never allowed lack of money to prevent me from going home at every opportunity.

John did manage to get into trouble more often than most of us I seem to remember. He was often not able to hold his tongue when the occasion warranted a cool head. He made some enemies along the way for this reason. He was demobbed about a month before me but did not go home to Kent at the finish of his RAF time. He had become sweet on a girl from a local village. Her name was Miriam and he was besotted!

In order to remain in the area he managed to acquire a small caravan on a site close by. As a way of making the caravan more comfortable, he took some small pieces of equipment, including a small rug, from his room on camp to use in the caravan. This was not a clever thing to do because all rooms are inspected and an inventory is taken when any person leaves any military base. This is all a part of the 'clearing camp' process when you leave.

At the inspection it was quickly discovered that a number of items were missing from his room. John tried to claim that they had gone missing over time, but rooms are also inspected at regular intervals, mostly by the SWO or one of the commissioned officers in the admin building where John worked. As I say, John had made a few enemies over time and there were people who had waited to see him in trouble. The items were retrieved when his caravan was inspected. He was charged with theft of RAF property. He wisely decided to accept the CO's punishment and was sentenced to just ten days in cells at RAF Raynham and a dishonourable discharge. This was about the minimum that could have been awarded under the circumstances because he had previously served three days clink for an earlier offence of insubordination.

John, of course, felt that he had been badly treated after his three years of 'unstinting' service to the Crown. I visited him during his short incarceration. He was well treated by the staff at Raynham and he, naturally, remained unrepentant to the end! The pity though, from my point of view, was that John could not get to my wedding because his period of incarceration did not end until two days after that blessed event. Thus it was that my best friend was not able to attend my wedding.

6
Bircham Newton – Beginnings!

I PRESENTED MYSELF at the door of the Adjutant, the squadron leader, and knocked. An airman, an SAC, opened the door and 'demanded' to know what I wanted. I gave my name and replied that W.O. Rubin had told me that the squadron leader had asked to see me.

"Wait!" was the peremptory response. The airman disappeared as he closed the door in my face. A few moments later he re-appeared and motioned me into the room. It was a small ante room where he apparently had a desk, a phone and a typewriter. He was clearly the adjutant's clerk typist and vetted, apparently officiously, whether by land or wire, all callers for his master. He moved towards a door set in the wall opposite so I followed him through.

"A/C Kreit, Sir, you wanted to see him."

I stood to attention in front of the desk at which the squadron leader sat. I did not salute because I was not wearing headgear. Squadron Leader 'B' was a younger man than I had expected him to be. He had fair hair; he was clean shaven and so did not sport an RAF handlebar moustache. He was slim and, as far as I could tell, in view if the fact that he was sitting down, he appeared to be quite tall.

"Stand easy!" he spoke the order softly and even smiled as he looked up at me. There was no invitation to sit down here! "So you're the crack shot of the 44th intake." He muttered, more to himself than to me. I was taken aback at this. Was it a joke, was he taking the mickey? I could not tell; all I knew was that I was no crack shot. As far as I was concerned, my marksman's badge was something I was very pleased with but it really only denoted a basic proficiency at accurate shooting with a 303 Lee Enfield rifle.

"It's true that I did get my marksman's badge at the first try sir." I replied diplomatically.

"So I see, so I see." As he spoke he was reading what appeared to be a report from a file that he had in front of him. He continued; "You did, in fact, shoot a very tight group at the first attempt and then repeated that quality of shooting when asked to have another go. I have the flight sergeant's report here." He waived the document that he had just been reading. "It's a very full report." The squadron leader sat back, as if waiting for me to say something. I grinned. "That's very decent sir for a man whose sergeant had just been under fire!" This attracted his attention. He sat bolt upright. "What do you mean by that?" And so I told him the full story of the shooting incident that occurred just before my turn on the 25 yard range at RAF Bridgnorth in my training summer of 1960.

It so happened that a very serious incident occurred during the very first batch of trainee 'riflemen's' attempts on that day. The R.A.F Regiment Sergeant was in the process of giving the first batch of 5 or 6 airmen their shooting instructions for the exercise. He had explained that there were no Butts on a short 25 yard range like this but that the targets could be retrieved by winding them back to the firing points on a wire. He had explained what the shooting position should be and how and when one should sight and breathe in order to get the best chance at a decent group on the target; a 'group' being a series of five shots as close together as possible on the target. We had all been instructed to listen carefully to these general

instructions, as the sergeant did not want to repeat them for each batch of 'shooters'.

I was not among the first selected to participate and I was glad of this, as I wanted to make certain that I had absorbed all of the possible issues before I had my go. I was both excited and very nervous to do well at this particular element of the training programme, the bulk of which was becoming a real and total pain in the arse as far as I was concerned.

The sergeant instructed the five men to lie down and assume a prone firing position. He continued......as he did so he remained on the range and continued to stride to and fro in front of the five, by now, anxious and eager young men. "I shall instruct you to engage the first round by easing the bolt back and pulling it into the chamber as you have been shown." No-one appeared to hear the sound of one bolt engaging at this point. There was too much general and excited background whispering going on. "I shall then count '1-2-3' Fire!", at which point a single shot, a shot that silenced all whispering; a very significant and unexpected shot, rang out, as if to shake the very ducks off the wall. At that moment exactly, I had my eyes on the sergeant. To this day I am convinced that he had a very near 'incontinence' moment, because the round passed within a few feet of him, as he magnificently strode the range before his minions. "Fuck!" was all he seemed able to mutter as the blood drained from his face. I guess that that was understandable because a 303 round, at a distance of just a few feet, might well have taken his leg off. It would have been very different from the John Wayne Western Scenario, where the hero gets a leg wound, has a bit of a moan, ties his neckerchief around the leg to stench the flow of blood, climbs on his loyal 'white' horse and rides off into the sunset.

The RAF Regiment Flight Lieutenant in charge of the range had witnessed the incident, both angrily and impotently, from his office at the rear and to one side of the range. He was not amused! The sergeant was ordered off the range and, I believe, suspended for

a disciplinary process to take place. His superior, a regiment flight sergeant was called in to take the rest of the trainee shooting programme.

"Well I'll be damned!" This was all the squadron leader could say as I finished my tale. After a few moments of sober thought, he went on to ask me if I would like to join his shooting group, using the 600 yard range at Swaffham, near RAF West Raynham, on Wednesday afternoons. He took pains to explain that joining the group was voluntary but that, once joined, he expected airmen to take the group seriously.

The squadron leader's plan was for the group to form the basis of a future station shooting team. I assured the officer that I was very keen to join and that I would be as committed to Wednesday afternoons as the service would permit. "You can leave that side of things to me." He said quite heavily. "The Group Captain is very much in favour of station sports teams. We have his full support." He sat back into his comfortable chair once again. "Mind you", he continued slowly. "We do not want any incidents like the one at Bridgnorth." "Amen to that sir!" It was all that I could think of to respond to that one. He suddenly brought the interview to a conclusion. "Right then, we begin next Wednesday. Meet up by the armoury at 14.00 hours." "Very good sir." I replied as I came back to attention, turned back towards the door and made my way out of 'the presence'. As I did so, I little knew, that my first afternoon with the newly formed Bircham Newton shooting team, was to be just as dramatic as had been my earlier shooting experience at RAF Bridgnorth had been!

The rest of my time over the first few days was spent in becoming familiarised with my work in the pay accounts section at my new place of work. I went home, as usual, for the weekend but did not have to hitch hike this time, as Norman offered me a lift on his motor bike, an ancient Royal Enfield Bullet. I'm afraid that I annoyed the hell out of Norman by referring to it as a Lee Enfield Bullet a couple of times. A poor joke I realise now but then I was young and that's my

only excuse. Maybe it was being asked to join the shooting team that had brought it on?

I realise that I do not refer in any detail to my weekends at home. This is no accident. They were personal and, in my mind, a separate universe to my time spent within the RAF. Joyce and I got married just three days after I left Bircham Newton for the last time. I left camp on 04-07-1962 and we married on the 7th July. That too was deliberate timing, although I was not officially de-mobbed until the 27th July. I had no intention of asking Joy to marry me whilst I was still subject to the disciplinary command structure of an organisation which would subject her, through me, to a vicarious portion of that discipline. We had been engaged for over three years by the time we got married.

I had one engagement prior to that next weekend home, more-over. It was my meeting with the Rabbi, this being the meeting that had been arranged by my section Warrant Officer, Mr. Rubin. I have to say, that despite my own initial prejudices on the subject; I found the RAF and its personnel to be far less anti-Semitic than I had antici-pated. Much less, in fact, than I later experienced when working for Lloyd's Bank in the City of London. RAF Bridgnorth had actually boasted a Jewish Prayer room, in reality a multi-faith room. I was given an HM Jewish Forces prayer book and an HM Forces book of Jewish thoughts, shortly after arriving there. I still possess both of these. They are both within reach as I write these words.

I was called up to the guard room shortly after 2pm on the Friday. WO Rubin actually walked to the guard room with me and walked us back to the sergeant's mess, once we had met with the Rabbi and introduced ourselves to him. Mr. 'R' left us to it, once he had settled us into a nice room and had instructed an airman attendant on the mess to provide us with tea and biscuits. When I first told my dad of the kindness that I had received from the two WOs I had, so far, met at Bircham Newton, I am certain that he thought that I was pulling his leg, 'big time'.

The Rabbi was a stocky man, in his mid to late forties, I guessed. He had driven over from Norwich, which was the nearest town with a Jewish Community. He was bearded and really enjoyed his tea and biscuits! He explained that he had been on the go all morning and had not yet had time for lunch. I suddenly realised that he had to be from a Liberal or Reform Jewish Community, because he responded favourably to my offer to try to get him some sandwiches. I had made the offer without thinking, but things quickly fell into place as I realised that no orthodox Rabbi would accept an offer of food, even biscuits, from a non-kosher kitchen.

I explained my own background to him and advised him that my Jewish family was an orthodox one but that my mother was not Jewish. This did not 'phase' him one bit, so I went on to explain that I had decided at a very young age that I was going to be Jewish, and regard myself as Jewish, whether the Jewish authorities liked it or not. This seemed to amuse him. I went on to explain, however, that war makes you grow up quickly. I did my early growing up through-out the war in bomb raided, bomb strewn London. I had had, even as a young boy after the war, when the truth about the 'final solution' became ever clearer, a personal and embryo realisation. I gradually became aware that, if the Germans had ever successfully crossed the channel, I would have gone along the same dark route, not fully understood by me at that time, as all others of my Jewish family, almost certainly my mother as well.

As I grew older and my understanding grew concomitantly, I also began to take a personal stand against the evil process that was depriving the world, not just of a people, but of a culture and all that goes with it; literature, language, philosophy. On frequent occasions I begged my father to teach me Yiddish but he would not hear of it. I did, however, gain some understanding of the language for myself, when, as an adult, I regained contact with my paternal grandmother, my Boobah.

Dad's mental, philosophical and social preoccupation was communism and the working class struggle for justice. In all reality he had left his Judaism behind him, although it would have been very rapidly brought back to confront him had he, God forbid, ever been captured by the Germans. My own determination, on the other hand, was hatched very early.

I amused the Rabbi further by telling him of an incident at school when I was about eight, and the teacher had called the morning register and I had told her that I was not a Christian and therefore did not have a 'Christian' name. To this day, I am convinced that she did not appreciate the significance of what I was saying, and that she felt that I was simply being rude. Rude or not, it is a stance that I have taken pretty much ever since that time.

The rabbi and I talked for a while. I discovered that he was married, obligatory for a Rabbi, even a Liberal or Progressive one! He had three children, all daughters, and that his wife was Spanish. He had first met her whilst fighting, as a very young man, against Franco in the Spanish Civil War. Best of all, though, he was a football fan. Even better than that! He was a Spurs supporter! We spent the next hour or so talking Spurs and football, and it was one of the best of times to do so, because the team from White Hart Lane was on top of the world!

We parted the best of friends and he promised to come to see me again, which he did. I seem to remember that he visited me on three more occasions during my time at Bircham Newton. Apart from the geniality of the visits they did me a wider favour. The Rabbi's visits gave the impression to others that I was more religious than was the case in fact. I did not take too much advantage of this, but it did come in handy, over such times as Jewish holidays when I asked for time off. Our section sergeant, later to be promoted to flight sergeant, actually did his best to try to accommodate me on those occasions.

The coming weekend passed only too quickly. On Wednesday, however, we were due to take our initial steps as the RAF Bircham

Newton shooting team, with the first ever practice afternoon at Swaffham range. What a session it was going to turn out to be!

I actually got to bed at a reasonable time on the Sunday evening, because Norman had given me a lift home and back as he lived quite close to my parents' home in Enfield. It was a long weekend too, because the sergeant had allowed us to leave camp on Friday evening rather than Saturday mid-day. I had not begun to change my attitude towards the RAF and compulsory military service yet, but things were certainly looking up domestically!

If I had gone home by train my return to camp would have been quite different. I would not have got to bed until about 3am-3.30am on the Monday morning. This was because the last train from Liverpool St. to King's Lynn did not leave until about half past midnight on the Sunday night. It arrived at King's Lynn at about 3 am. The bus that met it, however, served three air force stations; RAF Marham, RAF Sculthorpe and RAF Bircham Newton. Because of its position Sculthorpe, then a U.S. base was always served second, thus leaving Marham and Bircham Newton to be served either first or last. From that decision would mean a difference of about 45 minutes, either way, on the eventual time to get to bed.

Events were crowding in on me, for on a particular Monday evening, a group of us were due to meet up to celebrate the de-mob of a national serviceman 'T', who had served his time as a cook in the W.O's and senior NCO's mess. "A real cushy number" was all he would say when asked to describe his job.

We had arranged to pile down to a local pub for a few bevies and then to bring a few more of the same back to 'T's room, where we would enjoy them, together with piles of sandwiches and cakes, that he had 'arranged' to be laid on via his connections with the WOs' mess. I did not know T, but was quite happy to enjoy his hospitality, especially since it appeared quite likely that I would inherit his room. A very nice room at first glance, on the first floor of a block, and just across the internal camp road from the airmen's mess, and about a

100 yard or so, walk from the 'office'. As the evening wore on, however, the prospect of inheriting this particular room became less and less attractive.

It really is almost unbelievable just how badly the behaviour of otherwise rational young men can deteriorate when 'in their cups'. I had the opportunity to attend many de-mob parties during my period of national service and it was ever thus. Normally, I have a predilection for food to stay on the plate or on the table, when it is not actually on its way to the mouth. Flying food has always been an anathema to me, except on that occasion, both to my shame and to my cost. My new friend John, however, seemed to have no inhibitions as regards 'flying food'.

Egg and mayo sandwiches make quite a 'splat' when they hit the wall; boiled eggs do even better! Once one person begins to giggle, moreover, the pleasing effect is enhanced to fever pitch. As the walls yielded to a virtual bombardment, they became more and ever more peppered, spotted, hardly decorated, no certainly not decorated, by this fusillade of egg based projectiles. Even under the heavy influence of the drink, I began to realise that it might be wise to decline any offers of this particular room as my permanent home. Once again I was to reckon without warrant officer power!

I could not begin to understand why the SWO had singled me out to bear the benefit of his sarcasm the next morning. It was totally unfair, I thought to myself, when the pain in my head would permit me to think that is.

"Were you or were you not at the debauchery that produced this bloody shambles?"

I began to respond by reminding him that I was not the only one there, but caught the glint in his eye, when I had uttered just a few words in that direction.

"Yes sir" was my consequently meek reply.

"And who, just who, did you think was going to occupy this room after its present occupant had escaped my anger by leaving the bloody

service?" I had never heard him swear before, nor did I since that sad, undistinguished and indistinct morning after the night before.

"I didn't think......"

"No, you damned well didn't, did you? You did, though, manage to get so pie eyed and gormless as to help make yourself a lot of work."

Oh God, I thought. Here it comes...

"I do so hope that some of your recent drinking buddies will have the decency to help you to rectify the damage done to this room last night. When you are negotiating with them you can remind them, in my name that having your own room is a privilege that does not come to many ordinary airmen. We have plenty of barrack block accommodation on this camp, as you and they, all well know, and I will have you all back there faster than you can fart, if this room is not up to scratch by 8am tomorrow. This is now, pro-tem your room. If it does not pass my inspection by then, you are all back in barracks. You can tell your buddies that from me!" It is fair to say that the SWO was pretty damned angry and that his power was absolute on matters like this. The whole drinking group, together with help from some others, worked like mad for hours that evening to try to bring life back to the original colour scheme of my, perhaps temporary, room.

My interview with the SWO the next morning was not exactly plain sailing despite the fact we had all worked well into the night, in a combined effort to repair the damage to the room. There had been some stains, mainly in the corner of the room, opposite the door. We had all taken turns to apply 'elbow grease' to these stains, but complete success was not to be obtained. Egg and mayo is a formidable combination when applied to a wall at high speed. Some of these stains were still evident, although greatly reduced in intensity. I decided, finally, to try to reduce the unpleasing impact of those obstinate stains by moving the wardrobe to hide them. There were also a couple of stains on the ceiling, where projectile eggs had made their marks. The ceiling was white and so we eventually covered these fairly successfully with a judicious mixture of 'Blanco' and water. We

were all, more or less experts, with regard to the uses and application of Blanco of course.

The SWO did not seem to be impressed by our efforts. He gave off the air of a man who had seen it all before and was not going to be fooled by the mere moving of a wardrobe. He did not actually demand to look behind it, but he took his own slow time to inspect the room. He seemed, however, to have missed the erstwhile egg stain on the ceiling. I was beginning to congratulate myself on this when, at the end of his inquisition, he turned to me only to give me a stay of execution.

"I'm going to give you two more weeks to get this room fully back to its previous pristine state. You can use my name to get a can of paint from stores. That will give you another opportunity to move that wardrobe, won't it?"

"By the way....", he continued as he prepared to leave the room. It's good to see that you've found an ingenious use for Blanco...."

That was it; the inspection was over for the time being. I did have my own room, also for the time being, and a good chance of keeping it moreover, for I was quite a dab hand at DIY, as it came to be known across the country. I put the matter to the back of my mind for the while, though, as, that afternoon, being Wednesday afternoon, I was due to go off with the shooting team for our first session at Swaffham.

Over the next few days I took opportunities to walk around the camp and get my bearings. Time and again I was surprised, astonished in fact, at the lack of security. A public road truly did run right through it. There were no security barriers along the road to prevent unwanted intruders from simply wandering onto the camp. As I say in other places, my main worry in this regard was the armoury, which was almost totally unprotected from a determined encroachment. We had repeated low level warnings through 'Group' orders about IRA activity, although this, of course, had not reached anything like the level of the late 60s and the 70s through to the early 90s.

The main camp lay on roughly the western side of the road, where the guard room, the admin block and airmen's living quarters were situated. The armoury and officers' quarters lay on the other side of this road, together with other facilities, that I do not remember because I had little cause to cross over there, other than Wednesday afternoons, to gather at the armoury for shooting sessions or to inspect the armoury security when on 'picket' duty. My first taste of which was to begin on the coming Friday, for my first weekend on guard duty. During that weekend, I was to learn for the first time, about the 'Ghosts of Bircham Newton' and even establish one of my own!

7
Wednesday Afternoon is Sports Time!

IT WAS A little known fact amongst the general public that, both before and after the period 1960-62 of which I am writing, Wednesday afternoons were dedicated to sports activities between all the services as well as within services. This included the RAF, the Army, the Navy and also the Police Force. In this way sporting competitions between those services were made that much easier to organise.

After my meeting with the Rabbi and the weekend home, my next big moment then was the first meet of the station shooting team, as I had now come to think of it. I made sure that I was standing outside the armoury well before the appointed time on the next Wednesday afternoon. The squadron leader arrived just at 2pm or 1400 hours in military speak. He had arranged for an RAF regiment corporal to open up the armoury, to allocate weapons and to manage the ammunition during the afternoon. There were about eight airmen, a mixed batch of A/Cs, LACs and SACs. We were each allocated a Lee Enfield Rifle. The RAF regiment corporal made it very clear that we would each be responsible for the cleaning our allocated rifle on the drive back to camp and that he would inspect them before we would be allowed to leave the armoury.

The corporal also made it clear that he would manage the accounting, of and for, all ammunition. He little realised how onerous this task would prove to be. The squadron leader also authorised the issue of several sterling sub machine guns. He explained that this was in order to add some variety to the afternoon and to our shooting experience. I had never before seen or heard of this weapon. I almost never saw one again, nor wished to, after the more dramatic events later that afternoon!

The Swaffham range was situated about 20 or so miles, almost due south, from Bircham Newton. The range appeared huge compared with the tiny 25 yard range at Bridgenorth. As there were eight of us, the squadron leader split us into two groups of four. My group was selected to serve the first stint in "the butts". The butts section of a rifle range is the 'backstop' or the area behind the target into which a shot can fall safely. Outdoor and sometimes indoor ranges have earth or sand butts and sometimes concrete. A deep ditch or trench will run the length of the butts and in front of both this backstop and the targets themselves. The ditch looks rather like a WWI trench. This area is known as "the butts" and serves as a place in which to safely manage the targets for the shooters.

Modern day ranges are run on a very formal basis with range managers and people designated to work the targets and to manage them safely. On the occasion of which I am writing, however, this was undertaken much less formally. A series of target positions ran along the length of the trench. The targets could be easily run up and down on 'sliders' and poles [pointers] held by those working the butts. These could be raised to indicate the position of the shots to guide the shooter as to his accuracy. The top of the trench was well above head height, so that those serving in the trench were safe from the shots passing overhead. At the right hand end of the trench was a flag pole. One person working the butts had the responsibility to run flags up and down the pole to indicate when shooting could commence and when it must cease.

The squadron leader took some time to explain, very carefully, just how we were expected to behave on the range, and how to manage the butts when our turn came. He then explained to us, that we each had to 'zero' our rifle, and that that weapon would be assigned to that specific airman, whilst he remained a member of the group. And so we proceeded to the next stage, zeroing our rifles, whilst taking turns in the butts.

An important device that is mounted on the rifle is the sight. While there are many forms of rifle sight, they all perform a similar function, in that they permit the rifleman to set the angle between the bore of the rifle and the line of sight to the target. There is a geometric relationship between the line of sight and bore angle.

This relationship is determined through a process called "zeroing." The bore angle is set to ensure that a bullet on a parabolic trajectory will intersect the line of sight to the target at a specific range, 100 yards, at the time that I was doing it. A properly adjusted rifle barrel and sight are said to be "zeroed." I have taken the decision to briefly mention this necessary activity here, but it is a complicated process, which varies from rifle to rifle and about which many very expert chapters have been written. The paragraphs above are not technical. They simply indicate that there is a process, an important one, which has to be undertaken if one is going to shoot accurately at a target. It is possible to shoot a tight group without zeroing. To get the group close to the centre of the target, however, the rifle must be zeroed.

When the squadron leader was satisfied that we had zeroed our weapons, he allowed us to shoot a few targets each, whilst taking turns in the butts. I should say that we were shooting 'prone', without rests, but with rifle slings to hold the weapon steady and to aid reasonable shooting. In this, the rifle sling is slackened off to the comfort and requirements of the shooter, who slips his non trigger arm through the sling from its far side. He then grips the barrel, so that the sling is held tight against the arm, thus holding the rifle quite

firmly. Having made my first attempt at zeroing the rifle, I shot two targets from 100 yards. The groups were not too bad, but not as good as at Bridgenorth and the zeroing needed some attention. I did O.K. compared to the others, so I was not too downhearted. When we had all finished, we removed the clips from our weapons as well as the bolts. We then checked the barrels to make sure no stray bullets remained in our rifles.

At this stage we were all quite tired, but flushed, with what we saw as the success of our first afternoon's shooting as a team. The squadron leader then offered us the opportunity to try something a bit 'lighter'. No grouping, no zeroing, just the opportunity to familiarise ourselves with the Sterling sub machine gun. This was quite a light weapon with a folding shoulder stock, which, in the folded state, could almost be described as a machine pistol. Over the years there have been several 'marks' with a variety of features. Our guns held 30x 9mm rounds in a straight magazine. They were fairly accurate up to about 50 yards. It was to this distance from the targets that we moved for this part of the proceedings.

Accuracy with any machine gun depends on the shooter being able to fire the weapon in short bursts of 3-4 rounds at a time. It takes practice to be able to keep to that regime, and to mentally separate the opposite actions of tension and release of the trigger, and that was the focus of a dramatic and potentially serious incident, that suddenly erupted into our erstwhile happy afternoon.

We were shooting, one at a time, in the direction of the butts, just two at a time in the butts, to manage the targets for the one person shooting, just one magazine per person. The plan was that we would return to camp when everyone had had a go. Just two of our group of shooters were assigned to the butts. As it turned out they were in the safest place for the next few minutes.

It so happened that I went first and thoroughly enjoyed the experience. I got the hang of firing the weapon in short bursts and actually managed to get quite a number of shots on target. I removed the

magazine, checked that no rounds remained in the chamber of the barrel, and stepped back from the firing position. I was replaced by 'H' a national serviceman from the stores department. He was given the order to begin shooting but he seemed to hesitate. Suddenly he began to cry out "It's stuck Sir!" He was trying to say that his gun was jammed in the firing position. What had, in fact happened, was that his finger had tightened on the trigger and that mentally he could not release it. That would not have been a great problem if he had kept the gun pointed at the target.

The unfortunate airman did not have the presence of mind to do so, however. As he cried out, he turned round and towards the group including the officer, standing about fifteen yards behind him. I was just a few yards behind the man and dived forward to get as close to him as possible. Split seconds later I sensed, rather than saw, the others diving in all directions for the ground. There was no actual cover to be had. Fortunately for all of us, as he turned around, the barrel of his gun travelled in an elegant arc upwards as he swivelled uncomfortably to his right. The nerve shattering rat-tat-tat of the weapon lasted a few seconds only before the magazine was exhausted. The world though had become encased in a slow motion time loop, whereby you felt that you could hear each tiny explosion quite separately and clearly, and measure the intervals between them. By the Grace of God or our inestimable good luck, no-one was hurt over and above the impact of injured dignities hitting the ground hard. 'H' was excused from further activities with the shooting team!! I do not know if any further sanctions were imposed.

8
Picket duty with the ghosts of Bircham Newton

IT WAS NOT until long after I left the Air Force that I began to realise, that the station on which I had begun my very reluctant time as a very unwilling conscript, did and does occupy a very respectable place in the history of the R.A.F, one that far outweighs its size. It has, moreover, garnered many and diverse ghost stories during its illustrious life. Many of these stories were known to permanent staff at the unit. If they did not know them, they invented and embellished them, from snippets of stories they had gathered together.

When one remembers the geography of the base, it is easy to understand just how many of these stories had gathered momentum. I certainly needed no stimulation in order to conjure up my own night spectres. Bircham Newton was just about as isolated as one can imagine in England. At night time the darkness was tangible, for the lone serviceman on picket duty around the back of the huge hangars, or on the other side of 'the road that ran through it', when checking out the armoury. Certain guard corporals enjoyed regaling young national servicemen with nerve racking stories of ghosts and Ghoulies usually just before they set off into the night for their regular patrols around the camp.

One of these standards was not in fact a ghost story at all; it involved a wild and cynical story of possible IRA attacks, which would have the intention of gaining access to the armoury. The story usually involved a reminder that our sole means of defence was a heavy torch. My standard response to this was to reply, that if such an eventuality arose, I would put the torch to very good use by using it to lead the way to the armoury. At first I took these IRA warnings with a pinch of salt because, in the early 1960s, that particular organisation did not have the high profile that its later cowardly deeds were to gain for it, all over the U.K. in just a few years' time. It was not until one of my NCO chums showed me a current copy of Group Orders, which contained a warning to be aware of, and to be ready for, possible IRA attacks. It was at that point, that I mentally reaffirmed my decision, that the heavy torch would best serve its master, me, by guiding any invaders to anywhere they wanted to go. If my military masters could only see their way to providing me with a torch, albeit a heavy one, as my sole defence, then I would use it in the way that its manufacturers intended, to light the way!

As I threaded my way around the camp on cold, dark, winter evenings and nights, the stories often bounced around in my head. The IRA tales were easy to discard in those years. They had not yet become the national and international scourge, that which was to unfold in the late 60s the 70s, and so on until near the end of the century.

Other hot tales were, however, much easier to imagine, when the north east wind was piercing through your clothing into parts of your body that you would rather have forgotten about at that moment, whilst quietly doing your duty and protecting the camp. In spite of the benefits of the truly wonderful RAF greatcoat, the wind, I swear, came across the North Sea from the Arctic directly aimed at me. I tried pulling my beret down until it resembled an upside-down shallow pudding basin, whilst pulling my greatcoat collar up as far as I could, in a vain effort to persuade the two to meet and to keep my poor

neck warm. There always remained, however, a gap through which that wind carried its numbing message. A Balaclava helmet would have been very welcome, but tentative, hopeful, enquiries revealed the RAF had in fact issued such a garment but, apparently, only during the war and specifically to aircrew. It seemed that no-one in the air ministry had had a thought for poor little me, fighting my private battle against arctic winds during Norfolk's Januaries and Februaries.

I have often thought about those winter months of my first year, when the wind blew direct from the frozen north and the snow was so deep, that married airmen had great difficulty in making their way a couple of hundred yards to their married quarters. Those weekends of guard duty, in the enduring snow, only served to feed my hatred of the 'spiteful bugger' who had persisted in sending me those unwelcome letters of invitation from Her Majesty. I was a really sad, angry soul, with an axe to grind against the military system of compulsory national service. It was an axe that was all powerful and likely to engulf me.

That was the winter of 1960/61, when it had begun to snow on Christmas Eve and did not let up until well into March. It was the winter, when the SWO organised us into snow digging parties, aimed at digging and keeping clear a path to the married quarters. It was moreover the winter when an RAF regiment flight sergeant, managed to disable our sole mechanical piece of snow moving equipment. One of the Regiment Lorries, a powerful looking six wheeler, as I remember it, which could be fitted with an appropriately angled snow blade, which the flight sergeant endeavoured to snap permanently from its mounts on the forward frame of the vehicle. He did this by repeatedly ramming and reversing, ramming and reversing, into the same piled and hardened section of snow, in spite of the clear evidence that he was creating a wall of compacted snow, that quickly became so strong that the blade snapped almost clear of its mounts and frame.

The scene still lives dramatically in my memory. In other circumstances it would have been comical and quite at home in a 'Carry on

Sergeant' type film. If the SWO had had enough hair he would have been tearing it out in huge tufts. In my two years at the base I never once saw him quite as angry as that, on any other occasion. That flight sergeant was busy trying to make his excuses, which did nothing to calm the SWO. The flight sergeant's bluster took on a whole new dimension with the arrival of his guvnor, the RAF Regiment Flight Lieutenant. The danger that the SWO would explode, only receded to the extent that he could now drop that tragic NCO deep into the proverbial.

The front of the regiment lorry was a comical sight. The snow blade had been bolted onto twin frames at the front of the chassis. One of the bolted sections had broken clear away, but the structure would have been strong enough to support the blade from either end, if only the enthusiastic NCO had stopped ramming the lorry into already impacted ice, thereby forcing one end to break away. He did not stop, however, the result of this additional enthusiasm was that the remaining mount had bent horribly forcing the other end of the blade into the ground, so that when the unfortunate NCO tried to reverse away from his personally- created ice wall, he had actually begun to inflict damage onto the truck's chassis. He became less and less popular as the extent of his foolhardiness came to light. From the point of view of the digging team, moreover, worse was yet to come.

The flight sergeant was neither happy nor popular, particularly with that same crew, which included yours truly, designated to do the manual digging. Partly to pacify and largely in order to restore some feeling into frozen limbs and fingers, the SWO ordered that a warming tot or two of rum was to be issued to the digging party. A huge demijohn of inviting deep red liquid, reputedly containing some 7 gallons of finest navy rum, was long known to occupy its own shelf, in full view, but in the depths of the kitchen. This heavy container was moved, at the SWO's instructions, into the mess hall by several very willing volunteers. After some cheering, and unwanted advice,

the SWO removed the stopper and slurped a ration of the inviting nectar into a mug. He took a formal swig but immediately began to choke. One had experienced a great deal of foul language thus far in one's military carer but it came strangely from the lips of the usually calm SWO. "It... it's fucking Ribena!" Someone, never to be discovered which someone, had surreptitiously removed the rum and substituted a cleverly disguised concoction. The kitchen staff were immediately under suspicion. No-one owned up, needleless to say, or murders might well have been done.

If the SWO could have justified blaming the regiment flight sergeant I am convinced that he would have done so. That NCO could well have ended up as an addition to Bircham Newton's ghostly history....

That observation inevitably takes me back to my tales of picket duties and ghosts at Bircham Newton. I never did see a ghost, despite the repeated efforts of various mischievous guard corporals to induce me to do so. I have to admit, though, that there were times, at the rear of, and in the darkness of, the hangars near the airfield, when I felt the phantasmal presence of those stories.

Yes, it was easy to recall those stories in the dark shadows around the camp, when the winter winds played their own particular music in the structures of darkened buildings. I do not wish to be accused of plagiarism by inserting any details here, but the interested reader need only to google 'The Ghosts of Bircham Newton' to provide him/herself with the details.

Yes, indeed, you can read of the Bomber that crash-landed on the landing strip killing its entire crew. One tried hard not to think of their ghostly souls, when skirting the airfield, during very cursory checks among the shadows of the huge hangars on those dark, windy, and very cold, winter nights.

And there is the public road that runs through the base, to which is allied a story of noises and voices filtering up from beneath the road, and said to be the sounds of deceased airmen, whose ghosts are trapped in a former underground air raid shelter, the remains of

which are now located under the road as it runs part way through the camp.

There are more stories that are now in the public domain and available through your home computer. The third and final one, though that I wish to mention here, is, in my view, the easiest to believe, for it talks of a drunken airman who crashed his car into a hangar during the war, killing himself and his passengers. It is this story that I was thinking of in my robust exchange of words with a certain warrant officer at the end of the next chapter.

9
My Own Bircham Newton Ghost

GUARD DUTY, BETTER known locally as picket duty, was nothing like I ever imagined it would be. I had to report to the guardroom immediately after dinner on the Friday night. The guard NCOs were usually corporals from the RAF Regiment contingent on camp. I was happy to see that my first duty was to be with Corporal James. He greeted me quite warmly, recognising that this was all quite new to me.

"What's your first name?" he enquired. "You can call me Fred," he added helpfully, "considering that we're going to spend the weekend together."

As he sat there grinning at me, I was feeling slightly uplifted from my continual anti RAF gloom, by the realisation that this regiment corporal had asked me for my 'first' name and not my 'Christian' name. This was still by far the most common form of enquiry in those days and was usually followed by a look of bemused resentment, when I replied that 'I didn't have one', followed by the brief and deliberately unhelpful explanation that I was not a Christian.

Fred showed me round the guardroom, not that there was much to show. As far as I can remember it, there was the main room, with

a table in front of a large-ish window; to the left of this window and looking out of it, was the door through which I had just entered. At the back of the room were two cells and in the corner, diagonally opposite to the door, was a short corridor with a toilet at the far end. In the room itself was a table, on which were what looked like the means of making hot drinks.

I nodded towards this table and grinned. "All mod cons I see."

"We have to look after ourselves. The nights can be long - especially in the winter." He added the last bit, after a short pause, as if the winter were something special, in those parts.

I have to say that I rapidly grew to agree with him, on that point. Norfolk wears two hats; its summer hat and its winter one. In summer the living is easy, as the song goes. The days are long. The birds make babies and sing. The crops grow and get harvested, as the sounds and sweet smells of summer, entice one into a false sense of security. Norfolk in summer is a good place to be.

Then comes winter to shatter the dream and burst your bubble, as the icy winds sweep in from the sea, straight from the North Pole or from the frozen wastes of Eastern Europe. They tear into your clothing so that your bones and muscles lose their feeling and refuse to work; either with you or for you. The fierce, cold, winter wind chills your bones and rushes up your trouser leg, to freeze your vitals.

Norfolk is flat, you see! There is nothing to break the wind; no defence between you and those frozen Eastern wastelands that were the downfall of both Napoleon and Hitler. The winter winds of Norfolk make for an experience not to be repeated, especially in the dark, on the edge of a grass airfield, alone, and at all times of the night, and particularly when your guard corporal has spent an hour, at the beginning of the duty period, regaling you with a series of stories about the 'Ghosts of Bircham Newton.'

As I have mentioned previously, many ghost stories exist around this small RAF station. A range of sources are attributed, but they mostly date from the period of the Second World War and the post

War period. There were two, though, that had come my way via Fred before I set out on my first tour around the camp that night. It was quite a long stretch that I was required to cover on each round. I had to do this every couple of hours or so, through the night, and each tour, I discovered, would take about an hour, when done properly.

The first of Fred's tales came from the War years and was the one mentioned earlier and relating to a car full of drunken pilots, whose driver, also a pilot, managed to crash, his car, into a plane hangar thereby killing himself and his passengers. It is, of course, claimed, that the ghosts of these men still roam the base, even to this day. This was a comforting thought as I made my way through the camp, torch in hand, and threaded a path through barrack blocks, huts, and out towards the grass airfield, and thence to the dark side of the three large hangers.

I thanked Fred mentally, as I stood at the edge of the field, in that profound darkness, deepened because the moon was not yet in the sky. I naturally felt a sudden urge to do a pee. I even tried to do something about it, but, as I struggled with my woolly RAF gloves, then my thick RAF greatcoat, then my tunic jacket, I began to lose heart and the will to live, at the thought of finally fighting with the fly buttons of my RAF trousers. No zips in those days! I struggled to close it all up again, having decided finally, to 'bottle it' until I got back to the guardroom.

It was very dark on the airfield side of those hangars. My torch was of little use and limited comfort. I decided to make my way slowly down towards the administration offices, whilst weaving my way back between the various other buildings, towards the internal camp road and to the welcome street lighting there. I had been out on patrol for about a half hour by this time. I wandered slowly down towards the building where I spent most of my working life, and there, for the first time since I had been in the RAF, I witnessed what I regarded as a sensible piece of secure practice. The pay accounts safe, in my Flight Lieutenant's room, was in clear view with lights playing on it. It was

a heavy safe and I knew nothing of its quality as a safe, but the twin effect of being so well lit and in plain view, actually made it a much safer proposition than if it had been hidden away in a dark corner.

I finished my tour around that building. At this point, I needed to move over to the public road and to make my way along its edge, towards the armoury. In doing so, I would have the opportunity to check that side of the barrack blocks, to ensure that all seemed well, as far as they were concerned. The change of direction towards the public road, however, took me past the open pole barrier, the one I had noticed with some annoyance on my very first day at the camp. It really offended my sense of logic for this barrier to be open, just a few hundred yards from an exactly similar barrier; the closed one by the guardroom, and on the same camp road. I walked past the raised pole and actually walked on for about 10-20 yards, when my peevishness got the better of me. I stopped, and took one more look at the offending article. I strode back, pulled the pole down, pulled the clip over to hold it down, and strode away again, with a very satisfied feeling in my chest. I had made one small dent in this military world of security incompetence!

As I left the pole behind me, I looked back towards my tiny triumph. I was amazed. A sudden swirl of fog had drifted in from the sea across the airfield. I decided that I needed to get a move on, as I didn't want to be mooching around in the gloom behind the armoury, with fog adding its cloak of invisibility to the mix.

I made my way alongside the public road and Fred's second ghost story came flooding back into my mind. It was one that related to some very strange events, apparently reported by people driving along that very road. According to the story, the main ghostly effect occurred, when midway along the stretch of road running through the base, when a loud echoing could be heard by both drivers and passengers, beneath the road, for just a few seconds.

The tale explains further that there is a supposed hidden underground tunnel beneath the road, which had been used by air force

personnel during the war, in order to shelter from attack during bombing raids. This tale didn't seem to me to be as nerve racking, though, as other ghostly stories about the station, unless, of course, there was an implication that a bomb had actually struck the tunnel during a raid and had buried people alive. The noises would then be explained as the unearthly cries of the dead and would, therefore, be a true ghost story. Fred was not forthcoming on this point, when I cross questioned him.

My next main point of contact along my route was the armoury. Positioned on the eastern side of the road, this was a building that I knew well of course. I had never, though, had to approach it alone and in the dark. Before I left, Fred had 'taken pains' to remind me that there were warnings, even in those days, in Group Orders, about IRA activity. These were, in fact, low level warnings but still, they were there.

"What level of protection do I have if there is such a raid?" I asked the corporal.

"You have that heavy torch." He replied with a grin.

It was at that point that I made the instant decision, previously referred to, as to just how I would use the torch, under such trying circumstances. I reasoned, that if the RAF did not provide adequate security to a target, such as a reasonably well equipped armoury, it was beyond, well beyond, my pay grade for me to defend it with a torch, albeit a heavy one!

The fog had thickened considerably, by the time that I left the precincts of the armoury. I hurried back to the guardroom, which was not far away. As I entered the room, its warmth struck me and reminded just how cold I had begun to feel. The wind, of course, had dropped, which had allowed the fog to drift in from the sea. As it had done so, the temperature had seemed to drop by several degrees. Fred handed me a mug of steaming hot chocolate, but I was suddenly reminded by my lower regions that I badly needed to do a Jimmy Riddle. I was all fingers and thumbs, both cold and numb, as I tackled

the job of getting down to the necessary equipment. It's just another branch of Sod's law; I've decided over the years, that when you really need to complete a task quickly, as I did at that moment, everything conspires against you. I do not intend to go into any more detail than that but, suffice to say, that I made it only just in time to get away with my dignity intact.

Fred and I spent the next half hour or so chatting. We passed a very pleasant time, as I warmed up with the hot chocolate inside me. He suggested that I might like to read some of his copy of the Rubayat. I did so and that book quickly made its way onto my Christmas/ birthday list. The fog was swirling ever thicker and I was not keen to get out into it for my next turn around the camp. Thankfully that decision was still an hour away. It was about time for another brew. Fred felt so too and so I got up and made my way to the far corner of the room, in order to take my turn in 'doing the honours'. I had just reached the table, when the guardroom door was flung open, with such a loud bang that it rebounded on its hinges. I had not had time to turn around, when I heard those fiercely angry words. I can still hear them today as I write.

"What fucking idiot, bastard, moron, closed the barrier at the other end of camp?" It was a warrant officer that I recognised, but with whom I had had no direct contact. I cannot remember his name, nor do I want to.

Luckily I still had my back half turned away from the incensed source of that question. I used the split second of turning fully towards that source, to come to the speedy decision, that that was not the time for a George Washington moment! No Sir! In any case, George, dear George, had had natural familial lines of forgiveness to rely on. I did not know what or how this officer had been discomposed by 'my' barrier, but I did know, and instinctively felt, that no mere telling of the truth would mollify his anger.

"What has happened sir?" I asked, as calmly and politely as I could muster.

"What's happened? What's bloody happened? I've run into that fucking barrier in my new bloody car! That's what's happened!" He paused for breath at that moment, as if realising once again the enormity of the calamity that had just befallen him. He turned towards the corporal.

"You know Fred. You know just how long it has taken me to get that new car." Although he was talking to the corporal, he clearly had not forgotten me, because he kept glancing in my direction, as if to say,

"And I've not finished with you yet mate!"

I quickly decided that any further anger in my direction would be met by attack rather than submission. I was still very raw in my feelings towards the Royal Air Force, and this warrant officer was on much shakier ground than the last one I had tangled with. He rounded on me and, suddenly...

"Did you close the fucking barrier?" He was back to boiling point again. I tried to keep as calm as possible and the few seconds of respite had given me time to form a bit of a strategy.

"When I left the admin office to go towards the armoury, Sir, the barrier was still open. I have not been back there since."

It was a good strategy, I felt, to hide the lie behind a camouflage of truth. Before he could work out what I had done and rephrase the question, I decided that this was the time to go on the attack.

"Have you been drinking Sir?"

It was a dangerous strategy and the sudden look of panic on Fred's face indicated that he felt the same.

"Who the fucking hell do you think you're talking to boy?", "I'll have you on so many charges you won't know what's hit you."

I had no reason to want to be friends with this officer, so I continued with my attack.

"Well Sir, I can smell the drink from here, and as far as I can remember, barriers, closed or open, do not move about. A person might form the opinion, that you've driven into a perfectly stationery barrier, whilst under the influence."

He approached me menacingly; he came so close, that there was nowhere to duck from the spittle that exploded from his drunken mouth.

"You fucking young bastard. I'll have you for that. You're on a charge!"

Things had gone too far by now for me to allow him to continue with his bullying tactics.

"First of all Sir, if you swear at me again, I'm going to formally request that Corporal James should call the duty officer; and, unless you withdraw the threat of a charge, I shall do so anyway. I'll be very interested to see just how you would justify a charge against me. On what grounds? I have not threatened you; I have also asked my questions and replied to yours with courtesy."

I could see that my threat of the duty officer had made him think on. He would certainly not be able to continue his barrack room bullying approach in the presence of a superior officer. He may have also realised that, if I could smell drink, then so would the officer. It suddenly dawned on him, that he was on much weaker ground than he had thought. He went away very reluctantly, muttering as he went that the matter wasn't closed. I was simply glad to get him out of the room.

This incident was the only true attempt at bullying that I experienced during my two years in the RAF. I had differences with others for sure, some of them NCOs and even, on occasion, officers. These, though, were in the normal cut and thrust of military life and not personal. I am not happy about my part in the above incident, because I was reduced to lying over an action of mine that I still maintain was justified.

That warrant officer was also in the wrong. I would argue that he was much more at fault, because he was a drunk in charge of a car and had driven into a stationery object. He had, moreover, tried to bully me by using his military seniority. I am truly sorry about his car, however. I know from my own experience just how attached one can

become to a car. I also knew, though, that I would not have received a fair hearing from him, if I had told the truth right at the beginning. The brilliant idea of threatening him with the duty officer only occurred to me when we were well past the point where I could hold my hand up.

Fred tried to pump me after the W.O. had left.

"Well then, did you or did you not close the barrier?"

I was half expecting this.

"Look Fred. So far you've been an impartial witness to a really angry argument between me and a very senior member of camp staff. I don't want to answer that question either way, because I do not want to compromise your situation, if he tries to take the matter further."

"Fair enough! Still it was a brilliant idea to threaten him with the duty officer."

"Yeh!" I said as I turned away from him to return to making the tea; an activity that had been so forcefully interrupted not so long ago. Suddenly, though, a thought struck me that almost made me laugh out loud. It occurred to me, that when all was said and done, I could claim to have been responsible for creating my own Bircham Newton ghost; a lovely, dark green, brand new, but now battered Rover 100, so rendered by the ghostly pole-gate, one that seemingly closes itself, when the fog swirls landwards from the North Sea!

10
Flying High

IT IS A truly wonderful experience to see the country from the cockpit of a small aeroplane.

I came to use the Wednesday afternoons, initially, as an escape from what I saw as the tedium of my pay accounts work schedule. As time passed I found the work more and more of an emotional drag. Whilst on the other hand, my total hatred of my shanghaied status in the RAF had begun to lessen. I realise all this now, many years later. I was making friends, some good friends, and I had, at long last, learned that it was easier and more rewarding to 'go with the flow', than to try to do endless battle with an opponent as big as the RAF. I had the shooting at Swaffham. Then there came one further source of enjoyment, one that I had not expected in a hundred years.

The surprise came at the end of one Wednesday morning. We were just preparing to go to lunch, when an officer entered the room; one that I hardly recognised at first, then suddenly the penny dropped. It was the Group Captain, the station commander. One did not see him too often at our end of the corridor. It was not that I did not recognise him exactly; it was simply that to see him in our office was to put him out of context. The flight sergeant, however, must have spotted him immediately, for he virtually flew out of his chair at the end of the room.

"Good afternoon sir, how can I help you?" The officer grinned.

"I'm looking for a victim; one of the airmen, please Flight. We can't spare an NCO". Again he grinned, but I did not get his joke. The flight sergeant clearly knew what was coming.

"I'm sure that LAC Kreit would be happy to join you Sir." He looked towards me smiling wickedly. I had served over six months in pay accounts by this time and had been promoted to the heights of LAC [Leading Aircraftman]. This meant a small increase in pay after a short test supervised by our Warrant Officer Mr. Rubin.

The Flt. Sgt. excused himself from the officer and left the room, still grinning. "The Group Captain will explain Kreit." All very mysterious this! The Group Captain quickly explained his mission. I have to confess that, in spite of myself and my general attitude towards the RAF at that time, I was quite nervous as I crossed the room towards the man. I had never before been in a position to speak directly with such a high ranking officer and I had no idea what it was all about.

"How would you like to come flying with me this afternoon son?" I was very surprised at the informality of the question. During my service I had begun, slowly, to realise that, in some limited circumstances, senior staff would permit themselves a certain level of informality, whereas this was less the case with the lower ranks, both of commissioned officers as well as WOs and NCOs. My explanation of this phenomenon was and still is that senior personnel were so much more secure in their position of authority, that they didn't have the need to display it as regularly as lower ranks.

The Group Captain quickly explained that he was going to take one of the station 'Chipmunks' up after lunch and that he had room for a passenger. I jumped with some alacrity at this offer. I had never yet been in an aeroplane. This would be a very welcome first. He grinned at the eagerness of my acceptance.

"See you on the airfield at 2pm. don't eat too much, but do wear something warm." This was his parting advice.

During lunch I quizzed my colleagues about that offer by the C.O. It appeared that flying with the Group Captain could become quite hairy, once he'd learned to trust that you wouldn't be sick in his cockpit. That first time, though, I was glad of all advice not to eat too much for lunch. And, indeed, I did feel more than a bit queasy the first time we took off. He took the plane onto a very fast climb on take-off. I now believe, although he never did speak of it, that this was to avoid flying over the Royal Sandringham estate, which bordered close to the airfield at Bircham Newton.

That grass airfield around the runway had another more mundane but very useful claim to fame. It had a very productive mushroom patch. The productive quality of this mushroom patch was encouraged by members of the RAF regiment, who insisted in practicing fire drill on that particular part of the airfield. They maintained that the foam used, as part of practice drills, contained ox-blood and that mushrooms thrived on this mixture. I have no way of confirming or denying that claim, other than to confirm that the mushrooms harvested under their regime were delicious and that no-one died!

During the remaining 15 months or so of my time at Bircham Newton, I was invited to accompany the C.O. some 2 or 3 times on his Wednesday afternoon flying sessions. I was happy to accept these invitations, whenever they did not clash with shooting at Swaffham, although that itself did tail off during my second year at Bircham.

As I remember it, some three Chipmunk trainer planes were kept at the station. They were used to give some of the RAF apprentices and boy entrants a taste of flying. They were also kept for officers who had gained their 'wings' and were no longer on flying duties, but needed to log a certain amount of air time annually, in order to keep the pay allowance that went with those wings.

Even with my left wing politics, I could not bring myself to begrudge them these monies, nor this facility that was available to help them to keep their allowances. They were heroes to a man in my view. They had gained their wings by dint of hard effort and courage.

I also have to admit, that I was a beneficiary of the generosity of the tax payer, and the CO, in availing me of that opportunity to experience flight with a man of his expertise.

I have to acknowledge straight away, that I never did come close to learning to fly the aircraft, because my benefactor never showed me how to land it or to take off. Tricky bits both of these! I was surprised though, even on the first flight, he told me to take control and to get a 'feel' of handling the craft; a two seater, one behind the other with me seated in the front seat. In the few hours with this man and under his instruction, I learned how to keep the aircraft on an even keel; I learned how to bank both to the left and to the right. I was able to descend so as to view more clearly items of interest on the ground and then climb again. In short I could manoeuvre quite well, three dimensionally around the sky, but could neither take off nor land.

I do realise that these limited abilities would seem to be very small beer to a qualified pilot, but to me, a national service aircraftman in pay accounts, it enabled me to dip my toes into a world that may have been denied to me a few years earlier, by a politically biased selection system.

My poor words here cannot do justice to the experience of flying in a small aircraft, where you feel at first hand every gust of wind, every air pocket, small or large. I accept that I was operating in the best of all worlds and really only concerned with the joystick and the rudder pedals. The CO took care of everything else; nonetheless there were long moments when I truly felt that I was flying the aircraft.

On take-off the world began to open up in a way that I had not imagined. The chipmunk was a fully aerobatic monoplane that had been used as a first stage trainer by the RAF for some years. Flying north took us to the North Sea and to Brancaster Bay; banking slightly to the east and we were over Brancaster Staithe, with a view of the pub where I might be drinking later that night. One could see the seals on Scolt Head Island as well as on the beaches of Holkham

Bay. To the West lay Hunstanton and the Wash. This famous reach of water saw the sinking of the Mary Rose in 1545, a ship built for Henry VIII in 1511. That famous craft was apparently Henry's favourite ship. I never grew tired of seeing the sights of Norfolk from the clear vantage point offered by that small aircraft.

I was never capable of undertaking more serious and complicated manoeuvres in the sky, but the aircraft was, and so was the C.O, to whom aerobatics had literally been the stuff of life during his early flying career. "How do you feel about doing something a bit more exciting"? He asked me during my first flight. If you have ever been in a light aircraft doing a vertical loop, you have some idea as to what I experienced shortly after I agreed to this proposal. Sufficient to say, I was hugely grateful for the fact that I did manage to hold on to my lunch. We were at about one thousand feet and I was convinced that my stomach bounced up and down through all of them, by the time we had completed the manoeuvre.

A vertical loop in mid-air is all about stomach! That poor organ begins in the right place and makes valiant, but unsuccessful efforts, to stay anchored there whilst the manoeuvre is underway. As the plane descends to gain speed, the stomach gropes upwards towards your throat. At the bottom of the loop, it drops back close to where it began, but suffering slightly from shock. The worst, however, is yet to come. The climb begins, but this time, your senses begin to disobey both your need and your ability to control them. You climb towards the top of the loop at which point your stomach doesn't know if it's on its arse or its elbow, and you are beginning not to care about that, because your brain and eyes and the straps of your harness are telling you that you are hanging upside down, and you are seemingly gazing upwards at the ground, out through a Perspex window whilst your poor suffering stomach is being crushed against your spine. Slowly, oh so slowly, the aircraft begins its downward trajectory towards a horizontal path and your stomach finds the strength to reward you for treating it so badly. You are very grateful if you don't throw up!

As I said before, the Chipmunk was a fully aerobatic mono-plane. The CO was very keen to show me the full range of possibilities, once he realised that I had managed to avoid making a smelly mess of his aircraft. The barrel role, as I remember it after all these years, offered all the more exciting pleasures of the vertical loop as described above, except they were repeated, both at greater speed and more often, as he took the plane, and my stomach, into a forward plunge through the atmosphere and a series of corkscrew like twists.

There was also the time when, without warning, my demonic pilot turned the engine off. For fifteen or so seconds I was not able to enjoy the sudden peace. For me it was more panic than pleasure, until I heard his evil chuckle through my headset. At that point I realised, gratefully, that he was still in control. The silence was audible after the noise of the engine. It was the nearest thing, I believe, to the experience of flight in a glider.

I was grateful for my invite onto the first trip but I have to admit that my concern for my stomach contents did take the edge off of the enjoyment factor on that occasion. I was invited on two or three further flights with the CO and I was grateful, very grateful for each of those. There was always more demonstration of the Chipmunk's ability to torture and I did begin to get used to that. I was inured rather than happy at being turned upside down and inside out. It was, however, very exciting and my wider memories of the sessions are good. *Is that a case of time's healing power?* I enjoyed the sights I had of Norfolk from the cockpit of that small plane. It can be a beautiful and interesting county and for nearly two years, I had the opportunity to see it from a variety of vantage points.

There was never any indication that the Group Captain wanted to show me how to undertake either of the hairy manoeuvres, mentioned above. I was very glad of that, for I was barely able to sit through them, let alone try them out for myself. He also very clearly and very wisely had too much respect for his own safety.

Yes, indeed, you have not seen England until you have seen her from the cockpit of a small aeroplane or perhaps even better, a glider. In later years, with these thoughts in mind, together with the memory of my experiences of flying in a chipmunk at the invitation of the CO, I asked my children for a 'glider experience' day in Kent for my 70th birthday. When I happened to mention this forthcoming event to my GP, a few days before my birthday, I thought he was going to fall off his chair laughing.

I had just returned from a holiday in Spain, where I had suffered a heart problem that required the fitting of a pacemaker. I had come to the GP to ask, as per DVLC advice, if he was ok with me returning to driving my car. The GP was fine about me driving the car, but thought that the flying school might want something very special by way of insurance, bearing in mind that I was a very new user of a device designed to keep my heart pumping. With that response I decided to put the gliding on hold for a while. I am very sorry, now, to have made that decision, though, because I never did get back to it and I never did make enquiries to the flying school as to the insurance situation. It's the age old story in life, you should always 'strike while the iron is hot'. My own personal mantra being; the less you do, the less you're able to do. Nonetheless, I do still have the beautiful memories of my few hours in the cockpit of a small chipmunk airplane.

11
Additional Ventures

I WAS ALWAYS looking for ways to legitimately ease the boredom, as I saw it, of the work in pay accounts. I had already claimed membership of the station shooting team, as I insisted on calling it in the office, much to the sergeant's irritation; that alone being good reason for doing so, in my view, at the time. I had the protective umbrella of Squadron Leader 'B's keen enthusiasm, to be seen to be putting an effort into an activity-team of some sort. I had the sneaking feeling that he too liked to get away from time to time and, moreover, the Group Captain was in favour, which trumped all dissenters. It was great for me; for as far back as I could remember, I had wanted to shoot guns. It was an itch that I could now legitimately scratch and at the expense of HM Government; a real bonus that! Yet still I was always on the lookout for other ways to get out of the office. I had not yet begun to realise that my section Sergeant and Warrant Officer were both fairly decent men.

My friend Norman tried to do me a great favour before he was himself demobbed in the summer of 1961. He was a newly qualified accountant at the point when he received his kind royal invitation to serve his country. He therefore entered service in a mood almost as bolshie as mine had been, when I was shanghaied. Norman had, though, received an extracurricular and paid job that took him out

of the pay accounts office for a full afternoon each month. The job was to keep the books of the PSI fund at Bircham Newton; this refers to the President of the Service Institute Fund as it applied to RAF Bircham Newton. The aims of this fund are outlined below;

[The Service Institute Fund (SIF) is a corporate body that organises, through the SIF Committee and various other RAF Welfare Committees, all welfare and amenity activities at unit level for RAF personnel of the rank of Corporal and below.

The SIF Committee, through their President, is responsible for the proper administration of the SIF including the authorisation of all SIF Grants. SIF Grants, subject to the full approval of the SIF Committee, are available to all junior Service personnel to support a host of welfare activities or projects.]

Now then, the aims of the fund were laudable and apparent to me at once, from the moment that the Squadron Leader outlined them to me. He had, apparently, chosen me at Norman's recommendation. He ended our meeting by explaining that Norman would take me through the routine of the job and indicated what he saw as the advantages that would accrue for me. These were, firstly, that the job was a paid one, not hugely paid, but nonetheless an addition to my meagre RAF pay. Secondly, I would be allowed one half day a month to undertake the work. Third, in this batting order of privileges, I would be allowed to do the work in a room in the W.O. and Sergeants' mess. This was a real privilege, as Norman explained it, because one of the lower rank mess 'servants' would keep me well supplied with tea, biscuits and even cakes, when these were available and unlikely to be missed by the eagle-eyed Sergeant Cook. Finally the squadron leader saw it as appropriate that a person below the rank of corporal should be given this important function, bearing in mind the very creditable aims of the fund.

It seemed to me at once that this was an ideal niche for me, even though I hadn't a clue regarding 'double entry' bookkeeping, albeit after Norman took me through the basics. Each of the four benefits

outlined by the officer stood up to my immediate scrutiny as being 'just the job' for me. One further great bonus about this job, moreover, was that Norman, for reasons that were lost to me, had negotiated that the allocated half day would be on Thursdays. The Adjutant saw no reason to change this. I was, of course, fully in agreement with this arrangement.

As promised Norman did his best to explain the world of double entry bookkeeping to me. Even so it remained a very strange and foggy world as far as I was concerned. Norman tried very hard to help me to clear the fog from my addled brain, but it wasn't until some years later, when working in Lloyd's bank and doing my banking exams, that some very important pennies began to drop; far too late to help me to be a success at my job with the B.N. PSI fund. I held onto it for two glorious months before the squadron leader, no fool he, discovered that I was not keeping to the immaculate standard that Norman had set. He was very nice about my dismissal, so much so that I truly felt sorry for him, that I had not come up to scratch. Yet there were more goodies to come!

My section sergeant, by now a flight sergeant, failed to hide his satisfaction, even glee that I was now returned into his fold. His pleasure was short lived; however, for about two days later the squadron leader called me back into his office and offered me the job of running the newly inaugurated Camp Library supported, yet, by the PSI fund! I can only think that this level of consideration by the squadron leader to me for 'perky' type jobs was because of my steadfast attendance in his shooting team. I had been, in truth, one of the more committed members of that team and not merely because it got me away from the tedium of the pay accounts section. I really enjoyed that particular activity; one that only military service could have brought to me. I think that he was also impressed by my failure, as yet, to kill or injure anyone!

I need to explain at this point that, unfortunately, the shooting experience was winding down to a natural ending at about this time.

Firstly the squadron leader had lost some of his early volunteers because they had been National Servicemen who had completed their service time. Added to this was the fact that no further willing recruits were coming forward. The few of us who continued to be willing were becoming too few to merit the time that was being devoted by a senior officer.

Camp librarian, though, was a great position for me; much better than the ill-fated PSI fund job had been. I loved books and had actually been allowed a small float, supported as I say, by the PSI fund, to purchase appropriate books, when requested by servicemen. This included the RAF Apprentices and Boy Entrants. The library was to be opened for a few hours on Wednesday afternoons. I had, unfortunately, lost the privilege of working out of the office on one Thursday afternoon in four. I had, though, secured a new comfortable berth for my Wednesday afternoons.

I felt made up at the opportunity of that job. It was a position of trust that suited me fine, for those few hours in the week I was able to spend time in my very own domain, as that was how I came to regard it. There is only one negative mark on my reign as the camp librarian. It is staring at me even as I write these few words. It, the accusing finger from history, stares right at me from one of my own numerous bookshelves, even after all these more than fifty years. It looks innocent enough, being a scruffy green edition of Jerome K. Jerome's 'Three Men in a Boat' together with 'Three Men on The Bummel', all in one edition.

Scruffy indeed it is, but then, we are all beginning to show signs of scruffydom after all this time. Inside the front cover of my accuser is a stamp mark indicating that the book is the property of RAF Bircham Newton and it stares its denouncing gaze at me from just across my desk. I must have borrowed the book all those years ago, meaning to return it prior to my eagerly awaited demob. In spite of this denouncement from history I do not regard myself as a thief, although one of my current friends, Chris, still accuses me of stealing

his desk whilst he was on holiday and when I had been attached to his office on a training placement. He loses no opportunity to remind me of this dastardly action. Unnecessary meanness of spirit this, on his part, I have always thought.

I have to be honest. I never did feel overwhelmed by a rush of customers; two or three in an afternoon would have been a full session. These were mostly trainees; boy entrants or apprentices. The occasional regular staff from corporals down, very seldom a senior NCO or WO and never an officer. Imagine my surprise then, when one afternoon, I looked up to investigate the shadow that had just loomed over my reading matter, to see a commissioned officer, albeit a young Pilot Officer, glaring down at me, a very unhappy scowl on his face. "Good afternoon Sir" I attempted to dismantle the inexplicably icy atmosphere that pertained. No luck, no luck at all! It seemed that this young officer was not to be appeased by my cheery greeting. "Don't you stand up when an officer enters the room?" Oh god, one of those, I thought, but stood up immediately.

The young officer clearly wanted to make a meal of what he clearly regarded as my breach of military protocol. He ordered me to move from behind my desk and into the centre of the room, where he proceeded to walk around me as if on an inspection regime. It was quite embarrassing, which he obviously found appropriate to the situation, as he appeared to be enjoying himself. I was fuming inside and so, apart from trying to explain that I had neither seen nor heard him enter the room, I was damned if I was going to apologise. The inspection of yours-truly lasted for a couple of minutes I suppose, until he had satisfied his ego. With a final warning to me about my future behaviour he left the library without even looking at the books. That was not the end of my dealings with that young officer however. There came an opportunity for me to seek revenge but which ended much differently to my initial hope and plan.

Officers' pay in the RAF was not dealt with by the lower ranks like humble old me. They were handled, always, by the commissioned officer pay-accounts like my boss. We did, however, deal with some matters pertaining to officers' finances when they were transferred from one unit to another. These matters related to all moving expenses. We were responsible for viewing and checking all invoices and allowances claimed for the move. The orderly room staff were responsible for processing movement orders and bringing them, in the case of officers, to the attention of their commissioned officer.

In the aftermath of the incident in the library I felt bruised and unfairly treated. On the way back to my room, at the end of the afternoon, I concocted a number of revenge plans, each of which could be placed on a scale ranging from mildly bonkers to quite insane. Back at the block I sought out my friend, Tony, my equivalent in the orderly room. I related the incident to him, at which he agreed that the young officer was a right bastard. I then outlined some of my plans for revenge, the most dastardly of which was to intercept his movement documents and send them on to a remote early warning 'listening' station in the Outer Hebrides. At which, Tony pointed out in no uncertain terms, that I was a disaster seeking, bloody idiot and that the part that I had outlined for him to play was totally nuts and that he would have nothing to do with it. Mercifully that was an end to that particular conversation and that plan. I was forced to retreat into a world of sullen resentment and throw my rattle right out of the pram. My plans had fallen flat at the first hurdle but I was determined to keep the fire alight. My! Oh! My! I seem to have wandered into a world strewn with metaphors.

My feeling of resentment did not go away, but did abate somewhat as days passed. About two or three days later the old coals reignited, though, as I saw that same young officer striding along the corridor towards our office. For several moments I convinced myself that his mission must be to be to see our officer, whose office was next to ours at the end of the corridor. I took my eyes off of him for a moment to check something on my desk, but when I

looked up he was standing at the counter and looking at me across the room. I got up slowly from my desk and approached the man, my nemesis.

I was not wearing my beret and so could not salute. "Yes sir?" I asked. "How can I help you?" "I have come in to see if my removal and travel claim have been processed yet." At this I had an opportunity to ask his name, which he duly gave me. I checked our records and informed him that we had not yet received the documents in question. I did feel a slight pang of conscience, as one of my instruments for revenge had been to search out his documents and take action as outlined above. Tony had counselled wisely and forcefully against this action, on the grounds of the fierce retribution to follow if I were found out. He had also pointed out the practical problems arising from not knowing, at that time, the name of my erstwhile persecutor. Bircham Newton had a fairly high turnover of personnel, even of officers, as it was a re-training station for those officers needing such a service, and for a variety of other reasons.

The young officer was clearly disappointed, which, I admit, gave me a certain satisfaction at that point in the game. I advised him that these matters did often take a while to come through and that he could try again in a few days' time and that, if the documents came in earlier, I would send a message to the officers' mess. The same officer returned to the office a number of times after that, each time on a wasted errand and, each time, seeming more and more concerned about the delay in obtaining his money, much of which was related to expenses that he had already incurred and had paid for. He even began to ask for me and even allowed himself to let slip some details that made his situation appear more urgent.

He was young and married with a couple of young children. He did not say so, but I got the distinct impression that money was very tight. As time passed and his situation was not relieved, my attitude began to change; I even began to feel sorry for him. I urged him to speak to our Flight Lieutenant, as I felt certain that it would have been possible for the service to help him out. He was clearly very

reluctant to take that route. Finally I made a decision to take action, by way of speaking to my boss myself.

I was hesitant to take the action, because I was very aware that the pay accounts officer was a stickler for protocol, but then, I reasoned, what harm can it do? What can he do to me? I knocked on the door. I stood to attention in the 'presence'. One never received an invitation to sit down when in that office with the Flight Lieutenant.

The interview did not begin well. I explained to 'sir', as briefly as I could, the dilemma that the young officer was in. During this time the Flight Lieutenant did not even do me the courtesy of looking at me. His face remained studiously buried in his work. I finished and still he did not look up at once. There remained an uncomfortable few moments before condescension overcame plain rudeness. Finally, "Well then, firstly, this man is an officer and so his pay has got nothing to do with you and, secondly, there is nothing we can do about it until his documents arrive."

I had foreseen the first objection and so was ready with a response. "I realise that you deal with his pay, Sir, but I have been dealing with his enquiries at the desk. He has been coming in on numerous occasions and his situation is, I feel, now in need of an urgent resolution. Secondly, Sir, I can do nothing about it other than to bring it to your attention."

"Why do you presume that his needs are urgent?"

"We are both humans beings sir. I know that he is married and has children. In those circumstances money issues can become urgent."

"You are not yet married are you?"

"No, Sir, but my parents were." I tried hard not to emphasise the possessive determiner. I continued quickly by way of explanation. "I did not want to get married whilst I was in the forces. I did not want my wife to be subject, in any way, to the vagaries of military discipline or protocol." Well, I thought, 'you brought the bloody subject up mate.'

"Why did he not come direct to me?"

"I cannot say Sir. Perhaps he was nervous about bringing the matter to the attention of a senior officer?"

Now then, a Flight Lieutenant is not technically a senior officer but, as they say, a little flattery never goes amiss; it can sometimes truly oil the wheels...

"What do you propose that I do?" This came both as a sharp response as well as a surprise.

"Well sir, I thought that there might be some fund for emergencies that could be used to tide him over. He is after all an officer; surely his word could be taken as to the level of his expenses." I managed to say this without a hint of the sarcasm I felt when speaking to this particular officer. He had clearly had enough of me.

"You may go. I'll see what can be done."

I thought no more of the young officer nor of my attempt to involve my Flight Lieutenant. It was, after all, a ball that was much more in his court than mine.

The matter did not end there, however, for just a few days later the young officer appeared once more at the counter. I got up from my desk and prepared myself for the usual denial of receiving his documents but whoa! He did not have his usual woeful face. As I approached him he even began to smile. "I believe that I owe you a vote of thanks; Your Flight Lieutenant spoke to the Adjutant and they've agreed to tide me over until my documents arrive. God alone knows where they've got to."

I breathed an inner sigh of relief at this, that I had taken Tony's advice and had refrained from my intention to divert the documents myself; as it was I could accept his thanks with a clear conscience.

"That's fine sir," I replied, not knowing what else to day. I was, in fact, both pleased as well as hugely surprised at the thought that my stuffy Flt Lt. had bothered to mention my part in the event. As soon as that idea was born, though, its bubble was well and truly burst.

"Oh yes" he continued "The squadron leader mentioned your name and your part in the plan, thanks again."

Oh dear! How quickly can pleasant surprises be dashed by sudden reality!

Thus my Wednesday afternoons were now doubly protected as they had become pleasurable havens that ruptured the tedium of my RAF week in pay accounts. Earlier in my career I had had the occasional pleasure of an exciting flight in a small aircraft. I was looking forward to more of the same with huge anticipation; I had good reason for hoping that more of these would come my way. I had had a strong and established as well as enjoyable position in the shooting team. As explained, above, that was to come to end imminently. I had also had the temporary position with the PSI fund; not my finest hour, but by now I was fully established in the camp library. My friend Tony's wise counsel had diverted me from a course of action that could have ended in real disaster. Things were again looking up!

12
Times of fraud
and deception

ONE OF NORMAN'S tasks in the office was to audit the purchases of provisions for the station; that is with the exception of those destined for the officers' mess. That duty was performed by the accounts officer. We were underlings who had little to do with matters pertaining to our lords and masters. There was one illogical exception to this exclusion, as mentioned above, that being the calculation of staff allowances on transfer in from another station. This included officers' removal allowances.

On the day of which I am thinking, Norman had been studiously perusing the provisions manual for the junior ranks, RAF apprentices and Boy entrants' messes. It must have been in the summer of 1961 because Norman was about a year ahead of me in terms of the time he had served and I know that the events that I am about to relate took place in the summertime, as they were directly linked to the boys' summer holidays.

Like me, Norman could not wait for his release date to arrive, although, unlike me, he had been one of those poor souls who had constructed a 'tick the days off calendar' on which to view the passing of those days. I chose not to do this. My escape from tedium had

always been to engage myself in sundry extra-curricular schemes and activities to help me pass the time more quickly, or, should I say, less slowly. For me the construction of a 'termination' calendar would simply have emphasised the tedium.

Norman had been unusually absorbed that morning, by what had always seemed to be the 'tick box' duty of reviewing the provisions accounts. He had at first been absorbed, then in a frowning concentration, when suddenly a huge grin appeared and what can only be described as a whoop of what seemed like success. "Gotcher you bugger!" was all that he uttered, but it attracted the immediate attention of the flight sergeant. "What's got up your skirt Planter?" He grinned at his own witticism as he wandered over to Norman's desk.

"I think that it's serious Flight." He looked up at the NCO. "You need to call the Warrant Officer in on this one!"

"I'll decide what's to be done and who calls who, English grammar not being his forte. You just tell me what's afoot!"

"There are some serious discrepancies in the provisions accounts flight."

"The hell you say! - What makes you come to that conclusion?"

"I've been studying these accounts all morning. It's only just occurred to me Flight, after all the time that I've had this job, it's only just dawned on me that something is badly wrong."

"Don't keep us all in bloody suspense man! Tell us what you think you've discovered!"

"Well, they all go on holiday don't they, school terms...the boy entrants and apprentices?"

"You know they do, we all know they do, so what for God's sake?"

"Well he orders the same quantity of provision when they're all away from camp as when they're here. The holidays should only leave the permanent staff to feed and we're only about a quarter of the total, if that! On top of which, all of the permanent staff who deal directly with the boys, take their leave during those periods. Where do all those provisions go?"

The flight sergeant was dumfounded. "Are you sure of this Planter?"

"I'm dammed sure that he always orders the same quantities of provisions. I can't explain it, that's for others to decide. I think that begins with you Flight."

Norman handed the ledger over to the NCO with due deference and, in exaggerated fashion, he set about another piece of work. The flight sergeant looked around the office and managed to issue an appropriate but unnecessary order.

"Not a word of this outside of this office," he muttered, unnecessarily because all matters pertaining to accounts were by default, confidential. He took the ledger over to his desk and pretended to study it intently for about thirty minutes or so. He then took the now potent manual along the corridor to the office of the accounts section warrant officer, Mr Rubin, an experienced and very efficient senior member of the accounts team. Twenty minutes later Norman was called in to the consultation. I have to admit to a sudden feeling of envy at Norman's newfound ability to cause such a level of consternation in the upper ranks. The flight lieutenant was brought into the affair and, after a short period of further debate involving the Adjutant, at this point the C.O. himself was brought into the equation. On his instructions the Provost Marshall's office was informed.

"What fun!" was Norman's summing up of the matter.

The enquiry was short and sharp. I do not remember the final outcome for the culprit or culprits involved with this particular fraud, but fraud it was and those culpable would have been regarded as very, very naughty by the RAF and dealt with most severely. We came to understand that the extra rations ordered by the provisions NCO had been secreted away and sold in a local shop or shops owned by members of the culprit's family.

I must admit that I only remember the broad brushstrokes of those events. I do recall, however, that they happened and that Norman's accounting knowledge and experience had been needed in order to

bring it all to light. His perspective was also that of a comparative outsider to the world of RAF protocols and behaviours. That ability to view the matters from outside the window also helped. Even so he had been reviewing those provisions for some months before it quite suddenly occurred to him that something was not 'kosher'.

If anyone ever reads these pages I would ask you to try to remember the nature of the times in which we were living, in the late 50s and early 60s, when these frauds were perpetrated. Everyone on that camp had, in one way or another, been affected by the shortages that Second World War had imposed on everyone; even the youngest on camp, because food rationing had only been finally lifted in 1954 with the final de-regulation of sweets. Theft of food was still held by most people as the lowest form of crime and well 'beyond the pale'. It was difficult to see the actions of the provisions sergeant and his cronies as anything other than the theft of food and on the backs of school aged children at that.

Unfortunately, I was not at RAF Bircham Newton to follow the outcome of the provisions saga, for life suddenly changed for me, big time, because I was about to be unceremoniously whisked away from the scene of that particular crime into the hotbed of another even more serious setting of official naughtiness.

I was sitting at my desk, minding my own business and getting on with preparing my section of the pay accounts for Friday's pay parade, when W.O. Rubin entered the room. He strode directly over to my desk with a huge grin on his face.

"I've got some really great news for you." The grin worried me. Was it the grin of the cat just before he pounced on the mouse?

"Yes sir; what's that?" I was not hopeful that this news was going to be all that welcome.

"I've got you a month's attachment to the pay accounts section at RAF Uxbridge."

My heart sank, because I did not see or appreciate the kindness that lay behind this warrant officer's actions, in suggesting me for

the attachment. I was very comfortable at Bircham Newton. I had settled into just about the best posting there that I had heard of in all my discussions with other national servicemen over the past months.

"I don't want to leave Bircham Newton sir. I like it here."

Mr Rubin actually looked crestfallen, then angry. He had selected me for this temporary move, because he had thought that, being a Londoner, I would be really happy for a posting close to home. I had just thrown his decent action, and thought, right back in his face. The truth being that I did not trust his assertion that the posting was to be a temporary one. I was about to feel the strength of his resentment at my thoughtless response.

"My office now!" he commanded, then turned on his heels and strode out to the corridor and towards his own office. I rose from my desk slowly and caught the eye of the flight sergeant as I did so. He shook his head slowly and sucked air past his tongue in a way that suggested; "You've done it now laddie!"

I hurried along the corridor to where Warrant Officer Rubin was sitting at his desk in his office. He was furious.

"I'm sorry sir......." I began to apologise without yet realising what I had done wrong. I did not yet see the RAF as a benign element to my life. Two years were being stolen from me and all that I could think of was that Bircham Newton was the one saving grace amid all the negatives that I felt about my National Service.

"Stand to attention when you are talking to me." I shuffled myself into some sort of concordance with the order.

"Don't you ever talk to me again the way you did out there!... Do you hear me?"

This last came when I did not immediately respond to the first part. My problem was that I still did not see what all the fuss was about. I had only said that I didn't want to go to Uxbridge and that I liked it here. What was wrong with that. The warrant officer, though, was sitting on his pride and his hurt feelings. I was shrouded by the self-promoting attitude of youth. I was yet to understand that, even

in the RAF, NCOs and officers could perform actions solely out of kindness.

"I'm really sorry sir. It's just that I like it here. I like working in this office and this camp. I did not want to be transferred to RAF Uxbridge." That was indeed true. It would be too much like going back into the real RAF. That was represented in my mind by my training camps. That thought was all that I could think about.

"Firstly, the RAF is not a pick and mix self-service shop. If you are ordered to do something, then you bloody well do it. It's not an invitation. Do you understand?"

"Yes sir." There was nothing else to say. The penny had finally dropped. I had said too much already.

"Secondly;" the rest came out with more emphasis and with a further dose of the anger that Mr. Rubin clearly felt. "When did I use the term 'transferred'... did I use that term? Did you hear me say transferred?" He waited impatiently for my response whilst I racked my brain for an appropriate reply, because I could not truly remember his actual words.

"No sir. I didn't." This was the reply that he was clearly expecting to hear.

"What did I say then?" He had got me now because I could not remember his actual words. I had been overtaken by the horrible thought of being moved to RAF Uxbridge and away from the comfort of Bircham Newton. I hesitated because I did not want to exacerbate matters by quoting him wrongly. He allowed me some moments, too many moments, of discomfort.

"What I actually said was, I've got you a month's attachment to the pay accounts section at RAF Uxbridge." "Yes sir, thank you sir," I replied, without much conviction it has to be said, for I did not yet trust the RAF. My mood did pick up when I realised that there would be extra benefits to my meagre pay packet. I would be working in pay accounts of course and receiving 'living out' and travel allowances, because I did not have to 'bunk' at RAF Uxbridge. I could live at home

and travel each day on the tube to the station, returning the same way each evening. I did not even have to 'clear camp' at Bircham. All my belongings stayed in my room there. John assured me that he would keep an eye on everything.

It turned out to be a worthwhile, as well as an interesting break from Bircham Newton in the end, because work at Uxbridge meant a journey through almost the whole of the Piccadilly line, from Oakwood station to Uxbridge. It was worthwhile both for the extra money and the ability to live at home for a whole month, as well being able to see more of Joyce, without the necessity of travelling to and from Norfolk each weekend. This benefit was counterbalanced somewhat by my mum's same old and constant accusation that I was 'treating her home as a hotel'. An accusation recognised no doubt by every teenager and courting youngster in the history of the world. I'm sure we've all heard it. What made this worse for me was that the accusation had some real truth to it.

It was interesting at Uxbridge for two reasons. Firstly, for a whole month, I was able to watch as the London public revolved around me for an hour and a quarter twice a day on the tube. The variety of travellers in London is truly fascinating. The revolving snapshots of life in that great city, fully reflected Shakespeare's seven ages of man and more, because the variety alters according to the time of the day, as well as the area of London through which you are passing.

My journey gave me decent quantities of both time and variety of Londoner, as well as tourists; schoolchildren making reluctant passage to school, doctors and nurses, some going on shift, others going off shift. There were clerks and accountants competing to complete the 'Times' crossword, from which I have only ever managed one clue entirely on my own, in my whole life. Some of these diligents, however, strived to complete the task before they arrived at their destination station. This daily highlight always seemed very sad to me, but then I was very young, brash and only too ready to dismiss!

There were ladies of the night going off shift but still apparently willing to do business. Men there were, attempting to ogle innocuously, but unsuccessfully, around broadsheets. The occasional tramp carried his worldly goods, often odorously, with him wherever he went and often on the one ticket, round and round the system, begging a coin here and there. City men with bowlers and stiff, starched, collars attempted studiously not to sit near the tramp or the lady of the night, perhaps, sometimes, to exclude sudden and unwelcome recognition?

The pattern of London life thus rolled on around me, and by me, twice a day, five days a week, for one glorious month. The list is endless; I return nostalgically to it often, and always when I am on the tube in London.

The month at Uxbridge was interesting and thankfully did actually only last the promised month. It finally seeped down through the hierarchy, like the whispers in a tight village, that the entire section of the Uxbridge pay accounts team was under suspension, because someone or 'some-ones' had invented a complete 'Flight' of staff and was or were pocketing the pay of this virtual body of people. T'was a very healthy amount of cash if you can get away with it. I say no more. If this were truly the case one wonders just how the person or persons hoped to get away with it for any length of time at all.

I have thought about that month many times over the years. I was a very small cog in the wheel that revolved around that particular attempt at fraud and deception. My job, along with others, seconded, like me, on temporary attachments from across the nation, was simply to keep the pay accounts section at that camp running efficiently until a new, permanent, crew could be mustered. As I consider the situation, though, I cannot, for the life of me, understand just how the perpetrators hoped to get away with their crime. For crime it was.

I have no idea who, exactly, was involved, but my knowledge of the system gives me to think that they must have been either very foolish, or very desperate, or both, to have made the attempt. I do

not know the outcome for them; neither do I wish to know. I just know that, after all was said and done, I was very grateful to Warrant Officer Rubin for his kind thought, in making that attachment available to me. It was a period of one month that gave me, both new insight, and another perspective on London, that great city of my birth.

13
Nuclear Attack!! – The Four Minute Warning

"PICK THAT BLOODY stretcher up!" The dulcet tones of one of the RAF regiment corporals rang gratingly, through the clear spring air of 1961. A new season was on the point of beginning, and, with it, the annual farce of the AOC's inspection was near upon us. The theme this year, after the usual session of parade ground drill, performed by possibly the least efficient crew in the RAF, and never my favourite occupation in any case, was to be "Atom Bomb drill". Moreover, we, being the un-likeliest well-oiled machine in Europe, were to demonstrate before the great man just what could be done, within the Four Minute Warning allowed to us, before the Red Peril's missiles would descend upon us from their prescribed route over the arctic. Their route would then take them over Scotland, and so on down, towards the static air craft carrier that was East Anglia. I was still in a bloody minded frame of mind in those, my earlier days in the RAF. I was determined to co-operate with what I saw as damned tom-foolery as little as possible, in spite of the forthcoming 'presence' of the most senior officer in our immediate universe.

In the event, there was little with which to co-operate. The wider RAF, in the guise of the RAF Apprentices, was famously well able to organise, and produce, an acceptable drill and parade experience for the AOC. They were well used to that type of oper-ation. It seemed to me, though, that little effort had been put into any preparation for the optimum use of our final four minutes at RAF Bircham Newton! My own last efforts, moreover, would have been aimed at trying my damnedest to get a phone call through to Joyce!

The Great Man inspected, he also spoke to a few of the lower ranks, asking questions, and making observations, as he was well used to doing. As for the rest of the afternoon's treat, though, the response to a Nuclear Attack; there were men, designated as various types of wounded or dead. One cohort of such, having seemingly decided upon future careers as dramatic actors, were contenting themselves in making a range of 'wounded' noises, much to the aggravation of the regiment corporal in charge of the chaos. Others were enrolled as first aiders, with little or no logic as to the choice.

I had been designated as wounded and, apparently, also suffer-ing from probable radiation poisoning. It was urgent that I should proceed to the de-contamination area ASAP for treatment, although what the treatment might consist of was a mystery. It was as if that was something that was to be decided upon, after further consider-ation, sometime in the future. In fact it was totally something for the back burner. I very quickly decided that this farce would be a com-plete waste of the final four minutes of my life.

On the day in question, however, I was quite happy to lie where I was. The sun was warm, and the grass smelled of that hazy, new grassy, smell, as I lay there in the cosy spring sunshine. I did not want to move. I had done no harm to anyone. The poor corporal was having trouble organising his post-apocalypse scene! It was like something

from that legendary and somewhat proverbial military experience -
Fred Karno's Army – as in The First World War Song; I hummed the
refrain contentedly to myself, as I dosed in the warm sun.

> *"We are Fred Karno's Army,*
> *What bloody use are we?*
> *Etcetera, etcetera, etcetera,*
> *We cannot fight; we cannot shoot,*
> *Etcetera, etcetera,.....................*
> *Dum de dum de dum de dum.*

The strands of this refrain as well as those few intermittent words
that I could remember, wove persistently through my mind; I could
not get rid! It seemed so damned appropriate to the current exercise.
There had been no preparation beforehand; whereas most of us were
able to make some sort of an, albeit feeble, fist of the parade and drill
session. Those efforts were ably balanced, as previously indicated, by
the much more polished performance of the RAF Apprentices. The
poor contribution on our part carried with it the added, and considerable disadvantage, that none of us was either trained, or able, or fully
willing, to handle ourselves in the emergency that was now being put
before us. Thus there arose the recipe for chaos, and nobody enjoyed
chaos more than your average national-serviceman.

There had been no information dealing with the specifics of a
nuclear attack. What were the percussive strength, and effects, of
such a bomb at a range of distances from the centre? What was the
latest information regarding what one should really do, in the time
left to us, after the four minutes of warning had actually percolated
down to the 'other ranks'? I had, somewhat cynically, calculated that
we would probably receive news of the attack about fifteen minutes
after the bomb exploded!

There were many other such questions on cogent minds that were
left totally unanswered, largely, I suspect, either because no-one

actually knew the answers or, more probably, because the answers were so grim that they did not want to impart them. The whole of East Anglia was, as I say, a static air craft-carrier. We would probably be in the first line of such an attack if, God forbid, one should ever come. In truth, though, the lack of genuine information gave the whole business an air of an officially presented farce, to be enjoyed rather than endured. Many of the lower ranks very quickly began to see it in that light and to react accordingly. I was one of these.

"Pick that fucking stretcher up!" The change in emphasis, and tone, was sudden, and not to be totally ignored, if one wanted one's bloody mindedness to go the distance and prevail for the whole afternoon. I really did not like this particular corporal anyway. I can see him in my mind's eye, but I just cannot remember his name. He was one of those people who always looked dapper and smart in his uniform, no-matter what activity he might have been up to. He was not a big man, short-ish and slim, with a face like an out of tune fiddle that did not allow itself the benefits of humour. He simply took himself too seriously. Mind you, as I have said before, I have found that to be true of many people who are still on the lower rungs of power and on, what they would see, as the ladder on their particular route to success.

Corporals took themselves much more seriously than WOs, and junior commissioned officers were much more sensitive to the accoutrements of power, and discipline, than senior officers. Lower rung occupants' reactions were usually much more difficult to read and anticipate, than those who had had the power of senior office for years. Our dedicated corporal, adhering ferociously to this rule, was busy organising the 'dead and wounded', at a decibel level that was quite out of keeping with their 'sensitive' conditions in the role-play that they were supposed to be enacting.

I had been designated as one of the wounded - not walking wounded - and I was determined to take full advantage of that status. According to our noble NCO, I had suffered serious trauma,

as well as probable high doses of radiation exposure. In that role, I felt that it was not encumbered in me to ease the problems of the stretcher bearers! The season was spring, the weather was warm and sunny, and I, wounded and suffering, with almost certain radiation poisoning, was resting on the grass in the sunlight and not wanting to be disturbed by a bunch of idiots trying to get me onto a stretcher. The corporal, in totally pissed off mood, strode over to us to see what the problem was.

Things were not going well for him that afternoon. The parade for the AOC had not gone too badly, because the RAF Apprentices and Boy Entrants had been able to show off their newly learned 'Bull' and Parade Ground skills. They were impressive, to the point that they fully camouflaged the totally less than adequate abilities of the permanent staff, many of whom were national servicemen, who had forgotten as much, and as quickly as they could, of any parade skills that they had picked up on basic training.

The corporal, astute man that he was, promptly noticed that the main problem was me. He leaned over me in order to whisper something very unpleasant in my ear. Very Offensive! I rolled slightly to my right, to allow my bearers some space to slip the edge of the stretcher under me. As I did so, I noticed that our junior NCO genius had a very sensitive looking piece of equipment in his hand; it was a Geiger counter. I quickly began to formulate Nuclear Drill disruption plan No2!

Without too much more ado, I allowed my bearers to get me safely onto the stretcher and porter me, while puffing and blowing and complaining all the while, across the field to the old 'World War 2' war-time air raid shelter that had been brought into service as a field first aid station. All we 'wounded' were being brought there to receive 'treatment', after our experiences in the missile attack. As soon as I got there, and the corporal had left in order to bring other recalcitrant survivors under his control and authority, I began to make my preparations.

As I said, the actual parade had gone off not too badly, thanks to the younger generation. Like many of the others of my peers, I had no aspirations to excel in the field of parade ground drill. We must have been passable, as I have previously stated, because the AOC had gone off to the mess with the Group Captain and other senior officers in a relaxed mood. This was after having had it explained to him just what the current exercise was designed to achieve. I, like many of my friends, had wished that the same courtesy had been extended to us. I did not have the foggiest idea of what we were expecting to achieve. The whole plan, it seemed to me, had been conceived by the same committee as had designed the proverbial horse, that mysteriously become a camel!

Apparently, the camp was supposed to have been subject to a near miss by some sort of missile delivering a nuclear device. Little thought had been involved in just how powerful the device had been, nor exactly how far away it had struck. A couple of dozen, or so, of us had been positioned around the airfield, as victims of the attack. This was a farce in itself, because, for the majority of the time, we worked in offices well away from the grass airfield, and this was only used to support a couple of chipmunk trainers. These were provided largely for the benefit off ex aircrew and to provide the boy entrants and RAF apprentices with some flight familiarity. In normal times, the major injuries resulting from a nuclear attack that did not actually fry us, would have been those from collapsing buildings and flying glass; impact injuries of all sorts. We, the wounded, were to be taken to an unused brick building just off of the airfield that had been brought back into service as a quasi-air raid shelter and first aid post, although there was no tangible evidence of anyone present having any actual first aid knowledge, or experience.

After a rather bumpy ride, during which I was dropped from the stretcher only once, I was taken to this shelter and deposited unceremoniously on the floor by my unsympathetic comrades in arms. The corporal was still trying to supervise the comedy outside. He

was actually going from 'body' to 'body' with his Geiger counter checking for radiation, thereby indicating the intellectual level at which he was operating! He was, I thought mischievously, just the sort of person who might appreciate disruption plan No2! I immediately put the scheme into operation, with the aid of other 'wounded soldiers', who had been deposited in the shelter. We took a quick census of our watches, and selected 5 or 6 suitable examples. These were speedily handed over to me, and transferred to my left arm, to join company with my own watch, which was also a suitable model for this particular experiment in chaos promotion. Luckily, I was wearing a pair of RAF khaki overalls for this exercise, and so was able to roll my sleeves down, thus hiding the selection of borrowed time pieces!

The reason for all this subterfuge was quite simple really. The watches selected all had luminous painted dials. Luminous radium paint on dials was first used in the early part of the twentieth century, before the dangers of radioactivity were fully understood. Although health problems, in workers using radium paints, were noticed a decade or so after luminous paint first came into use, for 'glow in the dark' watch dials, radium paint continued to be used up until about 1950. There wasn't a suitable safer substitute available, and the military authorities continued to specify radium based paint for important applications such as, compasses, instruments, gun sights, and, of course, watches. The watches we had selected for our 'disruption' plan all had luminous dials, and were hand-me-down watches from parents or uncles, so that there was a good chance that they would not have come up to modern health and safety standards. That in deed, and indeed was our profound hope.

The corporal returned to the shelter to continue his round of 'inspection' for radioactivity among the victims of the nuclear attack. He seemed to have absorbed the absurdity of the role he was playing, as if it were reality. I had taken up a seated position on the floor, with my back to the wall; my chin resting on my knees, my head

turned sideways away from him, as if I were trying to sleep. He made his rounds of the airmen in the building and grinned each time he got a negative reading.

The Geiger counter had become a real hit with our sincere corporal. He was like a dad, who had just bought a new train set for his year old son; possessive to the core! Then he came round to me. I did not look at him at first, but I did hear his new toy spring into life. He ran the counter over me and the thing began to buzz away, like a wasp on heat! I looked up at him and demanded, "What have you done to me Corporal?" It's a bit of a cliché, but his face was a picture. There was the sudden realisation, writ large, that something different and unexpected had just happened. It was as if he had woken up from a dream, and could not understand his surroundings. Luckily for the continued success of the plan, he ran out of the shelter, shouting for the SWO to come to see what had developed.

I had expected that he would have become suspicious immediately and demanded to see what I had up my sleeve. I had expected, then, to be the subject of his embarrassment and anger. As I say though, he had become absorbed in the role play. We took advantage of his sudden disappearance to strip the watches from my arm, return them to their owners, and to await results.

The poor corporal returned, with the SWO puffing away some yards behind him. His physical training programme, in those days, mostly involved filling his pipe with tarred rope, and puffing away at the resultant pungent mixture. He did not appreciate the junior NCO's insistence on haste. The next few moments were a decided anti-climax for that unhappy junior NCO. He tested me, again and again, and once more to make sure. He examined the Geiger counter several times, moving switches and banging it, in the time honoured way of any man trying to 'fix' a technical problem that he does not understand. He glared at me, as if suddenly realising that it must all be my fault. He knew that I was at the bottom of his troubles, but could not put his finger on the 'hows' or 'whys'. The SWO tapped him

on the shoulder, just in time to prevent serious damage to the inno-cent piece of kit.

"Well?" he demanded. He then looked in my direction; glared at me for a few long seconds, and a penny seemed to drop. I suddenly realised that he had worked it out. I waited for the bombshell but it did not come. The SWO grinned, put his arm across the corporal's shoulders, made some casual remark, denigrating modern machin-ery and sympathising with the poor chap's bad luck. The SWO puffed again and again on his pipe as the two of them walked through the door, back to the uncontaminated fresh air, of Norfolk in the spring.

"Time for the NAAFI wagon." - His parting remark...

14
Last Man Standing

THE WEEKENDS WERE not predictable. We worked until lunch time on Saturdays, officially. The flight sergeant showed himself to be a decent fellow, though, and would occasionally give me the nod to leave on a Friday evening. Sometimes I would be able take the train home from King's Lynn to Liverpool Street London. I could do this if I had a rail warrant, available from my meagre annual allowance, or if I had managed to beg, borrow or steal one via another clandestine route. Sometimes even, I might have enough money to purchase a ticket using my RAF form 1250, [my ID card], to claim the reduction of price available to service personnel. Otherwise I would hitch-hike home. Once I got to Liverpool Street on the train, I was faced with a decision that ventured into the realm of family politics. My preference was always to take a bus direct to Edmonton, where I could meet up with Joy at the earliest moment. Whichever way, or however long my weekend, my prevailing intention was to get home to see Joy for as long as possible.

If the pressure of family politics prevailed, however, I would sometimes take a train from Liverpool Street, which would take me home to Enfield Town and my parents and my sister. I would have lunch there and exist on tender-hooks for a while in the hope that dad would agree to loan me his car, so that I could then drive round to

Joy's house for the afternoon and evening. There would often be frequent verbal charges during the whole weekend, to the effect that I never spent any time at home 'these days'. This was mostly from my Mum and all I'm afraid, very predictable, as well as very tiresome when one is courting and when available time is scarce.

The train to and from King's Lynn was always packed with service men, many of whom would be Americans from R.A.F. Sculthorpe, as well as airmen from R.A.F. Marham all travelling down to the 'smoke' for weekends packed with hope, lustful thoughts and the anticipation thereof. The Americans were universally a friendly bunch, happy at the thought of the carefree weekend to come, but they were mostly segregated and separated by colour, not seemingly by order, but by choice and custom.

At the time of which I am writing, this country had very a poor record of tolerance of difference of any kind, whether it be sex, gender, colour or ethnic difference. There were elements of society that had prejudices in any or all direction or directions available. One thing for which we can take some minor credit, however, is that we never did allow the type of social apartheid that the US forces wished to introduce, when they first came to be stationed in this country during WW2. This was such that black and white servicemen should not attend the same public functions, as with local dances and the like.

That type of official discrimination was never allowed, nor were there ever 'black' carriages or 'white only' carriages on public transport, such as trains and busses. This was the official position, although the U.S. servicemen themselves did impose their own 'voluntary' separation. It is a little known fact here, that when, on September 11, 1941, ground was broken in Arlington County, Virginia, for the huge new building that was to become The Pentagon, it was designed with exactly twice the number of loos that were needed for a building of that size. This was because the racist attitudes prevalent and widespread in the U.S. at that time, dictated that apartheid

of loo use had to be imposed i.e. 'white only' toilet facilities were an apparent necessity, leaving a separate allocation for black citizens. The then President, Franklin D. Roosevelt was incensed when this came to his attention, because he had ordered that no such provision should be made in public buildings. Thus the building is rich in loos, although, as it was probably designed by a man, it is most likely that women, black and white, will still need to queue from time to time!

It was but very rarely that one saw a white American airman sitting with black servicemen or vice versa. On one occasion, when I was sitting in a compartment with African Americans, they began to explain to me some of the more ridiculous forms of segregation that they experienced in the Army Air Force of the United States at the time. One example that is stuck in my memory was that a black military policeman was not authorized to arrest or detain any white servicemen suspected of committing an offense.

The African American resentment of these apartheid restrictions was profound and predicated on the fact that many of them were volunteers to the service and not conscripted or, drafted, as was their term. They reasoned that they had signed up for the service as a career and that the restrictions imposed upon them simply for being black amounted to a restraint of trade and a lack of recognition by the country of their birth, of their human rights.

I have thought on these conversations over the years and have realised that they took place at a time not too far removed from that when black men returning home from their World War Two duties had been hounded, brutalised, even lynched in some cases, and in certain states, for having fought against and killed white men during the war, albeit the Nazi enemy.

As I write this I am struck by the realisation that for the whole of my life, both my country and I have been on our own journeys through discrimination and our attitude towards it. For both of us each genre of discrimination has had a different timeframe. I believe, though,

that I can take the credit for beginning my travel towards at least two of the major forms of discrimination, long before my country began to address the issues.

I began my journey towards discounting and discarding racism at about the age of eight, when I began to make my own decision to regard myself as Jewish. Even at that young age, I realised that anti-Semitism was just another form of racism, and through this youthful way of reasoning, I came to the conclusion that if one form was evil then so were all forms, and levels of racism, evil.

I used to read a lot in those days, among which I read the works of some people like HC McNeill, otherwise known as 'Sapper', the works of Harriet Beecher Stowe and of the great American author Mark Twain. I began to realise that the works of different authors impacted differently on the situations of people subject to racial oppression.

On BBC radio in about 1949 I heard a recording of the black American singer Billie holiday, singing the song 'Strange Fruit' the words of which were written by the American Jewish writer and teacher, Abel Meeropol. It is an amazing song with very powerful words, when you hear it and understand the context. An early appreciation of the mixture of cultures that led to the creation of this song laid for me the cornerstone of a lifelong hatred of all things racist.

I have to say, however, that the United Kingdom was somewhat slower in confronting racial hatred. It wasn't until the 1960s and 1970s that legislators here began to address the subject with the initial attempts at legislation that, at first, began to change people's behaviour, and then slowly, as younger generations came onto the scene, to change people's attitudes. My own attitudes towards the feminist debate only began to change after Joyce and I were married in 1962 and I began the experience of making a family with her. I have to acknowledge that I have travelled slowly at first along this journey, but that I'm in a much better place now than I was in 1962.

Finally, the admission comes, that I only began the journey towards an acknowledgement and understanding of gay rights in more recent decades. It was during this period that I began to become aware of the injustices inflicted by society on this group, through association with Gay friends; nevertheless the journey continues.

After a while the weekends on the train became more frequent, due to the arrival of a period when I was able to obtain travel warrants more easily for one reason or another. I began to get to know some of the airmen from the US, if not by name, then by sight. They were friendly enough, as I say, and the occasional beer was exchanged between us during the two and a half hour journey to Liverpool Street, London. On one occasion, it must have been in the spring of 1961, I had arrived at the train on the platform at Kings Lynn puffing and blowing, and with just enough steam left in my boiler to jump on the train as it was about to pull out from the station. I walked along the corridor until I saw some faces that I recognized and realized that there was one seat left in the corner and so, very gratefully I sat myself down. They were all black Americans and treated me to huge grins of welcome as they recognized me.

We exchanged news about life and family, mostly girlfriends, for a few minutes, when slowly it began to dawn on me that one of their company was not joining in with the happy exchanges. He sat across diagonally opposite to me in the far corner by the window. He appeared to have some facial bruises, but even more apparently, his face was half covered by strips of sticking plaster. I looked at him, got his attention, and asked him if he'd had an accident. I was a bit concerned as he seemed that he might be in pain and looked to be quite miserable. As I asked the question, though, his friends all roared with laughter. This was quite unexpected and quite inappropriate, it seemed to me. Why would you laugh in such a way at a friend's misfortune? I looked around me, frowning at them, and received nothing back but huge grins and no explanation. Finally one guy took pity on me and deigned to explain.

It was not a long and complicated story but nonetheless it was an astounding one for my ears. It seemed that all the young men in the carriage were very keen on having a bet from time to time. The guy with the battered face in the far corner was also a keen boxer. They had devised a method of mixing the two in a quite bizarre fashion. The method required the presence of a number of idiots, each of whom was prepared to get into a ring blindfold. In the case of the man in the corner there had been nine others who climbed into the ring with him and allowed themselves to be blindfolded. Each one of the lunatics had to put $100 into a pot.

The name of the glorious game was.... wait for it...., 'last man standing', the aim of which being that the last one of this incredible crew remaining on his feet, after they had all swung and punched and puffed their very best, hoping to knock others over and out and so on repeatedly, until the last man standing could gratefully claim his pot of dollars. In Thursday's episode of this collective madness the lunatic in the corner had won the day. He was the one who had allowed himself to be blindfolded, though it did not immediately register with him when, eventually, all others had either fallen or given up, that he was in fact the one standing alone.

The madman's friends, and I use the term loosely, had decided that it would be fun to add a further dimension of torture and torment to the game. They tied boxing gloves onto long poles and kept him going for several more minutes by simply poking at him from outside of the ring. As they told the story there was much grinning and laughing and general good humour amongst the whole group of them. They were clearly of the opinion that the whole event had been a huge bundle of fun. As they were describing the mad event, I took repeated peeks at their victim, as he slunk lower and lower into his seat by the window in the corner. His face had become obscured from me by the collar of his greatcoat, so it took me a while to realize that he was laughing along with the rest of them. Perhaps, in the way he was laughing at them, his thoughts, perhaps, were on the thousand

dollars he had in his pocket. It was he after all who had had the courage to stand up in the ring in the first place. It was he after all who had had the distinction of being the last man standing! I guess that it became the perfect Tontine, but without the annuity!

15
My Only Form 252!

MY SECOND, AND personally memorable, experience on the train was on the journey home one Sunday night from Liverpool Street to King's Lynn. The train was the regular one that left Liverpool Street at 30 minutes past midnight during Sunday night/ Monday morning. Virtually the only passengers were servicemen returning to camp from weekends away in London. It was a time of tiredness and depression for most, at the thought of at least one more week before one could return home to loved ones once again.

The train made a couple of stops on the way to King's Lynn and at these places the majority of departing passengers were servicemen; so much so, that if all the UK and the USA servicemen in East Anglia at that time had jumped up in the air at the same moment, Norfolk and Suffolk would have snapped away from the rest of Great Britain when they landed.

By the time we got to King's Lynn it would have been about three in the morning. There was a regular contingent of servicemen from three camps remaining on the train by that time, these were; RAF Marham, RAF Sculthorpe (US) and RAF Bircham Newton. There was always a bus waiting at the station to deliver us back to our various camps. Sculthorpe was always the second station to be serviced by that bus; this meant that Bircham Newton would be last or first

depending upon which way the bus turned as it left the station. The difference meant the possibility of an extra three quarters of an hour or even an hour before one could finally get to bed. I can remember praying fervently as we left the station for the driver to turn towards Bircham Newton rather than Marham, so that I could get to bed as early as possible.

I also remember that RAF Sculthorpe always seemed to take its security more seriously than all of the RAF stations that I had known. This may have been due to the Americans natural inclination to take the security of their establishments as a firm given. They were, after all, in a foreign country, even though we all speak much the same language. I remember that as we approached the outer gates of the American camp, an armed serviceman would climb onto the bus, as it passed through the gate. He would check the identification of each of the Americans as they got down from the bus. He would then stay on the bus as it wound its way through the station to the back gate, where he would get down and allow us to pass through.

The American camp was in itself an eye-opener for all of us British servicemen. Instead of one tiny inconspicuous Naafi shop, as we had at Bircham Newton, the Americans and their wives had a long parade of shops at which they could spend their dollars quite comfortably. Wherever they were in the world American servicemen were paid in U.S. currency. Their wives, therefore, had the convenience of being able to shop as if they were at home. Some, of course, saw this as a real convenience, others may well have viewed it as a restriction of their ability and willingness to mix with, and to begin to understand local communities around the world. It meant, of course, that the wives and families of American servicemen had the facility offered to them to be able to remain in small-town America no, matter where they found themselves to be in this vast and interesting world in which we live. This is more the pity, because Americans generally seem to me, perhaps because of the huge size of their country, to be more isolationist and isolated from the wider world than many

societies allow themselves to be. Nonetheless, I can remember the tinge of envy with which we peered through the bus window at the grand array of shops available at RAF Sculthorpe.

On one of the journeys back from Liverpool Street, during one of those Sunday nights when I must have been particularly tired. I remember that the end of the weekend had not been so very pleasant. My parents, unfortunately, wanted to return to the theme of me spending more time at home. We had had a bit of a spat about this, as soon as I returned home from Joyce's house to gather my things and say goodbye to my parents, before going off to the station.

I did not like arguing with my parents, it always depressed me, so that on this occasion I returned to Liverpool Street in a low and foul mood. I had hoped that one or two of my friends on the train might be in a mood to exchange a few comforting words about mutual problems. No such luck however! It seemed that everyone in my carriage had had such a good weekend that all they wanted to do was to get their heads down and get some kip. They were in no mind to get into conversation, particularly a long moody conversation with me.

I nodded fitfully for a while, I do seem to remember, vaguely, the long and wailing cry of "Dowownaahm!" as we stopped at Downham-market, but by then I had relaxed enough to have yielded to the inevitable, and finally to have got myself off to sleep. It must've been very deep sleep, however, for although I did feel some shunting and clattering of the train when we arrived, I did not wake up until about 8 o'clock in the morning in the sidings at King's Lynn. My kind friends had left me to sleep on in the train and had tiptoed out of the carriage and out of the station to the bus.

I was now left with the problem of negotiating myself out of the train, along the track to the platform, and then with the task of phoning my section at the camp to explain that I would be late for duty on that Monday morning. I have to say that my flight sergeant, when I spoke to him, was much angrier than I had anticipated. He told me, in no uncertain terms, that I should get myself back to the camp

ASAP, that he would regard me as being AWOL and that I should not go straight to the section but report to the guard-room. I truly had not expected such an angry reaction and I tried to explain more fully what had happened, but it did not seem to interest him at that time. I realised later, that he was offended by what he saw as ill return by me for his frequent kindness to me, in allowing me to leave early for my weekends. I have to admit that he had some right on his side, although my lateness was far from intentional.

It took me a while to find out from the staff at the bus station nearby how I was going to get myself to the camp. It was therefore a couple of hours at least before I was able to report to the guard-room, where I was told that my section officer had issued a formal 252 charge sheet with my name on it. I was placed under arrest until I could be seen by the squadron leader admin, after lunch, which for me was to be taken in the guard room. I was supposed to be in a cell but the guard corporal assumed that I would not try to escape and so did not impose that indignity. He did not regard me as a hardened criminal. He actually allowed me to have my lunch as usual in the airmen's mess. At that point it did not feel like being under arrest.

Sometime after lunch the guard corporal received a call to say that the adjutant was ready to deal with me. Squadron Leader 'B' being the adjutant was also the officer who ran the station shooting team. I did not relish being paraded before him under these circumstances but, well, I had no choice.

An RAF regiment corporal appeared quite quickly at the guard room together with an LAC from that department and I was marched down to the admin block to the adjutant's office, at this juncture we waited in the corridor, where everyone who was interested could gawp at my predicament. At least that was what I kept thinking. In fact, no-one was interested in me.

After a while I was marched into the 'presence'. As we stopped in front of the officer's desk the order "Hats Off" was bellowed, the officer winced noticeably as my beret was dragged unceremoniously

from my head. I later asked why this was done and was told that it was in case I had been tempted to throw it at the officer when he imposed punishment. Damned nonsense! I remember thinking that there had been plenty of other, better, missiles in the room than my beret, if I had wanted an object to throw.

The charge was read out. I had to agree that what was alleged was true. I was asked if I had any explanation for being AWOL. I explained that I had fallen asleep on the train back from London and had woken up in the sidings at King's Lynn. I had had no intention of being AWOL and had phoned the unit as soon as I could find a phone at the station.

"Were there no friends on the train with you?" asked the officer.

"Yes sir. They chose not to disturb my sleep as they left the train." I endeavoured to sound as sarcastic as possible here.

He actually grinned at this. "You may need to speak to your friends?" I agreed wholeheartedly with him over that.

"Yes sir."

"Do you accept my punishment?" "Yes sir!"

"One week CB [confined to camp] and one extra guard duty during the 7 days."

Dammit! I thought. No going home this weekend!

I am happy to say that my 'friends' felt duly guilty when they realised that their 'joke' had resulted in me losing a weekend at home. I actually managed to do a swap for my extra guard duty with the airman who had been destined to do my punishment one. So another small victory and - No-one loses!

16
At Last! Moderate Sporting Success!

THIS IS TO be my final trip into the pleasures of Wednesday afternoons and the dedication of these periods, by the armed services, to sports events. It is a tradition that I sincerely hope persists to this day. For me, although I was never a dedicated participant in sports, it did give me access to a full six months of Wednesday afternoons shooting at Swaffham at the beginning of my time at Bircham Newton. By the time that the squadron leader decided that he had had enough, I had myself worked through my pre national service fascination for guns. Don't get me wrong, I still enjoyed the shooting and the afternoons of pleasurable activity with friends and comrades, but I had worked through the juvenile attraction that I had previously felt for guns per se. I was quite happy to go onto other things.

I tried tennis for a while. In doing so I ignored all advice and accepted an offer from Fred James the RAF regiment corporal to play a few sets with him. It was a mistake! I was 21 or 22 at the time and about as fit as I would ever be in my life, but Fred, a man some 20 years older, had me running ragged. I don't remember winning a whole game let alone a set. I may have picked up a few points here and there, but that would have been about the sum of it, and it would

have been Fred who would have lost the points rather than me winning them.

On the third Wednesday that we were due to play, Fred picked up some extra duty and had to call it off. I am convinced that we were both relieved at this; Fred, because I was not giving him a good enough game, and I, because he was too good and I was likely to be thrashed each week until I improved sufficiently to test him from time to time. At about this time, I lost my job book-keeping for the PSI fund but was given the job of looking after the small camp library on Wednesday afternoons. This I did, apart from the very occasional intervention of some other activity, until the end of my National Service.

Towards the end of my service, in the late spring or early summer of 1962, RAF Bircham Newton decided to put on its own sports day. I have to confess, like many of my memories, I can remember the event but not the details of how it came about. The CO was very keen that sports activities should play an important part in the camp curriculum, so the sports day may well have been inspired and promoted by him. I do not recall that any commissioned officers took part on competitive events against other ranks on the day, but the boy entrants and apprentices definitely took part in events against permanent staff.

The SWO, as usual, had the unenviable task of persuading, cajoling and even bullying permanent staff into taking part. As for me, I felt a distinct and very real sense of gratitude towards that particular officer for his recent award to me of the station's one and only Cup Final ticket. A not to be sniffed at event! Apart from that he had been a very decent influence in the camp generally during my nearly two years there. I also felt that he was due a bit of beneficial pay back, after the cavalier way we treated him on day one of the Uxbridge Group Sports day. For all of these reasons I actually volunteered to take part, long before the cajoling and bullying stage of the recruitment process.

I volunteered at an early stage, but I had no idea what event, in which I was going to try not to make a fool of myself. I reviewed all the possibilities and quickly ruled out any running events or, indeed, any event that required notable reserves of cardio vascular capacity at all; smoking my pipe and lack of any form of training had put paid to those options.

I had come to the conclusion, regarding my paucity of cardio vascular reserves, aptly demonstrated during an unfortunate test of my ability at tennis that Wednesday the previous autumn, against my erstwhile guard duty chum Corporal James as described above and with very little athletic credit to be awarded to me. One aim of this contest had been to help me with ongoing training for the sports day due the next spring. The main problem having been, that I had been too engrossed in my duties as Camp Librarian on Wednesday afternoons, until a couple of weeks before the event itself and the SWO was pushing me for a decision. I did not dare suggest inclusion in the tug of war team!

"You can only improve" was Fred's helpful advice whilst I was lying on the grass verge by the court, trying desperately to catch at least one more breath before I died. I tried to mouth the words "bugger off Fred" without success. Seeing my inability to put forward any argument that required using my vocal chords, he opined a suggestion that had some merit, I felt, after some breathless consideration. "You should try a throwing event he suggested. They require very little ability to run." And so it was settled. It would be brilliant. I would have a go at the discuss; I had had a brief acquaintance with that particular missile whilst at school. I did at least know how to hold it, which was a bloody good starting point as far as I was concerned. The SWO was delighted. He had not been swamped with volunteers thus far. My feeling, after speaking to him, was that he was about to do the rounds to inform a select group that they had volunteered and to inform them of their athletic choices.

I realised at once that I had made the better choice by volunteering "one volunteer being worth ten pressed men" and all that. I had, moreover, done some training in my chosen event, albeit some years in the past. The SWO had taken the nuclear route in his search for 'volunteers'. The moaning could be heard all around the mess at dinner that evening. "He can't force me, the old bugger" being the favourite and mild epithet used, for no-one disliked the SWO enough for violent bad language. They all knew, anyway, that an SWO can pretty much force people to do anything he likes, provided that it is half-way legal.

The great day arrived. All the 'athletes' gathered on the ancient grass airfield, away from the landing strip, where some markers had been painted in white to represent the lanes for the lucky selectees for the various running events. I perhaps use the word selectees unfairly, because some of those gathered had actually self- selected and had trained for their chosen events. These were mostly from the senior ranks of the RAF apprentice cohort.

I had thought, 'that those boys' would provide easy competition when discussing the matter in the pub the previous evening. Well, we had reasoned, you have to train somewhere! In the cold light of day, however, they looked tough and well prepared and were still doing preparation exercises; warm ups and the like. This did not bode well I thought. I had never harboured notions of winning my event. Suddenly though, I realised that I stood a strong chance of being humiliated by this juvenile opposition; not a heart-warming prospect that, for a man who was used to being called "staff" respectfully by these 'children'. By the time that I got to that thought though, I had had cold feet for some minutes. I even thought of feigning sudden illness, but the steely glint in the SWO's eye when dealing with a similar complaint from one of my erstwhile drinking buddies, convinced me quickly and very surely that that would not be a good route to take. I sometimes act foolishly, but I'm no fool!

The sports day had crept up on me with the only training under my belt having been the tennis humiliation by Corporal 'Fred' months

before, together with many nights in the pubs in Brancaster and Docking, drinking and thinking about it. Reality was now smacking me in the face. I tried unconvincingly to brace myself for the debacle to come.

There were about ten assorted members of camp personnel gathered for the event. Dear God. I thought, I'm about to come last from a group ten. That prospect made me even more nervous. The sergeant in charge of the event began to outline the structure under which we were expected to compete. It was fairly simple and designed to give any spectators an event that would last a decent amount of time and would probably not kill anyone, no dead spectators being the preference. It was due to begin at 2pm if my memory serves me right. We were to have three throws each in the first round, after which the six throwers [I will not repeat the abuse of the word 'athletes'] with the best throws would go through to the final and have a further three throws, during which the first, second, and third placed throwers would self-select by performance.

The first round took a surprisingly long time. What with a thrower's need to set himself for the throw, the throw itself, the measurement of the throw and the recording of same on the official 'performance' sheet, all taking about five minutes for each throw; the first round took nearly an hour.

I was totally gobsmacked to get through the first round in about fourth place, as far as I can remember. That I felt, was likely to be the height of my achievement that afternoon. The second round began with the throws of the first round still counting. Nothing changed for me during the first round of throws in this, the final. I put a real effort into the next round of throws and moved up to third place.

Before the final round of throws, my main thought was to pray that I would not lose my now, precious third place, a level of achievement that I had never dreamed of prior to that afternoon. I was therefore very nervous at the prospect of the final round but, miracle of miracles, far from losing my third place I actually gained one more

position and moved up to second place. I still have the second place trophy to prove my mighty athletic achievement at RAF Bircham Newton in the spring of 1962, just a couple of months before my demob. It stands on the shelf, rather shamefacedly, next to my ill-gotten copy of Jerome K Jerome's 'Three Men in a Boat' etc. My joy at my success was partially tempered by the realisation that the winner was a 16 year old RAF apprentice. Still, I thought, he hadn't had to do his training in the pubs of Brancaster and Docking!

17
Dental issues!

"SO WHAT'S YOUR problem then?"

That large and very imposing Squadron Leader Doctor was the first female officer I had met, or ever did meet, during my RAF career. She asked the question, moreover, in that tone of voice that indicated that she had 'heard it all before' and was not anybody's push over; not now, not ever!

Well then! I had had those teeth for years! Bloody wisdom teeth! They had been a problem ever since they began to erupt in my poor unsuspecting mouth; a period of about four years prior to that point. They did not come through in one sensible session as any respectable teeth should. No! Every four or five months during that period they had begun a new growth spurt and my mouth had exploded and turned itself into a home for vicious and painful ulcers. I had tried to suggest on several occasions, to my civilian dentist, that it would be a damned good idea to operate and to take them out. He simply would not hear of it. They weren't in his mouth after all! His response was always that the problem would abate in time and that I would appreciate the benefit of having those four new teeth.

I had been in the RAF for about six months by the time to which I am now referring, and my mouth had erupted once more. I was in a lot of pain, such that it was difficult to talk properly. My section

sergeant had been quite sympathetic when I explained that I needed to see the doctor. He even phoned the medical department to let them know that he was sending me up to see that worthy soul who now sat, imposingly and disbelievingly, before me.

I explained my problem to the Doctor who, all the time, looked back at me with a totally expressionless face. She made me quite uneasy with her apparent disbelief. She also gave me another problem, in that I did not know whether to call her 'Doctor' or 'Ma'am'.

"What do you expect me to do about it?" This was her quite unhelpful initial question to me, without even looking into my mouth, as I had stumbled towards the end of my sad tale.

"Well ma'am, I'd like you to refer me to an RAF dentist, so that I can ask him or her to remove them, so that I don't keep getting this trouble."

At this point she did decide to look into my mouth. Even she was impressed.

"Hell's Bells!" she exclaimed in a rather 'house and country' voice. "You really do have a collection there don't you?" She paused for a moment and sat back into her chair. To give her credit, her tone was altogether more sympathetic after she had looked into my ulcer factory.

"Look," she began to explain. "No dentist will be able to operate, even if they decide that that's the way to go, whilst you have that splendid set of ulcers. The danger of blood poisoning is far too great. Your mouth will have to be clear of them first."

I leaned forward with the intention of protesting. She held her hand up in clear signal for me to keep quiet.

"Today is Thursday. I'm going to refer you to the dental unit at the RAF Hospital Ely for next Tuesday. I'll organise a car to take you, so you'll have no trouble with transport. In the meantime, I'm ordering four days off work and a course of anti-biotics. ..You should be free of your mouth guests by the time you get to Ely. I have no idea if the dentist at the hospital will do what you want and take the teeth out, but I do think that it might be a good idea."

"By the way," she continued. "The four days off I've given you include the weekend, which means that you are confined to camp until you go to Ely on Tuesday." I did think of protesting at this but at no point had she given the impression of someone who would be prepared to discuss the point. I decided to quit whilst I was ahead!

That was the last time I saw that particular doctor. Despite her sarcasm, her brusque manner, and her original air of disbelief, though, I was grateful to her, for finally taking me seriously and for setting me up with the appointment at Ely hospital.

I made my way back to the section to give the sergeant the news and to hand him the chit from the doctor confirming my time off. I did make a half-hearted effort to offer to go into work the next day, if I began to feel better, but he would hear none of it. He looked up at me and smiled a resigned smile, "This is not like civvy street lad. This is the RAF and this..." He waived the chit at me, "is not just a chit from the doctor like at home. It's a chit from a squadron leader and tantamount to an order from a senior officer. No! You do exactly as she said. She wouldn't have given you the time off if she didn't think you needed it. She's not the type!"

I made my way back to my room rather slowly. I wasn't feeling too great, my mouth was hurting quite badly and, on top of that, I couldn't go home this weekend. I had managed to scrounge a fairly comfortable armchair for my room and a radio. I took the first of my pills and sat down in the chair, with every intention of listening to the radio and reading another chapter or two of 'The Storm' by Ilya Ehrenburg. It is a powerful Second World War story but proved to be too strong for me that afternoon. I quickly fell asleep and did not wake up until I was roused by people moving around, banging doors and so on, on their way back from morning work, and on their way to get some lunch. I usually enjoyed my lunch but did not feel at all hungry that day. I did, however, wander over to the mess, more to break the monotony of sitting alone in my room than with any intention of eating.

The walk to the mess was very quickly achieved, as the build-ing was only about eighty yards or so from my room. I still had little incentive to eat when I arrived. The cooks, though, had done us proud that day because they had conjured up a first course of mulligatawny soup. Just the job! I filled myself a large bowl of the divine liquid and sat myself down to enjoy it slowly, allowing the heat of the soup to momentarily ease the pain in my mouth and throat. I was first at the table but, as I sat there slowly sipping my lunch, others began to arrive. John Robinson was one of the first. He worked in the admin office in the same building as my section. He had heard of my visit to the doc and knew that I had got some time off work. He was just about the only one who did not make a comment such as 'lucky bug-ger' or something of that order.

I spent the weekend largely in somewhat lonely reading. Most of my friends made their various ways home. John hardly ever went home to Thanet where his family lived. He did pop in to keep me com-pany and to have a convivial smoke on his pipe from time to time, but he was not confined to camp as I was, and so took the opportunity to keep others company on trips to a variety of local pubs most eve-nings. From my point of view the time passed slowly. I enjoy reading but the confinement of having little else to do was something that I found quite wearing.

On the Saturday afternoon, WO Rubin, my section warrant officer, actually walked over from the married quarters to see me. I suppose that he could have been checking up on me, to see that I had indeed stayed on camp as instructed, but that would be too cynical, and any-way I did not get that impression. His attitude was quite solicitous. He sat with me in my room, chatting for about an hour. By this time in my service I had brought some of my painting equipment from home. He appeared to be genuinely interested in my enjoyment of painting as a hobby. His visit was as pleasant for me as it was unexpected.

We were approaching the end of what had been a hard winter. The weather at the end of February is rarely balmy on these islands

but the next day, the Sunday, was unusually bright and sunny, not warm but bright enough to induce me out of my room and to take a stroll around the camp. I even popped into the guard-room to scrounge a cup of coffee. The guard corporal was OK about the coffee but was not someone I knew well, so it did not become a coffee and a chat, just a coffee and 'off you go'! I wandered around for a while more but the camp was not a big one. It was also almost empty due to the weekend exodus. A few RAF apprentices and boy entrants were around, but they were no company for me and, in any case, association was not encouraged, between them and permanent staff.

By the Monday I was feeling much better. The anti-biotics were doing their job. I was also feeling bored. I wandered down to my section once again but the sergeant told me to clear off! He was not going to take any risks that I might have some kind of incident or accident when I was under orders to be off duty. I reluctantly returned to my room to a further day of reading, listening to the radio, as well as some painting, all interspersed by welcome breaks for mealtimes and company!

On the Tuesday morning I met with my transport. I still could not believe that the Doctor had arranged for me to be taken to the hospital by car. The car was a comfortable 'pool' car and the driver, an SAC, another national-serviceman, was a medical orderly who, he told me, was used from time to time to ferry 'patients' to a variety of appointments. His name was Bob - Bob Haynes. I queried with him this rather extravagant use of a car for a lowly airman. "It's this doc." he advised me. "As far as she's concerned you're a patient under treatment. Ely is across country from here - believe me it's a lot easier by car than by public transport, a lot better for you!"

I was quite ready to believe that but I still could not believe my luck that I had fallen into a Station such as Bircham Newton, in which to do my service. I still regarded myself as a press ganged man, but there were many times over those forthcoming months, the remains

of my two years, that I metaphorically pinched myself to confirm that it was all a reality to be on that particular camp.

The drive to the hospital took about an hour. It was not a long journey but was across country and the driver was, apparently, under strict orders to drive carefully, as he had 'pranged' two pool cars during the past year. The RAF regiment flight sergeant in charge of the motor section had taken great care to warn him of the dire consequences of any further mishaps to any of his cars. The message, however it was conveyed, had struck home. This driver was, therefore, a very careful chap! We arrived safely at the hospital and in good time for my appointment.

The first thing that struck me about the military hospital, that was RAF Ely at that time, was that peace and quiet reigned throughout. As I walked through its corridors, I began to realise that there was a very good reason for this peaceful ambiance. There were no patients! That observation was not quite true. I did spot one group of women, who, even with my, as then, untrained and inexperience eyes were certainly waiting for an ante-natal clinic. A few members of staff were to be seen making their way from here to there, but the walk through the hospital to my destination in the department of dentistry was akin to a walk in the countryside after a heavy fall of snow, it was unnaturally quiet. "This is the way to run a hospital properly". I thought. – 'sans' patients, the place was clearly running very smoothly!

Bob guided me to the reception desk, which was staffed by a very attractive and helpful young woman, who quickly directed me to 'dentistry'. She even 'phoned through to let them know I had arrived. My impression was that she was glad to have something to do to break the monotony of the morning. Bob offered to walk to the department with me but that didn't seem to be necessary. The directions were clear. On enquiring of Bob as to what he was going to do, it became clear to me that he had plans regarding his waiting time. The plan began with a trip into the city of Ely. Have car will travel! This

was a reasonable motto to have in the circumstances and would certainly have been my approach if the circumstance had been reversed. Having assured me that he would be back in very good time to take me back to Bircham Newton, he disappeared back to the car, leaving me to hope that the dentist would deal with me that day as I had hoped. I could not blame Bob for not wanting to wait for me for what was, at that stage, an undeterminable period of time, but I did curse a bit at the speed of his departure.

I made my way through the quiet corridors to the department of dentistry. I arrived in a state of real anxious anticipation. I was anxious because several dentists had previously ruled against relieving me of these troublesome teeth! As I entered the dental section, I conjured up a mental picture of being strapped to the dentist chair, whilst someone akin to Frankenstein worked on me totally oblivious to my cries of pain, with my screams of pain resounding around the erstwhile quiet corridors. Nothing fanciful then?

The dental receptionist met me almost at the door. She offered me a friendly grin which dispelled all thoughts of Frankenstein. A youngish man dressed in the uniform of a flight lieutenant was sitting across the room reading a newspaper. The receptionist introduced him as the dentist, Mr so and so, I cannot remember his name, but I do remember wondering why he would need to be wearing his day uniform. He had clearly had a really busy morning! There was not a sign of another patient, neither when I arrived, nor as I was leaving. He rose, reluctantly I thought, from his chair and ushered me into his torture chamber. My mental picture of Frankenstein re-appeared momentarily. There had been no smile of welcome, nothing to break the ice

"AC Kreit?" The question was abrupt.

"Yes sir." My response did not need any elaboration.

"You're demanding to have your wisdom teeth removed?"

"Sir! I think that 'hoping' would be a more correct expression." He was beginning to get on my tits! My appearance in his surgery had

clearly spoiled his day. Without further ado he ushered me brusquely into the chair. We were not intended to be bosom buddies, this ill-tempered grouch and me. Not that I wanted or expected anything like that but, you tell me, who wants to be treated by a dentist in a bad temper?

"Sir! Have I offended you in some way?"

"Are you being insolent?"

"Not at all. I just wondered if I should try going out and coming in again."

I saw the dental assistant's eyes widen in astonishment but his bad manners were rapidly burning through my own fuse. I decided that, in for a penny, in for a pound was going to be my 'kill or cure'. In any case, although the ulcers had disappeared, my teeth were hurting like billy-oh, which was not the best basis for this conversation.

"No-one likes going to the dentist sir, but one is usually greeted by some sort of welcome."

The flight lieutenant looked at me as if I were something out of a 'how do we handle difficult situations' training book. He turned sharply on his heels and walked over to a counter display of dental instruments. He called his assistant over in the same brusque manner that he had been using on me. Oh dear! I thought, he's turning on her now. He began to issue some instructions to her and, as he did so, the tone of his voice began to soften. He turned back to face me.

"You're right. Let's start again!" He did not apologise but 'start again' was good enough for me.

"Open up!" He began to examine my teeth; a few hissing intakes of breath later, to which he added a few tut tuts and quiet mutterings, then he spoke again. Not brusquely this time but firmly, and business-like.

"Your wisdom teeth can come out. They're not much use anyway- to anyone that is and they're ready to be pulled. I will have to take some x-rays first though." He paused for a few moments as if weighing the pros and cons of his next question.

"Would you like me to do the operation today?" It was like being part of a Jekyll and Hyde movie. I made my mind up very quickly and responded very politely.

"Yes please sir. That would be great!" The flight lieutenant., now back in dentist mode, nodded slowly.

"Right, we'll get the pictures taken then..." He paused again for another question. "Do you prefer gas or an injection?"

"Injection please sir." I reasoned that loading him up with a few sirs was appropriate in view of his extraordinary change of mood.

"Good – you can take a bit of light lunch and a cup of tea and we'll do the op after we've all had a break and I've checked the x-rays, just to make certain there are no complications indicated there."

The dental surgery was well equipped; he took the necessary pictures himself and told me to come back at 2pm. It was 12.30 by then so I had an hour and a half to kill.

I was surprised to find that there was a small but well supplied canteen open and ready for business. There were few customers when I arrived there. There was not, though, any sign of my driver. This was a bit disconcerting, but on the basis that he would be in big trouble if he went back to BN without me, I settled down to the hope that he was probably enjoying his afternoon more than I was about to do, after the lunch break. I did enjoy my light lunch during the moments when I could take my mind off coming events and, although the canteen did fill up considerably as time passed, I had no-one to talk to.

All too soon it was time for me to return to the department of dentistry. It was no consolation either that I had long wished for the time when I could persuade a dentist to rid me of these damned teeth. It seemed a long walk through the hospital corridors back towards the dental department. One could hear more in the way of hospital noises this time, although it could never be described as 'hustle and bustle'. RAF Hospital ELY was not, seemingly, in the business of 'hustle and bustle'! My footsteps still echoed along the route. I arrived at

the door of the dental department all too soon. My adversary was already there to greet me.

"Right?" he asked. "Ready to go?" Then, without waiting for my response he demanded

"By the way; when do you clean your teeth?"

I was really taken aback at the 'left field' aspect of this question. It seemed so out of context.

"In the evenings before I go to bed and when I wake up."

"Oh! So you clean your teeth according to your bedtimes rather than according to your mealtimes then?"

He smiled a superior smile, as if he had won a major point with a really decisive and incisive argument. He then went on to other things, thus leaving that issue entirely in the air. He offered no counter advice from his own expert knowledge.

The subject was never touched on again. I have, though, thought about this short exchange many times over the years, wondering sometimes if even he reflects upon it, from time to time, in the light of modern opinion on the subject. Many dentists nowadays actually advise against brushing teeth after meals, as the enamel is softened at that time. Before bed and on rising are, in fact, favoured times for brushing teeth. The episode still irritates me after all this time, over fifty years later, so much so that I am now in the process of aggravating you with it!

The rest of the session went much better than I had anticipated. The worst part as far as I was concerned was, in fact, receiving the injections. It was the usual process; injections that seemed to take forever with their pushing and probing, such that one's eyeballs felt as if they were about to be ejected from their sockets! My torturer did not ask me to leave the room for a while so that the injections could take hold. There would have been no point, as there were no more patients waiting in the wings.

The dentist prodded and poked from time to time as if to test the efficacy of the anaesthetic. Finally he was ready and the rest

was comparatively easy from my point of view. I had a bit of a struggle keeping my head and neck braced against the effort he was having to put in to pull the offending teeth from their strongholds but, one by one, they all 'pinged' into the metal dish. As the eventual success of the mission became more and more apparent, the young officer gradually, with each successful extraction, underwent a personality change; he became more solicitous of my feelings and my welfare.

A series of instructions regarding the care of the wound cavities accompanied this route change towards care and concern. I began to realise that some of his earlier abrasiveness had almost certainly been due to apprehension on his part regarding the operation itself, to extract the four teeth. Nonetheless he went ahead with it, very successfully from my point of view.

The officer gave me a prescription for strong painkillers to be filled by the hospital pharmacy before I left, and, advising me that my mouth and jaw would become quite painful, probably for several days once the anaesthetic wore off, he offered to write me up for a few more days off work. I think that I surprised him by refusing this offer. There was no way that I wanted a repeat of the boredom of the previous week. I told him that I would rather stick with the painkillers and go to work. Finally, as I took my leave, I thanked him profusely for removing my 'demons' of many years. He sealed his change in personality by actually shaking my hand and wishing me luck as I went away. My feelings of relief and general well-being were later tempered somewhat as the side effects of the strong painkillers began to kick in. I am now very wary of all codeine based products, as, apparently, codeine morphs into morphine in the body, which often causes real delays in the body's 'through' system!

To complete the successful outcome of the day's events, Bob, my driver, was waiting for me, a bored expression on his face as if he had been waiting all day, on a chair at reception. I could not accept his suggestion of a cup of tea or coffee before we left. One of my final

list of instructions as I was leaving the surgery was not to drink anything for about two hours to give the wounds time to congeal properly. We arrived back at BN in time for Bob to get his dinner. My jaw
was beginning to fight back from its war with the dentist. All I wanted
was a couple of strong painkillers!!

18
M y Manchester Diversion

I REALISE THAT I have refrained from discussing my trips home in any detail, but, for several reasons I feel that it is correct to make an exception regarding the circumstances under which I gained contact, for the first time in my life, with that part of my Jewish family residing in Manchester, my Boobah [my paternal grandmother] in particular.

I have placed this chapter of my RAF story close to the very end of my written thoughts regarding those two years for two reasons. Firstly I have to recognise that the events described here took place during those years and were indeed largely enabled by my temporary separation from my parents. Secondly, though, they are family experiences and so I did want there to be some separation of them from the major part of my national service story.

I have to say at the outset, that I have gained very little of the information I am about to set before you here, from my parents themselves. It has virtually all been gained from other members of my large family, both maternal and paternal, as well as from Joyce, who has compiled a family tree that has been really helpful. My aunt Joan, my mother's youngest sister, is now one of only two members of that generation, on either side of my family, who is still alive. The other is Sam Gontarsz, who is a cousin to my late father.

Joan has been a true friend to me all of my life. Only very recently she filled in some details relating to how and when my mum and dad got together. There are, however, some differences in the nuances of these early days according to who tells the story. In my view that makes it all the more interesting, but has left me with the task of filling in the gaps, from my understanding of how people in my family have 'ticked' over the years

For anyone who wishes to gain some understanding of the early history of my Jewish family, you only have to watch the film Fiddler on The Roof. The only difference really being, that the politics of family relationships in my family from those depicted in that great story, were enacted in their own style once my family was in this country, rather than in Eastern Europe as in the film.

They came over in 1906 from a town called Hrubeshief [Robishoyf, in Yiddish] now in Eastern Poland, but in those days a part of the Austro Hungarian Empire. Whatever the geography may be, it was then, and still is, one of the most ardently anti-Semitic regions on earth. My grandparents fled to this country in order to escape the regular Pogroms, these were life threatening purges, that were perpetrated there, and in other countries in Jewish European History. The abomination, to which Mrs Hitler had given life, the evil corporal, was about 17 years old at that time. Like Tevye, my grandparents came here with little, except hope for a future. They brought with them one babe in arms, my aunt Pearl.

My dad grew up in a largely dysfunctional, even crazy or, in Yiddish, 'meshuggeneh', family. He was born a few years before World War 1, at the age of about 19 or20, he met a young woman, not Jewish, at the Young Communist League, in Stamford Hill, North London. I do not know her name but Dad made it known to his family and told them that he intended to marry her. Again some pieces of the puzzle are missing and have now been lost in the depths of family history. The fact is, though, that his family, by one means or another, managed to scupper that relationship on the sole basis that the girl

was not Jewish. Apparently Dad was devastated. He disappeared to France for six months, travelling and working here and there to make his way, as well as to learn some of the language.

Dad returned to England and took up, once again, his membership of the Young Communist League in Stamford Hill. At this time, the family was living in Cannon Street Road, Whitechapel, in that section of North London known as the 'East End'. This is an area of London that has seen many waves of immigration over the years. After a time Dad met another young woman, my mother, also not Jewish. They fell in love, but this time, he decided that he was not going to advise his family. Mum and Dad arranged a registry office wedding without telling anyone on his side of the family, with, I believe, the exception of his older brother Harry. After the wedding he went back to the family and dropped his 'bombshell' on them. To say that it did not go down well would have been an understatement of the highest order. The Yiddish expression "Oy vay! Vi a gevalt!" would not nearly have covered it. The family, with the exceptions of Dad's older brother Harry and his younger brother Rueben, completely disowned him. They even said Kaddish for him at Synagogue, just as if he were dead. The Kaddish is known as the mourner's prayer and is used in times of mourning. It is, in fact, a prayer glorifying God's Holy Name.

Up until the time that I went into the RAF, I had had no personal contact with any of them, except for uncles Harry and Rueben, who were both good uncles, as well as good friends, to me for the whole of their lives. This obstinate refusal to make contact was maintained on both sides, even at family functions like bar-mitzvahs, where some of them might be present. My parents would not allow me to approach Boobah or to speak to her, nor was she apparently ever in the mood for me to try. In any case I never felt strong enough, in those days and in company, to defy my parents on the subject. A Bar Mitzvah is the ceremony which is held in Synagogue on the Saturday closest to a boy's thirteenth birthday. At this ceremony he takes on the religious duties of a man.

Going into the RAF, I had long decided, would give me the psychological elbow-room to make a contact with that part of my family. By that time they were all living in Manchester, including Harry, but with the exceptions of aunt Pearl, the oldest, and living with her husband Mark in Israel at that time, my uncle Rueben who was living in Hackney with his family, and my Uncle Lesley who had emigrated to Australia with his family just after the war.

My dad had had a large family of siblings; these were five girls and five boys, of these, I had only ever met the two uncles already mentioned. I contacted Uncle Harry by letter, to advise him of my intention and to ask him to facilitate the event. He was overjoyed and agreed that it would be best to say nothing to my parents beforehand; being away from home made this much easier for me. I simply said that I was going to be on guard duty that weekend. Joy, of course, was party to the intrigue.

My next task was to negotiate a long weekend away from camp. It was an awkward time of year in some ways, being winter time. For me to travel to the family on a Friday, I would have to leave early, so as to get to the house well before sunset. Shabbat, which is the Sabbath, comes in just as the first stars are, or would be if it were cloudy, shining in the sky. It lasts from Friday night to Saturday night. I did not want to make a bad impression by arriving by public transport, after Shabbat was under way.

I explained to my flight sergeant, that, due to a long lasting family argument between my parents and my paternal family, I had never met my paternal grandmother. I also explained about my need to get to the house before sunset. I asked him if there was any way I could take a day's leave for my mission. He said that he would see what he could do. That was on a Monday morning.

Once again I was to be surprised by the kindness and consideration shown to me by my now colleagues in the RAF. After lunch Mr Rubin called me into the office he shared with the warrant officer in charge of the orderly room and whose name I cannot remember.

"Flight Sergeant Lane has explained your problem to me." Was all he said as he handed me an envelope. I was gradually becoming aware that he loved a dramatic and mysterious gesture.

"Open it," this being all he would say in response to my quizzical look. I did so and inside was a travel warrant made out in my name for a return journey between King's Lynn and Manchester for the next weekend beginning on Friday morning. I was completely lost for words.

"I trust that you can make your trip this weekend. The flight sergeant has told me, that, in spite of your otherwise bolshie attitude, you have settled into your work well. I have authorised a compassionate leave of absence for this coming weekend including Friday."

I did not know what to say. My mind was in a whirl as to how I was going to organise myself and my family. So far the trip had been a totally theoretical proposition. Now all the ways and means had been handed to me on a plate and I was close to getting cold feet. I was in a mild funk as I muttered...

"Thank you sir, thank you very much."

I made as if to shake his hand but he waived me away with the biggest bunch of fingers I had ever seen on a man.

"Go away" - was all that he would add. I did, however, feel that I had caught sight of an embryo grin on his face or in his eyes before I turned towards the door.

I made the arrangements with my uncle Harry. I advised my parents that I would not be home that weekend and I let Joyce know that 'operation family' was due to take place on this coming weekend. Suddenly it was Friday morning and I was on the train on route to Manchester.

As I travelled my anxieties grew. How would they receive me? Would they receive me? I knew that Uncle Harry would be OK but I had never met or spoken with any of the others. I was aware that, apart from Boobah and Uncle Harry, several others - my Aunt Freda, my aunt Fay, and another uncle, older than Harry, my uncle Isaac, also

lived there. It had to be a large house, I thought, as I left the train at Manchester New Street. I felt a sigh of relief as I saw the familiar and friendly face of dear old Uncle Harry on the forecourt at the end of the platform. He waived to me and kept waiving well after he must have seen that I had noticed him. I'm not certain of this but I do think that we were both nervous. It's crazy I thought. I'm only going to meet my grandmother. What could happen? That, though, was the problem for me in a nutshell; I did not know what could happen.

I have to say, however, that the journey through central Manchester in my uncle's old Ford 'Popular' did an awful lot to take my mind off of the meeting with my family. My priority quickly switched to the imminent possibility of meeting my maker! I later found out that Harry had never passed a driving test, largely due to the fact that he had never bothered to apply! Ike [my uncle Isaac] I discovered later, had passed a test in the army driving trucks. Receiving your licence under those circumstances seemed to have relied on the supreme test, that if you didn't actually hit a wall or kill a pedestrian, you got your licence. Driving tests were under the supervision of a sergeant assigned to the task. Harry and Ike were at about the same level as far as their driving abilities were concerned. I later found out that riding with either one of them as a passenger required a supreme confidence in one's good standing with the almighty. I was greatly relieved when, at last, my driver pulled to a stuttering halt outside a large house in Howe Street, Salford.

As we walked up the steps and path towards the house, though, my nervousness rapidly switched back from the cliff-edge experience of the drive from the station to the immediate prospect of meeting my Boobah for the first time. How would she receive me? Would she receive me? Would she be angry with me at this invasion of her home, particularly on erev Shabbat? A veritable melange of disturbed and disturbing thoughts weighed heavily on my shoulders as we approached the door. Harry, however, appeared to be magnificently unaware that anything unusual was about to happen. He ushered me

through the front door with a forceful shove between the shoulder blades and a cheerful "C'mon son, let's get on with it."

I found myself in a large hallway, dark, undecorated, and uncared for, apparently for many years. That though was very much the least of my concerns at that moment. To my far right the stairs led up to the first and second floors. To my immediate right was a door that, I later discovered, was that of the front room. Below the stairs were another set of stairs apparently leading down to a basement. In front of me, slightly to my left, was a room into which I could not see, as it was so dark inside, but I later found out that it was my uncles' workroom. To the right of that room was a smaller room from which I could hear quiet voices. Harry guided me towards this room. "They're all in the dining room," he explained.

I did not see at first just how many people there were in the dining room, which was not a large room, but clearly served as the main family room in this large house. I looked round quickly in order to locate my grandmother. I was not interested in anyone else at that moment. I just wanted to see her reaction to me and to get over the tension I was feeling. I spotted her almost at once. She seemed to be as apprehensive as I was.

Boobah was sitting in an armchair across the small room and, in the tumult of emotions that I was feeling; her sudden reaction hit me like a bombshell. She sat still as a stone in her chair. She took one look at me and just burst into tears. She simply fell into a torrent of tears, her shoulders shaking visibly under the comforting ministrations of one of my aunts. I was totally unprepared for this, as was everyone else in the room. The other aunt immediately glared at me, as if blaming me totally, for this unexpected outcome. She began to shout something at me in a mixture of Yiddish and English.

I did not know who was who at that time, which made the situation that much more dramatic and uncertain for me. Through the melée I could see my grandmother, still in tears, beginning to waive everyone down from their initial panic. Nothing ventured, nothing

gained. I crossed the room so as to stand next to Boobah. Slowly she looked up at me and, without attempting to dry her eyes; she took me by the hand, but continued to sob gently. The tumult, the gevalt, died a natural death.

Many times over the years have I wondered at my grandmother's reaction, trying to assess the reasons for it. The best that I have ever come up with is that my dad was 22 years old when he left and was regarded as dead by some members of his family, especially Boobah. I was just a few weeks short of my twenty second birthday when I walked into her living room that Friday evening. I believe that this coincidence of circumstances was too much for her. She did not stand up, instead she pulled me down to her level to give me a long sobbing hug. I took that opportunity to regain some of my own composure. Had it come down to this? I thought sadly. All that family 'gehokteh tsuris', bitter trouble, all that real family suffering, perpetrated over all those years by religious bigotry, family pride and cultural difference. Does it all, in the final analysis, come down to the sobbing and tears of a frail old lady, who is suddenly confronted with all that she has missed, by the arrival of a total stranger? I suddenly felt real, deep sadness for both of us.

There were two women in the room, apart from my grandmother, whose names I already knew but not which was which. Freda, though, I soon discovered, had been the one who had looked as if she were quite prepared to blame me for having mischievously upset my Boobah. Fay was the calming influence. These discoveries gelled totally with verbal biographies I had received about these two ladies. My Uncle Ike sat behind where I stood beside Boobah; he stood up and put his arm round my shoulder. "A gut shabbos boychick" was all he had time to say before Fay began to light the candles on the table. I was not, though, fully aware of any of this because, I had just noticed a young boy sitting, dwarfed by his huge armchair, near to the door by the hallway. I must have walked right past him as I had made my way towards my grandmother. He was about 12 or 13 years

old and I had known absolutely nothing about his existence. I must have been staring at him.

"That's Shimmon" my Aunt Fay explained "he's my son, your cousin," she added somewhat unnecessarily. I was intrigued. I had suddenly added a whole new cousin to my already long list of relatives. I removed the flat cap that I had worn for the trip and donned a yarmulke, a skullcap, for the Shabbos meal. I do not habitually wear either garment except in Shul, Synagogue, but I had come prepared for this occasion. Uncle Ike then said the Shabbos prayers and we had all said the broches over the challah and the wine. They were surprised that I could do this, for broches are short prayers of thanks giving. Challah on the other hand is a braided bread, very rich and one of the few really great Jewish contributions to world cuisine. Harry took no part in the saying of prayers, for he, like my Dad, was a staunch communist.

The meal proper then began with the inevitable chicken soup, naturally. I managed to carry myself quite well through the meal without making any mistakes or faux pas, right to the end, that is, when tea was served. Without thinking I asked for milk in my tea. Boobah kept a kosher kitchen and we had just had a meat meal. I knew about kashrut from my reading of Jewish law but had never had the experience of living under the laws and behaviour of such a regime. My Aunt Freda took great pleasure in giving me the unexpurgated version, just as if I were a naughty child. I very quickly began to feel that she and I were not going to get along! The word kosher simply applies to that food which obeys the laws of Kashrut; the laws of which are far too complex to endeavour to explain here. They deal, in fact with the whole of Jewish life, much more than just food.

Jewish orthodox life is dominated by the laws of kashrut which, for our purposes here, focus on Jewish dietary laws, the main element of which, again for the purposes of this commentary, is the very strict separation of milk and meat in meals. The code of Jewish Law is derived directly from the bible, which is regarded as the written

word of the almighty. Biblical exhortations within the bible became interpreted and expounded upon by erudite rabbis over hundreds of years to become formulated into two learned and sacred books, the two Talmudim; the Babylonian and Jerusalem Talmudim, each of which identifies and explains rabbinical interpretations of biblical texts such as the one from which we receive the law to separate milk and meat.

"Thou shalt not seethe the kid in its own mother's milk."

There are several theories given for this injunction. Whether you are a believer that the bible is the direct 'word', or are of the view that it was more likely written by wise sages, who only wished to guide a recalcitrant people into an orderly path, there is one theory that most appeals to me. It is one that relies on a basis of concerned animal husbandry in that one should not offend the 'mother' twice, firstly by slaying her young and then, secondly, by using her own milk to cook it.

"Why milk?" I hear you ask. Remember that these ancient peoples were nomadic and that water was a precious commodity that had to be carried from water hole to water hole. To cook the meat in milk may well have been a convenient way of preparing it 'for the table'. These are my thoughts and do not reflect accepted Jewish Law.

This biblical text is regarded as being of particular importance to the almighty because it is stated no less than three times in the bible; twice in Exodus and once in Deuteronomy. For this reason the rabbis felt that it required more than usual attention and gave it a unique importance at the centre of Jewish family life.

There is a social hierarchy of 'kosher' that has inevitably developed in some elements of Jewish society, whereby people strive to be more 'kosher' than the next person. This may operate less at the truly, most orthodox strands of Jewish society, where everyone is at the same level, partly because the communities are so tight. Perhaps, though, I am less than qualified to talk about that. To declare my own perspective I am of the view that we should all live and let live.

When I enter a kosher house I behave accordingly. I know what I am doing in a kosher kitchen and would do nothing to devalue it. When pushed, though, I have to say that I am of the view that these particular laws of kashrus have the effect of tying women to the kitchen and to the home. To keep a truly kosher home is a full time occupation. I obey the biblical injunction to my own satisfaction by having never seethed a kid in its own mother's milk and will never do so unless, my life depended on it. I do not say this flippantly moreover.

When I thoughtlessly asked for milk in my tea at that meal, I failed to recognise that my Boobah's house would be a 'kosher' house. I settled for lemon in my tea, which I often take as a preference in any case.

The meal itself, though, passed off in good style with several glasses of wine. After the meal we sat and talked. Boobah actually asked me about Mum and Dad and my Sister Denise. I answered her questions as fully as I could, with Uncle Harry prompting me here and there as he saw fit. He did, of course, know us quite well, as he had made it his business never to lose contact with us. I discovered that Uncle Ike enjoyed reading science fiction books and that he had an old tea chest nearly full of ones that he had read. This news immediately established a bond between us, as I explained that I had just finished reading the Asimov 'Foundation Trilogy', which is still, I believe, one of the 'musts' among S.F. aficionados.

Uncle Ike asked me if I would like to go to Shul with him in the morning, to which I replied, quite honestly, that I would very much like to do so and to which my dear Uncle Harry snorted his disgust. He was made of the same communist building blocks as my dad, which is probably why there had always been such a strong affinity between them.

I went to Shul with my uncle the next morning after a quick breakfast of tea, challah and cream cheese. We met some of his old friends and I was greeted with genuine warmth. I explained that my Hebrew was 'weak', which, in fact, was not even the half of it. I

was then given the mitzvah, an act of merit, of opening the arc and 'undressing' the Torah scroll. A nice Kiddush was held after the service. The Kiddush, never to be confused with Kaddish, is the prayer and ceremony that sanctifies the Sabbath and Jewish Holy Days. We then returned to the house in good spirits chatting about the area, about Manchester, about science fiction books and authors we liked the most. Finally, after some considerable hesitation, he got around to his feelings about my dad and his behaviour when he got married.

It was a subject that I had hoped would not come up so soon, although, if it were to do so, I felt that Uncle Ike was the best one in the family to broach it with me. His view, he explained, was that my dad had been wrong in going off to get married in secret and then by dropping the bomb, as he saw it, on his mother. Marriage 'outside' as he put it, just was not possible in those days. "These days however,......" he paused as if preparing himself for something that he found difficult to express......"more is possible" He looked at me and clearly there was more that he wanted to say.

"Do you know what a Shidduch is?"

"Yes, it's an arranged marriage." What on earth was coming? I thought to myself.

"We have one we could do for you." It was like a bullet to the heart. Here was I, beginning to think that my first trip to my Manchester family was going so well when 'bam', I was suddenly being thrown back into family politics, potentially as complicated as those that I had come to Manchester to resolve. I turned and looked at my uncle; the look of astonishment must have been writ clear across my face. To do him credit he did show some embarrassment himself.

"You know that I'm engaged to be married to Joyce?" It was half question, half statement of fact. He responded without acknowledging my comment.

"The girl I'm talking about is a nice Jewish girl, good family, good prospects...err...financially." I sensed that his heart was not in this.

"Then why is she not already married and why, why on earth, would she want to marry me?"

"You should speak to Harry....." He managed to get this in just before we made our way into the house.

We had reached the house and I was becoming angrier by the minute. My family weekend had been hijacked in a most unexpected, unlikely and unwelcome manner. Just how and when this had all been cooked up I could not imagine. I had only arranged this visit with Uncle Harry during the past week. How on earth had they come up with this in such a short time? Manchester Jewish, off the peg, marriage service or what! I had to speak quietly to Uncle Harry to get to the bottom of this and to stop these thoughts from going any further. I wanted to try to do it without offending anyone if I could. Who was the shadchen here? Yes indeed who was the actual marriage broker?

Luckily I had already arranged with Harry to take a walk to a local market to have a 'mooch' around after Shul. Thankfully I did not have to argue down too strongly an offer of a lift in the car as it was Shabbat. I would have to accept a lift back to the station on Sunday but didn't want to load the dice too negatively, when I could avoid it. I took the route of pleading the 'Shabbos' case to Uncle Ike. We had, after all, only just returned from Shul. This argument was totally lost on my Uncle Harry. Nonetheless we agreed that to walk would be pleasant...

I was continuing to feel that after a fairly good start, my weekend had taken a very unexpected and unwelcome turn. I desperately wanted to get Uncle Harry on his own, so that I could quiz him on the latest turn of events. I did not want to offend anyone but, if that was what it would take, then so be it.

Unfortunately Harry was not as much help as I would have hoped. He seemed to think that the whole idea was close to a joke. Not a joke to me though! I pushed the questioning.

"Listen to me" he responded roughly after a series of questions from me. We were walking down the hill along Bury New Road

towards Manchester. "The whole idea of shiduchim, [arranged marriages plural], at any time, let alone these days, is crazy, immoral." That was all he would say on the subject, except for,

"You'll need to speak to Ike. He's the genius who thought this one up, to try to please your Boobah you understand. You'll need to keep your guard up though. He's ok but he's not speaking for himself."

After a while he added, "Do not raise this subject with your aunts. They're both as daft as three bob bits! " So then the shadchen was a collective of two!

That was it then; I felt as though I was being passed from one to the other. I now had to wait until I could get Uncle Ike alone, in order to kill the plan, if indeed there was an actual plan, at birth.

As my uncle and I walked on together, however, we began to chat on other subjects. He had been a feature in my life for as far back as I could remember. I began to realise, though, that I really knew very little about him. Whenever he had visited us he had always been pleasant but was, in reality, coming to visit Dad. My Uncle Harry was a bit of a loner. For many years he had been a merchant seaman. I got the strong feeling that this had been to get away from his 'meshuggeneh' family. I was certain then, and it became confirmed in later years, that my Dad was the only member of the family for whom he had a strong family feeling. According to my Uncle Rueben, his youngest brother, I took over that role when my father passed away, but that truly is another story.

"Mum doesn't speak much English." He volunteered this information a propos of nothing. "You'll have to learn some Yiddish yourself, as most of the talk around the table is in 'Mame Loshen' that's Yiddish in Yiddish," he grinned. In fact Mame Loshen means mother's language.

"Don't worry, though, we don't have deep intellectual conversations in this family. It's mostly 'pass me the salt' Yiddish. You'll have no trouble."

"You know?" he began after a short period of thoughtful walking. "One time, when I was in Israel, I went to live for a while with an orthodox and Yiddish speaking family. I really didn't think I'd have any trouble but I was way out of my depth. Their level of the language went way beyond me. They actually had conversations about politics and things; didn't talk much about passing the salt!"

He grinned as we walked on down the road as we passed the ominous walls of the Strangeways Prison. "Not far now" he informed me. I glanced back over my shoulder. We had come quite a way from the house and it was all uphill on the way back.

The 'market' when we reached it, wasn't much more than a small collection of stalls just back from the main road. Still Harry seemed to enjoy the experience, as he took himself slowly from one to the other, chatting casually to each stall-holder as he did so. He didn't seem intent on buying anything, whereas I actually found a few items I would have bought if I had had the spare cash. I did, eventually, end up with one book, science fiction, which I had not read but, in truth, I was hoping that my Uncle Ike had not read it, on the basis that it would be something with which to break the ice, before I pressed him about the Shidduch. My two uncles were apparently playing 'pass the parcel' with that one, and with me…

They were all there, waiting for us it seemed. We were offered tea, which I accepted gratefully, as the walk had given me quite a thirst. It seemed that I could have either lemon or milk on this occasion because we had reached a neutral point in time between meals when milk could be taken with the tea. I do not intend to go into the details of that here. Enough to say that I was getting the full story from Aunt Freda as I was coming through the door, as I was taking my coat off, as I was saying hello again to everyone and explaining where we had been and what we had done and as I was sitting down. She was one of these people who can [a] talk much faster than 18 to the dozen and [b] keep her concentration fixed steadfastly on to her

theme, no-matter whatever else was going on in the room. She was a phenomenon.

We all drank tea, milky, and engaged in quiet conversation once Freda had exhausted her 'flayshdich – milshdich'mini lecture. I took this quiet opportunity, really for the first time, to begin to take in my surroundings. I have to admit, although I take no pride in doing so, that they were not prepossessing and that is to say the least. Beyond the small dining room I could see, through a door in the opposite corner from where I sat, a glimpse of a small kitchen or scullery. It may be kosher, I thought sadly, but it's not particularly clean. The dining room come lounge in which we all sat was scruffy and not well appointed with material possessions. The floor was covered with a sad, beige lino. Worst of all, however, several chickens roamed the room, apparently quite confident that they were welcome and that no-one would put them out of the house. I began to realise that this house was truly meshuggeneh rather than homely. Boobah did seem to have all her marbles but had lost both maternal and material control over this 'bag of cats'. The chickens were, apparently, the property of my uncle Harry. He insisted that they provided a 'homely' atmosphere!

There had been ten siblings, of whom four still lived 'at home', plus Boobah and my newly acquired cousin, Shimmon. They lived, but there was little love in evidence in that house. There was a series of underlying tensions that I only began, poorly, to sense, let alone unravel, at that time. Any details, that I am able to give here, are as a result of the knowledge and familiarity that I gained subsequently, over the years.

The youngest of the four siblings living with my grandmother at that time was my aunt Fay [Feygeleh]. She was a woman, then in her early forties. I had just discovered that she had a son, Shimon, the latest acquisition to my fairly long list of cousins on both sides of my family. She was still married to Shimon's father, although he had been neither a steadfast husband nor an attentive father. By the time

that I came to visit the family she was, in fact, engaged in the second period of marriage to that same man. Max and Fay had met when Fay had made Aliya to Israel a few years after it declared statehood in 1948. She became pregnant and they got married, in that order, in Israel, where Shimon was born.

Max demonstrated his feckless attitude to both marriage and fatherhood very early on, both as a wastrel and a 'shpieler' i.e. an inveterate gambler. Any money that the man earned through his often successful business enterprises throughout his life, he squandered away at the tables. He demonstrated the total fallacy of at least one old saying by being a total nothing, both at cards and as a lover. Fay and Max parted company shortly after Shimon was born. It would be a more accurate description to say that Max parted from them! Mother and son came back to England where she obtained a civil divorce, but Max refused to allow her a 'Get' under Jewish law which meant that she could never re-marry as a Jewish woman in Synagogue. The word 'Get' meaning 'cutting off' and is used to indicate divorce.

There is total inequality, however, in Jewish law as laid down in the Talmud, as when a man initiates divorce he has to free his wife from the marriage in the form of a written document known as the 'Get'. If the man refuses this document he can re-marry but she cannot; not if she wants to live a Jewish life. She is then known as 'agunah' [anchored]. This was absolutely the position that aunt Fay was in because Max had refused to consider a religious divorce, whereas Fay had obtained only a civil divorce, due to Max's abandonment of his family and continued refusal to have anything much to do with them. After a period of some years, however, she gave in to what she saw as the inevitable and re-married him in a second civil ceremony. According to my dad, though, when discussing his family in later years, Max's insistence on re-marriage had been for sordid tax reasons. Nonetheless, they were re-married by the time that I first met my aunt Fay.

It has just occurred to me as I write here, that my oldest paternal aunt dad's sister Pearl, [Polly], was actually declared 'agunah' by a religious court when her first husband 'died'. This man was also a Max and Polly married him sometime in the thirties. He later became a merchant seaman and served during the war on the transports to Russia, a well-known and very hazardous field of endeavour during that period of our history.

In any event Max's ship was sunk and he was declared 'lost' at sea. That description was not good enough for the religious authorities and so she was advised that she could never marry in synagogue unless her first husband's death could be verified. The implications for an orthodox woman of ignoring this injunction are usually very serious, for her, and for any children that she might have as a result of a new and 'forbidden' union. The children become 'mamzerim' [bastards], which means in Jewish law a child of any unlawful union, and not a child simply born out of wedlock. 'Mamzerim' are not able to enter into Jewish life in any meaningful way, not ever!

After the war Polly moved to Israel where she met a man, yet another Max, who was a survivor from the 'camps' and who's whole family, wife and four children, had been murdered by the Germans. Polly and Max3 decided that they wanted to get married but, of course, a Jewish marriage was out of the question for her and so they went over to Cyprus and engaged in a civil marriage there. They knew that there was no question for them of having children due to age and personal circumstances but wanted to live together as man and wife. Many years later, after Max3 had passed away and Polly was living back in Manchester with the family, I heard her refer to the civil ceremony. "As far as we were concerned, she smiled; the religious authorities could go hang!"

My uncle Ike is the one who I know least about. He was not a tall man. In fact no-one in that family was tall. The men averaged about 5'7" – 5'8". My lasting memory of Ike was that he was the one who, on my grandmother's insistence, tried to arrange a quite unlikely and

very unwanted marriage for me. I never asked for the details but was told that the poor young woman in question was, by local standards, 'on the shelf'. Her father was a rich man in the community and was prepared to 'arrange' a quick conversion for me followed by an even quicker marriage for the pair of us. Apparently 'my prospects would have been good' if I had been prepared to play ball. For all sorts of reasons, Joyce certainly being the main one, it was an arrangement that I could never have even looked at. I never even saw the woman in question.

Apart from that 'barn pot' plan, however, Ike always seemed to me to be a kindly and quiet man. He was short and stocky and wore an almost permanent smile on his face, as well as a Trilby hat on his head, under which he also wore a yarmulke. He also wore a Tzitzit Katan which is a short vest-like garment with ritual fringes. These garments were regularly worn by Jewish men in those days but are less common nowadays, except by more religious men. Shimon was the only other one of my male relatives who I ever knew to wear one. I met with Ike perhaps a half dozen times during my trips to Manchester and each time he invited me to attend services with him. I always agreed readily to do so, as I have always enjoyed the informality of what is, in fact, a ritualised service. Everything according to a well understood and established order.

My aunt Freda was a bird of a very different feather, however. I really do not think that I ever saw her smile. Nor, now that I think about it, did I ever see or hear my uncle Harry speak to her. Many years later, when Shimon was grown, married and working as the Chazzan, the [Cantor], at the great synagogue in Cologne, I discovered from him the reason for both of these family tensions.

Freda was well into her forties by the time that I first met her at the house in Manchester. Of all those in the house she was the least friendly towards me, or to anyone for that matter. She was, as far as I was concerned, a most unprepossessing character. Her glass was not simply always half empty, it rarely reached a quarter full! She was by

far the meanest personality and moaniest person I ever met in my life. It was not until I learned from Shimon of some of the events of her early life, many years later, that I began to put her attitude into a more balanced perspective.

Freda had an unkempt and unwashed appearance. She made no effort to make the best of herself. Added to her defects of character and personality, her face was physically disfigured as if she had had a stroke, from which she had been left with this permanent and cruel affliction. I was told by my grandmother, and supported by others in the room at the time, that when Freda was a child she had been inclined to make faces at others and that, in spite of being warned of the dire consequences, she had been in the act of doing this one day when the wind had changed and she had been left with this terrible result. I could not tell at the time whether this tale was just a way of telling me to mind my own business or whether they actually expected me to believe that rubbish, a real Boobah-Myseh, an old wives' tale. Whatever that case may have been I was not interested enough, at that time, to pursue the matter.

Many years later, about thirty years later in fact, in 1991, I was passing some eight days in the apartment occupied by Shimon and his then wife Hedvah, in the Cologne synagogue, when I learned more of the true story from him. The story that unfolded from Shimon, with Hedvah adding her own acidic embroidery, was one of tragedy afflicting a young girl in accordance with the very ignorant public mores of those times; the 1930s.

It seems that Freda, when still a young girl of 14 years of age, was made pregnant by a religion teacher, who had taken to visiting the family to teach the younger boys their bar-mitzvah. As I heard the story I realised that I was hearing an early tale of very serious sexual grooming. The family reacted badly and totally unsupportive of Freda; who they blamed entirely for the 'embarrassing' circumstances. They decided that she would have to have an abortion which, in those days, meant a back street grope with a knitting needle. The

baby was aborted but poor Freda was left with both psychological as well as physical injuries.

From what I gathered from Shimon, I learned that she had developed some form of blood poisoning from the incompetent treatment she had received. She nearly died. I know nothing of the medical treatment she would have received but, suffice it to say, it was the effects of the abortion and not the changing of the wind that had wrought havoc on that young girl's health and appearance. No-wonder, I thought, that her glass was never even partially full.

As Shimon and, to my growing anger, Hedvah, related the story, it became clear that they still regarded Freda as being totally at fault over this incident, as she had brought shame on the family which was the reason why Harry, 'understandably', refused to speak to his younger sister even decades after the event.

At this point I had my one and only serious argument with Shimon; he was after all my cousin and had become my friend over the years. I pointed out, very angrily, that as a religious man and religion teacher himself, he should realise that the family had committed a huge injustice, a sin as I put it to him, against that little girl who, in the cultural bubble in which she lived, probably did not even know what was happening to her when that 'pig' raped her. I used the Yiddish/Hebrew word 'chazer' thus making clear what I thought of the visiting chazzan who had, apparently, extricated himself totally free, and without blemish, from the situation.

I made it clear that I thought that the family had been spineless in their lack of support of Freda; Harry in particular. It would have been no sin, I reminded Shimon, in the Jewish Law that he so revered, for Freda, a child herself, unknowingly, to have brought a child into the world out of wedlock. What was definitely a sin in Jewish law, though, was to 'murder' an innocent unborn child. I was just sorry that I was not able to make my feelings known to other members of the family who had, sadly, all passed away by the time that we three were having that conversation.

I have often thought of Freda over the years and of the anguish that she must have felt as a young girl in a situation that she could not have fully understood; born into a family so unsupportive and ignorant. I am both sorry and very ashamed, for her, of that episode in my family's history.

Whenever now I think of my Uncle Harry, I am reminded of the adage that even good men can do bad things. For having behaved so badly, for so many years, towards his sister, I cannot forgive him. Yet it was a strange family, twisted by tensions that are past understanding in this day and age. In all my dealings with him he was a kindly and quiet spoken man. During the short periods of time that I was in the house in Manchester, together with both him and Freda, I did not really recognise the extent of his refusal to speak to her. As I say, by the time that Shimon spoke to me in his apartment in Cologne all the relevant parties had passed away.

Yes, Harry was kind, a quiet spoken and thoughtful man and yet Shimon had one last disturbing recollection of our uncle that disturbed me just as much as his revelation regarding his attitude towards his sister Freda. It seems that Harry, in a quasi-parental role in the absence of Shimon's father, took it upon himself to discipline Shimon when he, Harry, felt that it was necessary. The form of discipline that he favoured was to shut the boy, for varying periods of time, in the cellar below the house. This cellar was accessed from the hallway. It was dark and dingy when I saw it and cluttered with old furniture, sewing machines of various types, no longer usable, as well as various other forms of junk. It was no 'playground' experience for a young and frightened boy in the deep dark gloom of that cellar. These tales by my cousin made me realise that, for him, his boyhood had not been a happy experience. For having behaved so badly, for so many years, towards his nephew, yet again I cannot forgive my Uncle Harry. It was no wonder that Shimon took the only way out of that house that he could, as soon as he could, by going to Yeshiva and studying religion to become a Chazzan. For some years in the 70s he

studied at Jews' College in London, where he and I met up from time to time for tea or coffee and, sometimes, a bun. On infrequent occasions he came over to see me in Whitechapel where we would have lunch in a kosher fish restaurant.

How do I explain this abhorrent behaviour by an uncle of whom both Shimon and I remained so fond? I can do so but only after much hesitation. Suffice it to say, that, in spite of Harry's outward calm and quiet persona, there was always an anxious tension within him. He was not a happy man. He was pursued mentally by the idea of marriage and family and this tortured him, to the extent that he would rarely speak of any relationships, past or present. Over the years I became quite convinced that he was gay. I do not mention this to explain his terrible behaviour, far from it. I put it into the mix both as an explanation and description of the tortured soul of a man who could not declare his true feelings, at a time and within a culture, wherein 'coming out' just was not an option. After considerable reflexion on the subject, I am convinced that it is this enforced imprisonment of his true self that, at least in part, explains the extreme nature of his behaviour towards the young girl, his sister, and the young boy, his nephew.

In the later years of Harry's life I am the one who came to be the closest to him. This all began to develop after Dad died. I remember my Uncle Rueben once saying to me, when we were chatting in the office of his factory in Hackney road, "You know, Tony, now your Dad is no longer with us Harry only comes to London to see you. He never comes to see me and I'm his brother." There was no rancour in his words, just a sad statement of fact.

My main reason for my trip to Manchester in the first place had been to see my grandmother and, perhaps, to make up some of the ground that had been lost between us over the years. This was, of course, a forlorn hope. My vision had been blurred by the really good and loving relationship I had with my maternal grandmother. To build anything like that was, naturally, a hope too far. Firstly, they were

very different characters. My Boobah never behaved towards Shimon in the way my maternal grandmother behaved towards her grandchildren. She had always been demonstrative of her feelings, both loving and disciplinary. She was quite prepared to give you the unexpected cuddle; sometimes unwelcome to a teenage boy but she did not care.

I can still remember, as a young boy, being half suffocated in her ample bosom as she gave me a hug. I can also remember, still with affection, the day when I was being nagged, in her front room, by Nan and a couple of my aunts. I was about 14 at the time, the oldest grandchild and 'flexing my muscles' in the family. I turned on Nan and shouted at her to "Shut up!" The next thing I knew I was flat on my back with a sore face and a much bruised ego. She had fetched me a 'backhander 'that took me quite off my feet. It was the only time that I can remember her hitting me but I never ever shouted at her again.

In all the times that I visited my family in Manchester I never saw a sign of demonstrative love or affection between Boobah and Shimon. As far as I was concerned I could not have expected to build the relationship with her that can only develop through close association between adult and child through the early years and throughout the child's life. I think that I can claim, though, to have built a bridge whereby we actually got on very well. The twin hurdles of culture and language were always there of course.

Boobah began to soften towards me when she realised that I was quite knowledgeable on Jewish culture and religion, even though I was not a religious person myself. I also made a point of learning some Yiddish. I would never claim to speak the language but that was not needed in that house. There was not much in-depth conversation or discussion between adults in that house. 'Pass the salt' was all that was needed in order to please her and to convince all of them that, together with my general knowledge of things Jewish, my 'Yiddishkayt' was up to standard.

I had one more memorable experience with which to end my first weekend in Manchester. It was occasioned by an argument between

my two uncles, as to which of them was to take me back to the station. I don't know how he did it, for he rarely gained one over his brother, but Ike won the day; he only won on points, however, because Harry decided to come with us and, moreover, to sit in the passenger seat beside Ike. Well, I can only say that that trip to the station remains one of the most dramatic, even terrifying, events of my life. The car behaved as if it were being driven by a committee! Which, in essence it was, a short committee of two. It was a relief to get to the station and it quite removed from me any emotion of regret that the weekend was over. Further emotions were aroused the next day, though, when I received an angry 'phone call from my dad. He had actually managed to get through to the accounts section at RAF Bircham Newton. Harry had 'phoned' him the previous evening to let him know what a great weekend we had all had together!

At this point I need to explain my feelings towards my own claim and assertion that I am Jewish for, of course, according to Orthodox Jewish law I am not. The fact is that I began to take up the mantel of being Jewish from about the age of eight. For all sorts of reasons you grow up quickly during a war and I was beginning to realise what had taken place in Europe during and before the war. It gradually dawned on me just what Hitler and his 'mamzerim' ['bastard'] cronies had perpetrated on the world, on the Jewish people and on my family. It also filtered down to me that, if the Germans had crossed the Channel, I would have been subject to the same fate as all Jews. I also began to realise at that early age the full meaning of 'final solution'.

In my small and child-like way I decided, over a period of time, that I would declare myself as Jewish, so as to make up, in very small part, for some of the evil that had been done and for all of those who had been murdered. It may have been a childish intention but it was and is, heartfelt. In later years I went before a panel of Liberal Jewish Rabbis at the Synagogue in St. John's Wood to discuss my Jewish knowledge. This revolved around my 'Yiddishkayt' rather than my religious competence. Perhaps this was to my advantage, because I

walked out of that building as a full member of the Liberal Jewish Community.

I am not displeased with myself for the stand I began to take regarding my early decision to think of myself as Jewish. I have always regarded that decision as being between myself and both my perished family, as well as all the other victims of that, the most terrible state sponsored terrorism, that was the Holocaust. It was a decision based upon ethnicity rather than a religious belief. Shimmon once pointed out to me that I was in fact allowing 'Hitler' to decide my identity. By this he meant, of course, my religious identity. My response to him was as a question, "Who then, in the twentieth century had a greater impact on who was or was not a Jew?" I took public charge of my decision very early. It was at school during the calling of the register; the teacher asked my Christian name for some reason that I cannot remember. I do remember, though, that I had summoned the courage to point out that I did not have a Christian name as I was not a Christian, that I was Jewish. That was my own version of 'coming out'. That was in 1947 or 48. I do not remember exactly.

19

The 'servicing' of Dad's car NXY 705

I AM NOW approaching my last few weeks of National service. I was at home one Saturday lunchtime, together with my parents. We were chatting about the past two years and I was explaining how I had come to dislike the service much less and that I had made some good friends. I mentioned several of them and one in particular, Ralph from South London, who happened to work in the motor pool.

I had noted that some of the permanent staff always had their cars serviced there for free. The motor pool staff often had time to fit the work in between their regular duties. I saw Dad's ears prick up at this and suddenly the conversation switched towards his own car. It appeared that NXY 705 badly needed a service and as Dad pointed out, it would be handy for me to have the car at camp to help me bring home some of my gradually acquired list of belongings. I readily saw the sense in this. I had been dreading the chore of somehow getting it all home on public transport services.

We agreed that I would make enquiries during the coming week and, if I got the go ahead from the motor pool mob, I would take the car back with me the following weekend. I rapidly became anxious to get the project under way ASAP, as I had to leave the camp in just a

few weeks' time. I could not bear the thought of the dreaded consequences if something went wrong with the work and I could not drive
the car home before my release date. I would not easily have been
able to stay in Norfolk to see the work through after my due date
because Joy and I were getting married just three days later. I rapidly
began to regret mentioning the motor pool at all.

At the time of my national service Dad's car was a Ford Anglia,
black as per the Henry Ford dictum; "You can have any colour....etc."
Dad was almost the first person in our road to own his own car, which
he bought new in about 1955; registration NXY 705. Sad, really, I can
remember the registration of that car, but not any other of sometimes lovely cars that I have owned over the years, other than the
latest. He was very proud of the car but was also generous about
allowing me to use it quite often.

Dad had his own driving style. It was one that pretty much
reflected his attitude to life in general. Wherever he was and whenever he was driving, he always obeyed the speed limit. He did this
largely out of pure stubbornness, for he also did his best to make
sure anyone behind him on the road was going to do the same and
stay behind him. This must have been really frustrating for anyone
trying to get to work in the morning in a hurry, having got up late and
trying to make up time; or anyone else for that matter that happened
to possess a simple, normal, level of frustration-tolerance.

Dad's method was to drive in the middle of the road at the speed
limit; a procedure designed to drive anyone behind him fighting mad
in suburban London during rush hour, where opportunities to pass
such a maddening individual were extremely limited. He must have
had his own personal lucky driving star hovering just above him every
time he took to the wheel, because no-one ever managed to get into
a position to confront him face to face. He did though promote some
angry horn work on his travels.

Dad had two further personal foibles re his driving. As soon as
he bought the car he joined the AA. He refused even to consider the

RAC because he felt that that was too posh. He didn't like the attachment of the word 'Royal' and, besides, the AA men gave you and your AA car badge a salute when you drove past them, sitting on their motor bikes, uniform and side-car displaying their AA credentials. He loved it!

Dad actually taught me to drive and was as pleased as Punch when I managed to pass first time. This was all the more so, simply because he was the one who taught me. In fact, as I remember it these many years later, it was the one solid and really positive activity that we accomplished together in those later years of my life at home. I say that I 'managed' to pass first time for good reason because I made two small mistakes that might well have failed me nowadays. I truly believe that it was the fact that I drove very confidently that got me through.

I very nearly drove my dad to utter and understandable rage a mere couple of days before my test though. I had spent the afternoon and evening at Joy's house and had stayed later than I had intended. I often walked home but realised that to walk home at that time of night would simply resurrect the old, "where have you been to this time of night?" confrontation from my mum. Even though I was 21 years old she would still be awake when I arrived home.

Without thinking I asked my future brother-in-law Sid, Joyce's brother, if I could borrow his car. Sid usually had a car around, although he never showed any interest in obtaining a driving licence or road tax or insurance! The current one was an old Austin shooting brake. Sid readily handed over the keys and showed me where the light switches etc. were. I set off home but as I turned into Lincoln road the nearside door flew open just as I was about to drive into the dip in the road under the railway bridge spanning the road.

The next few seconds were quite exciting, as I tried to drive one-handed whilst stretching across the car to struggle with the door, which, as was often the case in those days, was hinged at the back rather than the front as is usual nowadays. I could not stop the car

because there was little room and, as I was in a dip, I was all-but invisible to cars coming up behind me. With what seemed to me to be a heroic effort I managed to complete this driving challenge very successfully by closing the door without killing anyone.

A bit later that evening I was proudly relating to my parents just how clever I had been when my father nearly exploded. "Bloody Fool" was actually the worst language used, but his facial and body language left me in no doubt as to his true feelings and anger level, that, just two days before my driving test, I would take such a risk. It was beyond his understanding. The penny dropped very quickly, that I had thoughtlessly driven home without a driving licence and perhaps more importantly, without proper insurance cover. He pointed out that I could have lost my licence at the point of possibly gaining it. I could even have had a more serious penalty due to the lack of insurance. Yes, indeed, Dad was not at all pleased with me that night.

It was sad but true that, even apart from the above, my parents and I were going through a bad patch and that finally I was not as sorry as I might otherwise have been, when I had been forced to yield to the inevitable when given my final ultimatum from HM government. My mum and dad were intent on me going into a respectable career and one that would take me far away from the drudgery that clouded Dad's life, the 'rag trade'. He was a ladies' fashion pattern cutter of some considerable skill but, like all dads, I guess, wanted something better for his children. I was the oldest, my sister being eight years younger than I; the War and two miscarriages can be blamed for that. My parents' ideal choice of career for me was medicine.

Dad, like any good Jewish dad of those times wanted me to be a doctor. Unfortunately for domestic harmony, I preferred languages, my parents, however, could not see any future in that and so, in fact, they effectively chose the subjects I would study at 'A' level. Instead of French, German and English I was offered maths, chemistry and physics. I was even offered a place at the Charring Cross teaching hospital after an interview. Unfortunately for the plan my interview

skills were superior to my exam skills. In the exams I only passed maths and even that was no mean achievement for me.

I did attend Enfield Polytechnic for a further year in order to make a final attempt at the exams. I made the attempt but with little commitment; I have to admit that I put more effort into perfecting my 'bridge' game than my exams. After this final disappointment for my parents, I got a job at Chase Farm Hospital in Enfield as an operating theatre technician. That lasted a full year before the RAF finally got me. It was actually very interesting but it's also another story! It was during this period that I passed my driving test.

You will, perhaps, have noticed that my dad features more than my mum in the above paragraphs. That is because he took the lead when it came to matters of employment. This was the case even when it came to Mum's situation. She often expressed the desire to go out to work. This was not because we particularly needed the money but rather it was because she frankly found that being solely a housewife did not fulfil her needs. I realised much later how truly cruel was this confinement to housewifery for Mum. After Dad died she showed how capable she was of much more interesting endeavours. Again, though, that is another story.

Whenever the discussion came up Dad would not argue the point, he simply forbade it. There is no other way of putting it. He said 'no' and he meant it. I am very clear that he was a man of his time and saw a working wife as a slight to his own masculinity. He could not bring himself to be ahead of the times and be one of the first to move into the second half of the twentieth century.

In modern terms NXY 705 was a little beast of a car. It needed a gadget called a choke to help the engine to fire. This element was well named because too much use of it did make the engine 'choke', due to the fuel mixture in the carburettor becoming too rich. The engine also had to be physically turned over to make it fire. This was accomplished by the use of a starting handle that fitted through the bottom of the front grill, into the engine. This handle then needed

to be forcefully turned clockwise and with appropriate choke, with appropriate force and with the wind behind you the engine might fire. One more thing, one had to take great care to get the mix of those factors correctly balanced, for, if you didn't, then the engine might backfire, thus forcing the handle to rebound sharply anti-clockwise which could lead to a damaged or even a broken thumb. This procedure was not for the fainthearted, particularly in winter! No indeed, assuredly not for the faint hearted in winter!

The car had no heater other than the possibility of flask of hot tea and a blanket for the occupants. I have known my dad to actually drive the little beast with a blanket over his knees in winter. NXY 705 had neither radio nor window heaters. There was a warm air system that rose from the engine to help keep the windscreen clear of steam. This, however, relied on the warmth of the engine, a commodity that could take quite a time to arrive on cold days. Moreover, it was not at all efficient and you often had to drive with the side window open, even in the rain, to keep the windscreen from becoming totally opaque.

Nonetheless that little black car was my dad's pride and joy and I, notwithstanding the previous two paragraphs, remember that car with great affection, which is probably the reason that I still remember its registration number after all these years. Joyce and I did quite a bit of our courting in that car. We enjoyed trips out to the coast on a number of occasions. We even took Joyce's brother Sid and his then girlfriend, later to become his wife, for a trip out to Frinton-on-sea one weekend day before I was called up. Siddy was called up a few months after me.

Dad was quite generous when I asked to use the car at the weekends. Mum of course made regular acid comments that I only set foot in her home to pick up my clean washing and sometimes to borrow Dad's car! As I grow older and, I hope, wiser in the ways of the world, and families, I begin to realise that she led a disastrously boring existence from her point of view.

Dad would never relent his decision that she could not go out to work, yet her life at home was increasingly and mind numbingly boring, particularly with me in the process of living away from home and not intending to live at home after the RAF. I now realise that this is an emotional process that all parents must face. Dad of course was at work, and this for longer and longer days as their increasingly poor relationship continued to spiral downwards as if out of control.

There is no other way of putting it. My parents lived a life of open warfare. That situation existed as far back as I can remember. I recall that, as a child, I dreaded going to bed, because as soon as I went up the stairs [the wooden hill to Bedfordshire as the old saying goes] the battle began. To this day, I cannot explain the existence of this open warfare. I am sure, though, that its foundations spread far wider and deeper than Dad's refusal to let Mum go out to work, although that would not have helped the awful level of antagonism that existed between them. Individually they were both lovely people but together they were a disaster. Home should be a refuge from strife and blatant anger; for my parents it was neither, as the verbal battles frequently struggled on into the small hours.

When I finally succumbed to Her Majesty's kind invitation for me to bolster her military forces and bring them up to scratch for two years, I have long realised that I left one person to face this barrage alone. To my everlasting regret, my young sister was left at home to bear the brunt of our parents' internecine battles. She had a bad time of it and it is one of the major regrets in my life, that in my callow and shallow, youthful lack of understanding, I did not become aware of my sister's unhappiness until I was much older and it was far too late.

From conversations throughout our lives, I have come to understand that my sister had a much unhappier time of it even than I did. An added sadness for me is that she seems to have very few happy memories of her childhood, whereas I lived a Huckleberry Finn life for much if the time. It was the bedtimes that were largely unhappy

times. I am able to separate good times from bad, whereas she does not seem to have many good memories at all.

Getting back to the story in hand, however, I drove the car up to Norfolk, three weekends before the Wednesday that I was due to leave the RAF, and Bircham Newton, my home for nearly two years of my life. As I drove into the camp that Sunday afternoon, through the very pole gate that I had so innocently but determinedly and devastatingly closed many months beforehand, I realised that it was with very mixed feelings, that I was contemplating my imminent and permanent departure. At no point now did I consider making my RAF career a lasting career choice, yet I had made friends during my service. Among those friends was Bircham Newton camp and even the RAF itself. For me that had become a shocking realisation. If only I had been assigned to a trade more to my liking then, who knows, the end result might have been quite different. Mind you, the way that successive governments have treated our armed services..........

I handed my dad's beloved car over to my friends in the motor pool that Sunday evening. I returned to see the progress on the Monday evening after work and my heart sank and my gorge rose as I viewed the scene. To me there was nothing but the appearance of devastation. I had asked my mates to give a full service to my dad's old friend, for that is how he saw the car. I had said nothing about stripping the engine. The evidence of which now lay before me no longer where it should be, in the bloody car! The engine was out of the car and on a work bench with its bits strewn about that bench. I'm afraid that I raised my voice at this uncalled for vandalism.

The resulting exchange of views began to take a quite nasty turn. My energy being powered by thoughts of my explanations to my father and his views on the matter, when I took his dearest possession back to him on the back of a truck, still in bits but with an appropriate manual, complete with expanded diagrams to help him put her back together. My mood was not improved when one of the options

preferred by one of the vandals actually came very close to actually offering me the 'do it yourself' option. He was very lucky to live through those moments unscathed, but, just at the right moment my friend Ralph, the lad from South London, calmed me with the assurance that all would be well and that it would all be back together by the next evening. "They do this sort of thing all the time," he assured me.

Needless to say things did not work out as smoothly as Ralph had promised me. I returned to the motor pool after work on the Tuesday, with my insides churning in a mixture of hope and apprehension. Sad to say the expectation powered by apprehension trumped the version powered by hope. It was clear even to me that nothing had been done since the previous evening. Again I was re-visualising my dad's response when I returned the various parts of his car to him on the back of that truck. That particular eventuality had seemingly loomed just a fraction closer.

I was about to walk away from the workbench in that disheartened frame of mind, when I happened to glance into the bonnet cavity of the car. I was astonished to see that the whole interior of that inside front end of the car had been painted in rustproof paint. It was no longer black but was now clearly protected from weathering in the future. The paint-job, moreover, had been done neatly and to a decent standard. This was not, though, what I had asked the motor pool team to do and I remained concerned about the schedule. There seemed a lot to do to get the engine back together, to re-time and re-tune it, now that the pistons had been buffed and cleaned.

Less depressed, but still with my fingers crossed, I walked slowly back to the permanent staff junior ranks' mess to enjoy my dinner. Strange I thought, not for the first time, not at all for the first time, that with all the dire warnings both from my dad and Joyce's dad about military food, I could not remember even one unpleasant meal served up in the RAF.

They were all sitting together as usual, the motor pool team. They looked so smug that I felt forced to prick their bubble, just a bit. I spoke to my south London friend.

"I'm a bit worried Ralphie. There still seems a lot to do."

"I don't know," he responded "When do you intend going home."

"You know bloody well, you dick, I'm giving you a lift."

"Oh yeh, Saturday morning. Still got four whole days, no probs."

That was Tuesday evening. I went to bed that night after a few bevvies at a pub in Docking just a couple of miles away; just a nice walk on a summer evening when you want to clear your head and didn't I want to do just that! Trying as hard as I could, I simply could not rid myself of the thought of disappointing Dad by not being able to take his car back to him as promised, this coming weekend! And what the hell did Ralphie mean, four whole days? The terrible thought struck me that he might have made the error of thinking he had one more day than was actually available.

By the Wednesday afternoon I was quite nervous, as to what was going to greet me as I approached the motor pool after work and before dinner. I remember praying that I would be able to enjoy my dinner without the shadow of the car hanging over my shoulder like a fallen angel. I entered the hangar with some trepidation only to see that the car was, in fact, apparently intact. The engine was no longer sitting on the bench and, as I approached NXY705, I could see that there it was, in its proper place, sitting happily and squarely in the engine compartment.

The car, however, was still up on blocks. The motor pool crew hastened to advise me that they were simply finishing the service by examining the braking system; that all would be well by early the next morning. I ate my dinner and went to bed with a quiet heart and a clear mind for the first time that week. All too soon however! My reluctant chickens had not yet hatched!

It appeared that all was not well early the next morning. We are now in Thursday morning. The flight sergeant saw that I was

becoming anxious about the car and had sent me over to the motor pool, so as to get my anxiety out of his hair. He simply grinned when I said "Thanks Flight".

I was greeted by worried and frowning foreheads as I approached Dad's car. It looked OK to me. The wheels were back on but... why were there worried heads crowding around the car. I asked the obvious question; "What the f...ing hell is going on?" Then another; "Why are you tits standing around looking as if you'd just lost a winning pools ticket?"

Ralph looked at me and tried an unsuccessful grin. "Just a small problem about tuning the bugger in Tone, nothing to worry about." "Then why do you all look so bloody worried?" "Well, it's just that we didn't have a new set of spark plugs to fit so we cleaned the old ones. That should have been OK but we seem to have changed the gaps during the cleaning and we don't have a works manual for this car. It's running very rough at the moment."

I could not believe my ears. "You mean to say that you started out on a full service of my dad's car without a manual? You can't be serious, he'll kill me.... slowly. What the hell you goner do now?" My friend Ralph gave the distinct impression that he did not yet know the answer to that question. I was beginning to wish that the flight sergeant had not given me time off to check on progress in the motor pool. That way I could have lived a couple more hours in sublime hope and expectation.

"Why aren't you worrying?" I asked Ralph quietly. He grinned, a smart bugger grin. "Well, I've just got hold of a manual from Corporal Tucker. He also works here in the motor pool and he used to own one of these." He pointed at the car. I could have thumped him, cheerfully. He waived his set of feeler gauges at me and proceeded to get back under the car bonnet. "Won't be a tick." This was his parting message as he disappeared inside the car. A few minutes and considerable swearing later he emerged. "Job done." He advised me confidently. "Try it."

I got into the driver's seat and prepared to pull the choke whilst Ralph wound the starting handle. To give him credit it fired first time. It sounded a bit rough but he assured me that this was simply the pistons 'bedding in' after the full service. I was not totally convinced but I was extremely relieved to hear that old car running. I could not wait to get it back home.

Well we had got the car started, just, to my satisfaction and I arranged to meet Ralph in the motor pool the Saturday morning, after breakfast, for the trip home. Both our teams had given us the morning off. I used Friday evening to load the car with all the belongings that I needed to take home with me. We met as arranged on the Saturday morning. Ralph already had the car started. We loaded up with the rest of his gear and set off onto the road though 'my gate'. We had not travelled a hundred yards though when there came an awful noise from the nearside rear of the car and a terrible wobbling sensation from that end of the vehicle. Poor old NXY705 was in trouble.

I got out and viewed a very worrying scene. The nearside rear wheel was at an angle and barely still on its bolts. Some silly, negligent, bugger had not tightened the wheel nuts properly. The wheel had begun to wobble which had rapidly worsened, almost shredding the thread on the bolts. We only just managed to get the jack under the car in the reduced space left by the unusual tilt of the wheel. I managed not to express my true feelings to my companion. I was too concerned as to what could now be done to get us home, where I could get the car looked at in a proper garage. I glared at my now reluctant sidekick, raising my arms in a 'what now' expression.

Once we had the car up safely on the jack Ralph reviewed the damage and, more importantly, the next course of action. Finally, after several very long minutes rubbing his chin and making unhelpful and unconvincing noises he did begin to look hopeful. "Look," he began.... "We get the wheel and nuts in position as tight as we can on what's left of the threads. I will then centre pop all the bolts with

a cold chisel and that should hold the nuts until you get the car into a garage in London to get the bolts and probably the nuts changed."

There came a long pause at that point whilst we looked at each other. He was my friend but I didn't feel too friendly towards him at that moment. Still he had been trying to help all week and it probably was not he who had failed to tighten the bolts properly. This was definitely not the time to express my true sentiments. Ralph raised his arms sideways to indicate truly that there was no more that he could do. He had to run back to the motor pool to get the tools he needed for the job. He returned in about fifteen minutes, red of cheek and puffing like a train. I got the distinct impression that he had taken a bit extra time in order that certain 'bollockings' could be delivered.

Ralph completed the running repair in double quick time. He assured me that it would hold OK to get us to London and so we set off again, with some initial trepidation, but with only about 45 minutes having been lost. We drove to London in comparative silence. I had agreed to drop him off in South London. He lived not far from Borough Market, so I let him off just across London Bridge. I needed to get the car to a garage quickly, and Ralph said he could easily walk the short distance home from there.

I set off again towards Enfield and home, but firstly towards a garage now owned and run by an old school friend, Martin. I was hoping firmly that he would be still open by the time I got there. Many garages only opened a half day on Saturdays. To my great relief he was there. He had just been finishing a job before knocking off for the weekend. Luckily, also, he remembered me from school and more to the point, he listened to my car story with considerable amusement. He told me to go for a walk whilst he got on with it. I did offer to help but he shoo-ed me away, whilst muttering something about 'bloody amateurs' having done enough already.

I went for a short walk along the Ridgeway, returning in about a half hour, not expecting the job to be finished but too anxious to

stay away longer. There she was though, standing squarely on all four wheels. What a beautiful and welcome sight!

Martin approached me grinning. "By the way" he said. "I've also adjusted your spark plug gaps. Whoever set them must have been using his finger nails to do the job." Martin started the car and sure enough the engine was now running as sweet as a nut, a walnut, not a wheel-nut!! Martin, moreover, refused to take any money from me. "Old times sake". This was a great boon because I didn't have much. I did thank him though, profusely I hope. I would, moreover, like to take this opportunity to thank him once again over fifty years later. I have not met with Martin since that day but I hope very sincerely that he has had a successful and happy life. Many Thanks!

At the end of a very long day I finally had the car back home with my dad reviewing the work done on his beloved NXY705. He saw the immaculate new look engine compartment and listened to the now sweet running of the engine and, by the look on his face I saw that he was 'well pleased'.

I'm really sorry, Dad, if I've beefed up your level of satisfaction as to what you saw and heard from your car at that point, for we both know differently. That, though, is truly how I would have liked this part of my story to end. It would have been my great pleasure for you to have had a really good ending and so that is how I have made it here. Nonetheless NXY705 did survive to fight another day and for many days after that.

20
The final Few Days-
Avoidable tragedies

HAVING RETURNED DAD'S car home I returned to camp with only one remaining weekend left of my official time in the RAF. It was a time of mixed emotions. Joyce and I were planning to marry on the 7th July and so I was looking forward to that very much. There were, though, friends to leave behind and as reality tells us, that those partings would be forever. We did of course make promises to keep in touch but those would prove to be as fickle as the sun in February.

There was one exception. John Robinson and his wife Nina and I did keep in touch for many years. They did in fact come to our twenty fifth wedding anniversary get-together at our home. John was not, though, available to come to our wedding because he had got himself in trouble once again with the RAF police and was detained by them. A few others however did get down for the wedding day and we were very glad to see them. One, Tony Haynes, actually met his future wife, Barbara, at our wedding reception. She was the daughter of an old friend of my dad. We did not, inevitably and unfortunately; manage to keep in touch with them after our wedding.

As my time approached I became more and more aware that I had no job to go to after the wedding. I had had an interview with Lloyds Bank but had not yet heard the result of the interview.

I have to admit that, despite my natural desire to say goodbye to the RAF and to get on with my life, my attitude towards the service had changed considerably over my two years;

Very shortly after the time of my final leaving of the RAF a major incident was coming to a boil in our turbulent world. It was the Cuban Missile Crisis October 1962. There was of course talk of Britain becoming involved, as usual. Shortly after we were both discharged my brother-in-law was in fact put on alert that he might be recalled should the need arise; he did his time in the army as a paramedic. I received no such alert notice for which I was very thankful but then... who needs an extra pay accounts clerk in an emergency?

Finally as a postscript. Not long ago I read that RAF Bircham Newton had closed as an RAF base in December 1962. It was sad reading for me and, at the same time, the creation of a fond memory. I had begun my RAF career in anger and extreme resentment at the thought that my country was about to steal two years of my life. I had been very lucky, however, that I had landed up at Bircham Newton.

For more than 18 months I had had my own room and had been allowed to personalise it. I did not like having been allocated to pay accounts but I had to admit that the staff there had made me very welcome and had given me as much freedom as they possibly could under the regime of a military base. There were however some inevitable negatives as there always are in large organisations. I have not dwelled on these here because the positives had far outweighed the negatives for me. They do however have to be mentioned.

The RAF in 1960 to 62 was a very masculine dominated society. In fact the only woman that I met during my two years was the doctor at RAF Bircham Newton. It was she who had examined me when I had the serious batch of mouth ulcers and then sent me to Ely and the wonderful RAF hospital of few patients and wonderful staff. In both

the NAAFI and in the mess there were frequent lewd jokes and references to women workers there and about women. Even in those days
I found these references distasteful. As time has passed and with
the changing attitudes over the years I realise that they were quite
wrong and destructive in any society.

On a similar vein "queer bashing" was quite common. It was unfortunately almost a given in many largely male societies of that time
and of the military in particular. This behaviour continued according
to press reports over the years and decades to follow. It is perhaps
a sign of the changing times that the word 'queer' has now thankfully largely dropped out or public usage. Young people in particular
seem to have grasped the nettle of equal treatment to all levels and
all peoples in society. It is to be hoped that this change in attitude
largely adopted by the young people in our society will effect a uni-
versal change over the coming decades.

I did not see much evidence of actual direct bullying during my
two years in the RAF. One did hear of it however and I suppose that
unfortunately it can often be evident where large groups of people,
particularly young men, are gathered together in an imposed social
relationship. This can be the case in such places as boarding schools,
Scouts, Guides, the Police, Prisons and of course the Military of which
we are talking at the moment. In all these social arrangements there
are people with power and there are others without this power and
therefore lacking protection from bullying. In such circumstances the
bullies will attempt to abuse their power to the detriment of weaker
individuals.

In the RAF that I entered there was parade ground bullying by
NCOs who saw this as the only way they can get the job done in the
short time available to them. This type of bullying was in general
accepted and tolerated in good humour by most new recruited servicemen. There were some however for whom the bullying and rag-
ging by unscrupulous NCOs was intolerable. There were some who
had to seek medical discharge on this basis. Some indeed made the

final gesture of suicide to relieve themselves of this bane on their lives.

Parade ground bullying was something that I actually witnessed myself from time to time but not at the level where a person had to seek medical help. I now have to talk about a more extreme form of bullying which is one that I did not witness myself and I sincerely hope that I would have intervened had I been present. This was the case or perhaps I should say cases of boy entrants and RAF apprentices who were subjected to initiation ceremonies when they began their association with the RAF.

The standard furniture for an RAF airmen, apprentice, or boy entrant at that time was a small chest of drawers and tall wardrobe shaped like a narrow phone box. I actually heard of a case of a novice RAF apprentice who in his first few days, or should I say nights, was actually forced into one of these wardrobes which was then thrown out of a first-floor window. On impact with the ground the wardrobe shattered and a shaft of wood broke off and pierced the boy's chest and killed him. As I say I did not witness this; I heard about it through the general scuttlebutt that pervades all such societies as the RAF. I hope in fact that it was just that, scuttlebutt, and totally untrue. I have to say though that there was something of the attitudes pervading at some levels of military society, and with the sometimes poor level of Jr NCO management of young people, boys in particular, that I do believe that it was, unfortunately, believable.

The final incident that I intend to report here was the tragedy of one young apprentice who died during an ill-advised expedition into the North Sea by canoe of several young boys supervised by a young RAF officer. They did not of course go out far into the North Sea; the intention was to stick close to the shoreline. As I remember it however, this was in January and the North Sea in winter, even by the shoreline, is not kind to ill-prepared young people in canoes. As a result of this lack of judgement one boy died. I felt such sorrow at the time for the young person, even also for the young officer but most

importantly for the poor father who was a serving warrant officer in the RAF at the time. I can only imagine his grief and anger when he made the terrible journey to RAF Bircham Newton to retrieve his son's body.

As I said at the beginning of this short section I do not wish to make too much of these the negatives that I saw, heard of, or witnessed during my two years national service, for in contrast to my negative thoughts and frame of mind when I first entered the RAF my two years had provided me with far more in the way of positives than negatives. I did not expect this when I first went for that comical medical assessment prior to my entry into the RAF, nor did I allow any positive thoughts to enter my head or my heart during the first five or six months of my national service. It was my gradual realisation not only that the RAF was bigger than I was and could easily manage my reactionary frame of mind. It was also an appreciation that the people around me were not out to get me but were quite helpful and decent people and to just wanted to get through the day without too many problems.

At the time that I was due to leave the RAF, the system of national service was winding down. In fact the last national servicemen were entering the service at about the time that I was due to leave. Numerous men were being discharged during the same period that I became discharged. One side-effect of this was that there were numerous leaving parties during my last few weeks at Bircham Newton. Consequently one spent many days nurturing a hangover from the night before. I was no exception to this, in spite of the fact that I knew full well that was due to be married in in a few weeks' time and I still had the age old ceremony of the stag party to survive.

Joyce's brother Sid was due to be my best man and I knew at the back of my mind that he had something special in mind for my stag party.[Sorry but this too is another story]. Nonetheless I did not allow this to inhibit me during the leaving parties of the few friends who left the RAF during the weeks prior to my own discharge. I must have

spent much of those weeks in a kind of subdued fog. I could have expected some reproach from my flight Sgt. He however was at some of the parties himself. He was probably more used to it than I was and so did not show any loss of form at work. I'm not sure that I could claim the same for myself. I do not remember any particular leaving party, they seem all to have accumulated and merged into one; as did the pubs, they left me in the afore-mentioned foggy state right up to the last day when I was due to go down to London to meet Joyce so that we might buy the ring together in the Strand. That day was one that neither she nor I shall ever forget.

21
The last train home

THE TIME CAME then for me to say my last goodbyes at RAF Bircham Newton and set out for the future and my wife to be. Maurice Rubin my section warrant officer suggested that as he was travelling down to London that day we could travel together. He also suggested that I should call him by his first name now that I was leaving the service. He had always been friendly but now he was suggesting that we could travel on that, my final train to London as friends. I accepted his suggestion with some pleasure I have to say. This acceptance by me was a measure of my own length of travel during the previous two years. I could never have imagined doing so or wanting to do so when I first entered the service.

It actually took me quite a while to say my final farewells but I did eventually come to the point where I could load my final belongings into the boot of Maurice's car. He was going to drive us to King's Lynn station and to leave his car there for collection by him on his return from London. I have to admit to some feelings of sadness as we drove out through my own 'adopted' pole gate. Once through, however, my feelings began to change from sadness to joy and then into ones of real anticipation for the coming events of the next few days.

When we arrived at King's Lynn station the train was already on the platform and puffing away gently. It was of course an old-style

train with compartments within the carriage, each having two oppo-site facing bench seats to seat four people. The doors were heavy hinged slam-dunk doors. They got this name due to the fact that in order to close them you needed to slam the door and if the window needed to be open you used a leather strap inside the door to allow the window to slide down into a compartment within the door, thus dunking it.

I made to enter the train but Maurice clearly had a plan of action in mind. He ushered me gently towards the restaurant car which had a very adequately supplied bar and some comfortable chairs in which one could sit and have a nice drink and some good conversation. Part of Maurice's plan of action was that he would not allow me to buy any drinks although he was clearly not intent on stinting that part of the operation. He kept the drinks coming and the conversation going throughout the whole journey. He spoke about his wife and about his career in the RAF, of which he was very proud. I can understand this because to reach the rank of warrant officer in any of the armed services is an achievement of which one can be, and should be, proud, even though I myself would have chosen almost any other part than pay accounts in which to serve.

The journey to London had one great advantage, bearing in mind Maurice's plan was to ply me with the much drink as I could take on board. The advantage being that it was a journey from one terminus, King's Lynn to another terminus Liverpool Street. That way there was no chance of missing the last stop and going on to somewhere com-pletely unintended.

From Liverpool Street we took the tube to Charring Cross underground station with the intention of walking along the Strand towards the Holborn end where I had arranged to meet Joyce dur-ing her lunch hour. She was working in the civil service at that time, in Holborn. I realised that I had plenty of time to kill before I was due to meet her. Maurice elected to walk along the road with me. We were of course both much the worse for wear due to the drink we

had consumed on the train. Maurice was clearly not put off by this however because as we made our way along the Strand he noticed a promising looking hostelry where we could perhaps finish off his campaign to provide me with as much drink as I could possibly bear. What a kindly soul!

The hostelry in question was called, perhaps appropriately, the Coal Hole. This was a former coal cellar for the Savoy Hotel in the Strand and as you entered it is clearly deserved its name. In those days as I remember it was not well lit, being quite dark and very smoky as most people in such establishments in those days were keen smokers. There was a heady mixture of cigarette, cigar and pipe smoke hanging in the air. One thought little of this at that time; it was just part of the normal territory of social existence.

The Coal Hole was quite close to the jeweller's shop in which Joyce had seen a selection of rings that suited our purse and so I had no compunction in descending into that hostelry to continue our drinking until the time came for my meeting with Joyce. Inevitably, however, what with the drink and the conversation and the gradual dimming of my senses the time for my meeting with Joyce came and went almost unnoticed until I happened to glance at clock behind the bar and with sudden horror, guilt and panic I hurried Maurice up the stairs and back into the Strand to the nearby jeweller's shop hoping that Joyce would be merciful and not kill me.

Maurice elected to come with me, which was just as well as walking unaided and without support was becoming a matter of considerable difficulty for both of us. Maurice wanted to meet Joyce before he went off to conduct his own business of the day the like of which I cannot remember; I'm not even sure that Maurice had other business than to see me safely into civvy Street. It was with great relief that I saw Joyce hovering nervously outside the shop apparently unsure as to whether or not I was going to make our rendezvous. We caught sight of each other at about the same time and her face lit up momentarily into a relieved smile, when she saw however the

delicate way in which the two of us were proceeding along the road her face wrapped itself into a frown.

I cannot say in all honesty that I feel guilty about my behaviour that day because I truly enjoyed that trip from Bircham Newton to that jeweller's shop in the Strand. I am sorry though that I caused Joyce even a moment's anxiety as she was forced to wait 15 min into her precious lunch hour waiting for a pair of drunks! She was then, and always has been, a hard worker and a strong support for me throughout our long happy life together. It was she who had supported me financially to a certain extent throughout my two years in the RAF. It was also she I'm ashamed to say who had saved the money for the ring that we were about to purchase.

Despite being annoyed with me for the delay and the state in which I had arrived at our rendezvous she greeted Maurice with the warm welcome and allowed him give her a hug and kiss on the cheek even though she was keen to get into the shop and make a choice from the sadly limited range of rings that were within our budget. I was quite alarmed at first when Maurice moved over to Joyce for this greeting because I was temporarily left unsupported; this situation was reversed when Maurice left off holding Joyce and I was able to grab her to support me. I then managed a final goodbye to Maurice. I did not expect to ever see him again and that has proven to be the case. That last day however is one that I shall remember and, in fact, treasure to the day I die for the humour of it does not escape me. I have to say, though, I'm not at all sure that Joyce remembers that meeting with any affection at all. She may have some memories of the humour and stupidity of two grown men, approaching her, apparently needing to support each other while simply walking along the Strand.

Joyce and I entered the jeweller's with the intention that we would choose the ring together. I have to admit though that the choosing of the ring was largely accomplished by Joyce herself as I

was in no capacity to do other than agree to her selection. I would certainly, though, never change that ring for any other on this planet.

We left the shop but realised we had another dilemma on our hands; that was what to do with me in my state when Joyce had to go back to work for the afternoon. She guided me back to Lincoln's Inn Fields which was quite close to her place of work. She herself was very close to the end of her lunch hour and was anxious to make her way quickly back to work and so she left me at the entrance to Lincoln's Inn Fields with the firm instruction to stay there until she could come to get me at the end of her working day.

Luckily it was a beautiful summer's day. I was able, just, to remain upright without falling, but staggering somewhat, I made my way towards a range of deckchairs. I even had the presence of mind to drag one of those deckchairs over towards a public toilet and to place the chair strategically close and within staggering distance of those welcome conveniences. This was good forward planning on my part because I must have worn a deep furrow that afternoon from that deckchair, on and off, to those toilets!

As I say it was a nice warm day and I did manage to catch some welcome shuteye in the hours before Joyce came to collect me. I'm also very happy to say that the worst of my deteriorated condition had dissipated during the afternoon and when Joyce came to collect me I was able, thankfully, to walk unaided. So thus and sadly I come to the end of my memories of a short career in the RAF and of my last, my final journey, home from RAF Bircham Newton, on the fourth of July 1962.

Printed in Great Britain
by Amazon

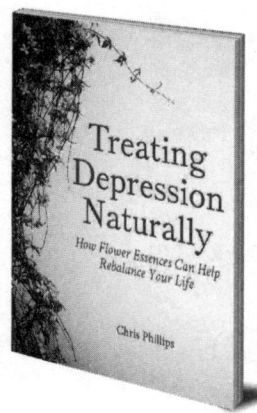 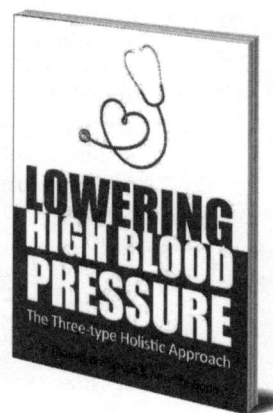 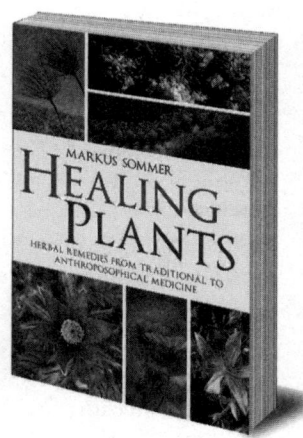
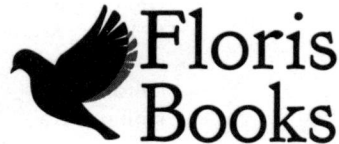